Cardiovascular Pathology
Clinicopathologic Correlations and Pathogenetic Mechanisms

UNITED STATES AND CANADIAN ACADEMY OF PATHOLOGY, INC.

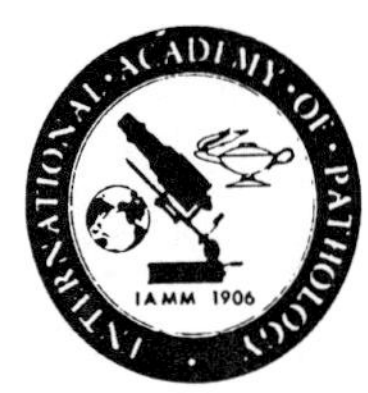

MONOGRAPHS IN PATHOLOGY

SERIES EDITOR, F. Stephen Vogel, M.D.
Secretary-Treasurer

UNITED STATES AND CANADIAN ACADEMY OF PATHOLOGY, INC.

Cardiovascular Pathology Clinicopathologic Correlations and Pathogenetic Mechanisms

EDITED BY

FREDERICK J. SCHOEN, M.D., Ph.D.

Department of Pathology
Brigham and Women's Hospital
Boston, Massachusetts

and

MICHAEL A. GIMBRONE, JR., M.D.

Department of Pathology
Brigham and Women's Hospital
Boston, Massachusetts

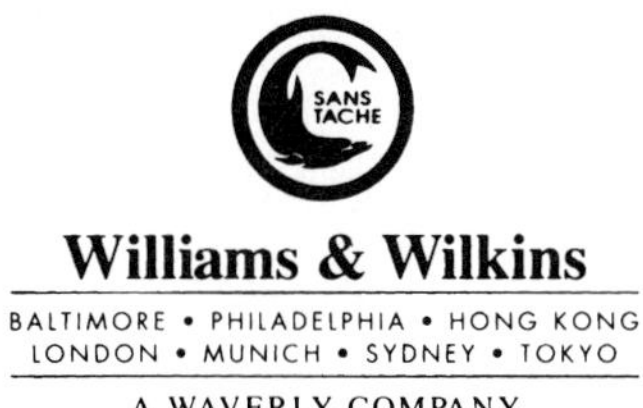

Williams & Wilkins

BALTIMORE • PHILADELPHIA • HONG KONG
LONDON • MUNICH • SYDNEY • TOKYO

A WAVERLY COMPANY

Foreword

The practice of pathology serves as a constant reminder of the clinical significance of cardiovascular disease in human health. Nevertheless, it is not unusual that pathologists focus disproportionate attention upon other subject areas, such as the recognition and classification of neoplasms. It is natural to respond to immediacy.

Wisely, the Education Committee and the Council of the United States and Canadian Academy of Pathology appreciated the necessity that pathologists remain current in the rapidly evolving knowledge of diseases of the cardiovascular system and selected this topic as the subject for the Long Course of the annual meeting in San Francisco, March 1994. This decision was strengthened by an awareness that pathologic anatomy serves as the foundation for the clinical practice of cardiology.

Drs. Fred Schoen and Michael Gimbrone were invited to serve as course directors. They graciously accepted, assembled an outstanding faculty, moderated the course, and in a very timely manner, edited the present monograph.

The Academy wishes to express its sincere appreciation to Drs. Schoen and Gimbrone, to the distinguished faculty who contributed to the content of this monograph, and to Williams and Wilkins who brought the text into published form.

F. STEPHEN VOGEL, M.D.
Series Editor

Preface

This volume comprises the manuscripts derived from the presentations at the US-Canadian Academy of Pathology's 1994 Long-Course: "Cardiovascular Pathology: Clinicopathologic Correlations and Pathogenetic Mechanisms". Since the previous Long-Course on this subject, approximately two decades ago, there has been considerable growth and maturation of cardiovascular pathology as a discipline. During this time, and largely as a consequence of major developments in cardiac and vascular surgery, invasive and interventional cardiology, cardiovascular imaging and cell and molecular biology, there have been numerous advances in our understanding of cardiovascular diseases, as well as expansion of the role of the cardiac pathologist as diagnostician. Cardiovascular pathology has not only been launched into the forefront of patient care, but the clinical progress has created an immense need for validation of the efficacy and safety of diagnostic tests and therapeutic techniques, procedures and devices, including balloon angioplasty, coronary artery bypass graft surgery, cardiac transplantation, endomyocardial biopsy and a wide array of prosthetic devices. This need also has stimulated formation of the Society for Cardiovascular Pathology, now in its 10th year, with over 250 members worldwide. The Society holds companion meetings with the USCAP and it sponsors a journal entitled CARDIOVASCULAR PATHOLOGY.

The objective of this course was to provide a contemporary approach to cardiovascular pathology that integrates practical areas of diagnostic importance with evolving basic science concepts. Although primary and secondary prevention efforts as well as advances in the treatment of myocardial infarction have decreased the incidence of cardiovascular disease as a fraction of total mortality, over the past two or more decades, cardiovascular disease remains the predominant cause of mortality and morbidity in the developed world. The first three chapters of the book therefore emphasize our expanding understanding of atherogenesis and endothelial cell dysfunction, the role of plaque disruption in the initiation of acute myocardial infarction and the myocardial response to ischemic injury. In recognition of the expanding role of the cardiac pathologist in patient management, the following three chapters address the differential diagnosis of cardiac valvular lesions, interpretation of endomyocardial biopsies, approaches to cardiac tumors, pathologic considerations in cardiac transplantation and the diagnosis of vascular inflammatory disease. New developments in vascular pathophysiology comprise the following two chapters, summarizing the pathogenesis of vascular inflammation, especially the diagnostic and potential mechanistic role of antinuclear cytoplasmic autoantibodies (ANCA), and the fascinating evolution of our knowledge of the genetic basis of aortic aneurysms, especially the role of the connective tissue protein fibrillin in the Marfan syndrome. The final two chapters review the differential diagnosis of sudden cardiac death, and the pathology of substitute heart valves and other prosthetic devices.

It was both gratifying and enjoyable for us to have the opportunity to organize this course and edit the resulting contributions. We hope that the reader will find this volume a useful overview of several important diagnostic and interesting basic science issues in cardiovascular pathology. Its completion would not have been possible without the enthusiastic efforts of the course participants and the work of Dr. Stephen Vogel and others at the US-Canadian Academy of Pathology, and Ms. Susan O'Donnell and others at Williams and Wilkins. We are grateful to each of them.

FREDERICK J. SCHOEN, M.D., Ph.D.
MICHAEL A. GIMBRONE, JR., M.D.

Contributors

MARGARET E. BILLINGHAM, M.B., B.S., F.R.C. PATH.
Department of Pathology, Stanford University Medical School, Stanford, California

ALLEN P. BURKE, M.D.
Department of Cardiovascular Pathology, Armed Forces Institute of Pathology, Washington, DC

HARRY C. DIETZ, M.D.
Division of Pediatric Cardiology, Johns Hopkins University School of Medicine, Baltimore, Maryland

WILLIAM D. EDWARDS, M.D.
Division of Anatomic Pathology, Mayo Clinic, Rochester, Minnesota

RONALD J. FALK, M.D.
Department of Medicine, The University of North Carolina at Chapel Hill School of Medicine, Chapel Hill, North Carolina

ANDREW FARB, M.D.
Department of Cardiovascular Pathology, Armed Forces Institute of Pathology, Washington, DC

MICHAEL A. GIMBRONE, JR., M.D.
Vascular Research Division, Department of Pathology, Brigham and Women's Hospital, Boston, Massachusetts

J. CHARLES JENNETTE, M.D.
Department of Pathology, The University of North Carolina at Chapel Hill School of Medicine, Chapel Hill, North Carolina

ROBERT B. JENNINGS, M.D.
Department of Pathology, Duke University Medical Center, Durham, North Carolina

J.T. LIE, M.D.
Department of Pathology, University of California Davis Medical Center, Sacramento, California

KEITH A. REIMER, M.D., PH.D.
Department of Pathology, Duke University Medical Center, Durham, North Carolina

FREDERICK J. SCHOEN, M.D., PH.D.
*Department of Pathology, Brigham and Women's Hospital,
Boston, Massachusetts*

JOHN SMIALEK, M.D.
*Department of Cardiovascular Pathology, Armed Forces Institute of
Pathology, Washington, DC*

CHARLES STEENBERGEN, JR., M.D., PH.D.
*Department of Pathology, Duke University Medical Center, Durham,
North Carolina*

HENRY D. TAZELAAR, M.D.
Division of Anatomic Pathology, Mayo Clinic, Rochester, Minnesota

RENU VIRMANI, M.D.
*Department of Cardiovascular Pathology, Armed Forces Institute of
Pathology, Washington, DC*

Contents

Chapter 1

Atherogenesis: Current Concepts

MICHAEL A. GIMBRONE, JR.

Atherosclerosis is the most common form of large-vessel pathology responsible for syndromes of vital organ ischemia (*e.g.*, myocardial and cerebral infarction) and, as such, is the leading cause of mortality and morbidity in most industrialized societies.[1] Although its histopathologic features have been appreciated for more than a century,[2] mechanistic insights into its pathogenesis have come only recently. Indeed, attempting to infer the origins of atherosclerosis from the examination of a thrombosed, scarred coronary artery might be likened to performing an autopsy on an Egyptian mummy. However, from a series of *in vivo* and *in vitro* experimental pathological, cell biological, and molecular genetic approaches, coupled with recent multidisciplinary studies of early lesions in children and young adults,[3,4] a dynamic picture of atherogenesis at the cellular and molecular level has emerged.[5] With this knowledge has come the awareness that atherosclerosis, despite its diverse clinical presentations and risk factor associations, may share certain basic pathogenetic mechanisms with other vascular disease processes, both naturally occurring and iatrogenic. These pathogenetic insights, in turn, have suggested exciting new strategies for diagnostic, therapeutic, and preventive measures.

Several comprehensive reviews have been published recently on atherosclerosis that address the complex interplay of cellular interactions, humoral mediators, and biochemical risk factors in lesion initiation and progression.[6–14] In addition, other chapters in this volume will treat the pathophysiology of the unstable coronary artery plaque and its "downstream" ischemic complications, as well as the pathobiology of related vascular disease processes (*e.g.*, transplant arteriosclerosis). In this chapter, we will briefly review the origins of the current working concepts of atherogenesis, and then highlight recent advances in our understanding of certain pathogenetic mechanisms at the cellular and molecular level.

THE "RESPONSE-TO-INJURY HYPOTHESIS" REVISITED

A useful organizing concept that has stimulated much fruitful research in this field is the "Response-to-Injury Hypothesis." Although its origins can be traced to the writings of Virchow[15] and von Rokitansky,[2] as later modified by French,[16] this hypothesis was formally proposed essentially in its current form in the early 1970s by Ross and coworkers[17–19] and subsequently modified and developed by many laboratories. Simply stated, it suggests that the lesions of atherosclerosis represent a chronic form of inflammatory-fibroproliferative response of the artery wall to various injurious stimuli—a protective response that, in excess, becomes the disease process.[9] As a working concept for atherogenesis, it has a number of useful features. First, it acknowledges the basic multifactorial nature of this disease entity, which involves several well-defined but apparently dissimilar risk factors; the interaction of multiple cell types, both vascular and blood-derived; and an ever-increasing list of autacoids, cytokines, and growth factors that have been implicated as mediators. Second, it attempts to explain the prolonged time course and episodic nature of progression (and regression) that are typical of the natural history of atherosclerotic lesions. Third, it suggests that, at a basic level, atherosclerosis, inflammation, thrombosis, and wound healing may share a common set (or multiple subsets) of cellular and molecular mechanisms. Finally, and perhaps most importantly, it suggests a number of experimental lines of investigation and provides a conceptual framework for data analysis and interpretation.

As originally formulated,[17,18] the Response-to-Injury Hypothesis postulated that the initiating event in the atherogenic process was some form of overt injury to the initmal endothelial lining, induced by toxic substances (*e.g.*, oxidized cholesterol, agents in cigarette smoke, homocystinemia, catecholamines, hyperglycemia, *etc.*) or altered physical forces (*e.g.*, hemodynamic disturbances secondary to hypertension). These putative noxious stimuli, which are related to various of the recognized risk factors for atherosclerosis, were thought to result in morphologically detectable endothelial damage, manifest as loss of permeability barrier integrity, surface membrane blebbing, and even frank desquamation. The latter event was then envisioned as the inciting stimulus for platelet adhesion to the injured vascular wall and the local release of platelet-derived growth factors. These substances would then elicit migration, phenotypic modulation, and proliferation of medial vascular smooth muscle cells, thus forming a fibromuscular plaque. The experimental demonstration that this sequence of events could be induced by simple denudation of the intima by an intravascular balloon catheter or other mechanical device lent further support to the response-to-injury concept.[20–22]

This balloon injury model, which has been studied in a variety of animal species from rodents to primates, has revealed a number of interesting biological and pathological insights.[23] First, the normally well-differentiated contractile element of muscular and elastic arteries, the medial smooth muscle cell, is capable of dramatic ""phenotypic modulation" to an actively motile, biosynthetic, and secretory state.[24] The hyperplastic, extracellular matrix-rich nature of early intimal lesions reflects this functional change in the smooth muscle cell. Second, the experimental characterization of the various growth factors that can act on vascular smooth muscle—their cellular origins, genetic regulation, and molecular mechanisms of target cell action—has contributed in a major way to our understanding of growth factor biology.[5,25–27] For example, it was the purification and sequence of platelet-derived growth factor, the first well-defined vascular smooth muscle mitogen, that led to the discovery of its homology with a simian sarcoma virus oncogene product (v-*cis*), thus linking the biology of wound healing and cancer at a fundamental level.[28] The similarities in intimal hyperplastic response to experimental balloon denudation, and the clinical problem of postangioplasty restenosis, also suggest a commonality in cellular and molecular mechanisms of vessel wall responses to injury.[23,29]

Further investigation of these fibromuscular proliferative phenomena has revealed an abundance of cytokines, growth factors, and other vasoactive agonists that appear to form a network of overlapping cascades, potentially triggered by diverse stimuli, but ultimately resulting in an orchestrated pattern of vascular smooth muscle migration, proliferation, and extracellular matrix secretion.[5] These include such distinct types of mediators as *platelet-derived growth factor* (actually two distinct gene products, PDGF-A and PDGF-B), a potent mesenchymal cell mitogen secreted by several cell types (*e.g.,* endothelium, macrophages, platelets, and even smooth muscle) that can mediate chemotaxis and vasoconstriction; *thrombin,* a key protease in the coagulation cascade that can also mediate multiple effects, including growth stimulation, secretagogue action, and chemotaxis, via activation of receptors on various target cells (*e.g.,* platelets, endothelium, smooth muscle); *angiotensin,* a classic vasoconstrictor peptide, generated by the renin-angiotensin system, that also appears to play a role in smooth muscle cell hypertrophy and hyperplasia; and *interleukin-1 (IL-1)* and *tumor necrosis factor*-α *(TNF*-α), immunoregulatory cytokines, produced in large quantities by activated monocyte/macrophages and other cell types, that can, directly or indirectly, mediate smooth muscle proliferation. A major conceptual advance in our understanding of these and other growth stimulatory substances was the discovery that these potent agents could be generated locally within the "injured" vessel wall by endothelial cells, smooth muscle cells, and various blood-derived leukocytes (monocyte/macrophages, T-lymphocytes). Furthermore, these so-called "autocrine" or "paracrine" loops of *intrinsic vessel wall growth stimulators* appeared to be held in balance by a comparable set of locally generated *vessel wall growth inhibitors*. The latter group of mediators includes cytokines such as transforming growth factor-β[27] which, in addition to stimulating the synthesis of connective tissue matrix components, is a potent inhibitor of smooth muscle replication, and various heparin-like proteoglycans and related substances.[30] Thus, the experimental study of the reparative response of the vessel wall (in particular, the aorta and its large tributaries) to a defined form of "injury" (balloon catheter or other mechanically mediated endothelial denudation) has provided valuable insights into the stimulatory molecules and cellular responses potentially involved in the fibromuscular proliferative component of atherosclerotic lesion formation.

ENDOTHELIAL INJURY/DYSFUNCTION: AN EVOLVING CONCEPT

Although experimental denudation of the intimal lining is sufficient to elicit a complex response-to-injury response, this form of mechanical damage is not especially relevant to "natural" atherosclerosis. Indeed, careful examination of the early lesions of atherosclerosis in diet-induced animal models typically fails to reveal any overt endothelial injury.[14] With the appreciation that the endothelial cell is a dynamic, interactive element that supports multiple vital functions, it has become apparent that the functional status of the vascular lining may be as important as its anatomic integrity.[31] The term *endothelial dysfunction* has been introduced[32] to connote phenotypic modulation of this cell to a nonadaptive functional state. This might entail the loss of nonthrombogenic surface properties (as manifested by increased platelet adherence and/or triggering of intrinsic or extrinsic coagulation pathways), or a serious imbalance between endothelial-dependent procoagulant and anticoagulant mechanisms.[32] The result conceivably could be manifested as an acute, localized thrombotic event, a more chronic thrombotic tendency, or disease of the vessel wall *per se* as in atherosclerosis. Other manifestations of endothelial dysfunction might involve decreased production of vasorelaxor substances, such as endothelium-derived relaxing factor (nitric oxide), with a resultant vasospastic tendency, as observed in hypercholesterolemia and early atherosclerosis.[33] Another pathophysiologically important change in endothelial phenotype is its modulation to a "proinflammatory state," with up-regulation of cell surface adhesion molecules and chemoattractant factors that promote leukocyte recruitment and activation,[34] as discussed in more detail below.

Various types of stimuli of endothelial dysfunction have been identified including immunoregulatory substances such as tumor necrosis factor and interleukin-1, viral infection and transformation, bacterial toxins, cholesterol, and oxidatively modified lipoprotein.[35] At a molecular level, perhaps the best studied paradigm is the "activation" of endothelial cells by inflammatory cytokines, such as TNF and IL-1, and bacterial products, such as lipopolysaccharide (endotoxin).[36] This process involves a coordinated sequence of events, initiated by cell surface receptor activation, that culminates in a pattern of gene expression that typically is characteristic for a particular cytokine or mixture of cytokines. At the level of the nucleus, a number of these stimuli appear to converge into final common pathways of transcriptional regulatory factors, such as the nuclear factor-kB system.[37] In addition to these soluble cytokine stimuli, biochemical forces generated by the pulsatile flow of blood through the branched arterial tree, such as oscillating wall shear stresses and cyclic stretching, can also influence a variety of endothelial functions.[38] Certain of these biomechanically induced effects appear to involve the modulation of endothelial gene expression at the transcriptional level. Recently, a shear stress response element has been discovered in the PDGF-B chain gene that appears to be involved in these processes. This *cis*-acting transcriptional element has been shown by deletion analysis to be necessary for shear-induced activation of the PDGF-B chain gene, and interestingly, is also present in the promoters of several other shear-inducible endothelial genes.[39] The ability of hemodynamic forces directly to influence endothelial gene expression may explain, in part, the nonrandom distribution of atherosclerotic lesions, which tend to occur near branch points and other vascular geometries associated with altered flow patterns. Further analysis of the transduction mechanisms that link these diverse stimuli, humoral and mechanical, to genetic regulatory events within the endothelial cell may provide fundamental insights into the mechanisms and consequences of endothelial dysfunction.

ENDOTHELIUM-DEPENDENT MECHANISMS OF LEUKOCYTE RECRUITMENT IN ATHEROGENESIS: THE ATHERO-ELAM HYPOTHESIS

Perhaps the earliest morphologically detectable cellular event in atherogenesis is the adherence of circulating blood monocytes to the intact intimal surface of large arteries.[40–42] These adherent cells then migrate across the endothelium into the intima, where they tend to accumulate, undergo limited replication, and become transformed into lipid-laden foam cells. Once present in the intima, in addition to accumulating cholesterol esters (the lipid "hallmark" of the early fatty streak lesion), this differentiating monocyte-macrophage population can promote lesion progression through the local generation of cytokines (*e.g.,* interleukin-1, tumor necrosis factor); growth factors (*e.g.,* platelet-derived growth factor, fibroblast growth factor, heparin-binding epidermal growth factor-like growth factor); various procoagulant and fibrinolytic components; eicosanoids; and toxic oxygen products.[5] Recently, considerable attention has also been focused on the presence, in more developed lesions, of T-lymphocytes that have the capacity to generate other cytokines (*e.g.,* γ-interferon, interleukin-4) through both immune and nonimmune triggered pathways. These lymphocyte-derived products add further complexity to the local cytokine milieu and the potential activation states of vessel wall cells (endothelium and smooth muscle) and other components of the developing atherosclerotic lesion.[43]

The localized, leukocyte-selective nature of this mononuclear recruitment process suggests that endothelium-dependent adhesion mechanisms analogous to those recently described in acute and chronic inflammation might be responsible.[44] This has led to the hypothesis that these localized mononuclear leukoycte-endothelial interactions reflect specific molecular changes in the adhesive properties of the endothelial surface, involving "athero-ELAMs" inducible endothelial-leukocyte adhesion molecules (ELAMs) expressed in atherosclerotic lesions.[45] According to this hypothesis, a candidate athero-ELAM should (1) support mononuclear (but not necessarily polymorphonuclear) leukocyte adhesion, (2) be inducibly expressed on the endothelial surface, and (3) be detectable in early atherosclerotic lesions (or in areas with a predilection for developing lesions).

An experimental search for molecules satisfying these criteria was undertaken in the rabbit,[45] a species in which dietary and genetic models of atherosclerosis are well described. Initially, leukocyte-endothelial interactions were examined *in vitro,* using cultured normal rabbit aortic endothelial cells. Treatment of these endothelial monolayers with a nonspecific activator, such as bacterial endotoxin, resulted in a hyperadhesive surface change that was detectable upon incubation with blood monocytes and monocyte-like cell lines. This endothelial surface adhesive change was dependent upon protein synthesis, and was detectable after a lag of 1–2 hours, reached a maximum within 6–12 hours, and then remained manifest for at least 96 hours. Murine monoclonal antibodies produced to these endotoxin-activated rabbit endothelial cells detected various inducible surface antigens, some of which exhibited a temporal profile similar to that of the adhesive surface change for blood leukocytes. In adhesion assays, pretreatment of activated endothelial monolayers with saturating concentrations of certain of these monoclonal antibodies significantly inhibited mononuclear leukocyte attachment. Comparative studies with various types of leukocytes showed that this inhibition was selective for mononuclear, but not polymorphonuclear, leukocyte attachment. These *in vitro* studies thus identified an inducible adhesion molecule that could selectively support mononuclear leukocyte lesion to activated arterial endothelial cells, thereby satisfying two of the experimental criteria for an athero-ELAM.

The expression of this inducible, mononuclear leukocyte-selective adhesion molecule was then examined during experimental atherogenesis. In rabbits fed a 1% cholesterol diet, and in Watanabe heritable hyperlipidemic rabbits, which have severe hypercholesterolemia, specific monoclonal antibody staining was localized to aortic endothelium covering foam cell-rich intimal lesions. Staining was also evident at various stages of lesion development, ranging from focal regions with very small intimal accumulations of foam cells to near-circumferential lesions with abundant foam cells. Often, staining extended beyond the edges of intimal lesions; however, in the same hypercholesterolemic animals, endothelium in adjacent, uninvolved regions of the aorta did not stain. These *in vivo* immunohistochemical observations thus satisfied the third experimental criterion for an athero-ELAM, its expression by endothelium during early lesion formation and progression.

Molecular characterization of this rabbit athero-ELAM through a combination of immunochemical and molecular cloning approaches revealed its homology to a human leukocyte adhesion molecule, intercellular adhesion molecule-110, previously identified as an inducible endothelial receptor for lymphocytes,[46] and expression cloned from a cytokine-induced endothelial library, as vascular cell adhesion molecule-1 (VCAM-1).[47] This cytokine-activated gene is a member of the immunoglobulin superfamily and is expressed on the surface of human and rabbit vascular endothelium in at least two molecular forms, presumably derived by alternative splicing.[48] Both forms can interact with heterodimeric integrin receptor, termed VLA-4 or $\alpha_4\beta_1$, a member of the β-1 subfamily of integrins, which is differentially expressed on certain leukocytes, including blood monocytes and lymphocytes, but not on polymorphonuclear leukocytes.[49,50] This matching of endothelium-expressed VCAM-1 with mononuclear leukocyte-expressed VLA-4 therefore provides a functional counterreceptor pair that can mediate a selective adhesion event.

Interestingly, when the rabbit aorta is carefully examined in a dietary model of atherogenesis,[51] endothelial expression of VCAM-1 appears to be detectable *before* mononuclear leukocyte recruitment into the arterial wall. Because one of the earliest changes during atherogenesis in cholesterol-fed animal models is the focal accumulation and oxidative modification of low-density lipoprotein

(LDL) in the intima,[52,53] it is reasonable to hypothesize that oxidatively modified LDL, or one of its components, might be an initial stimulus for VCAM-1 induction in this setting. Recent *in vitro* studies with lysophosphatidylcholine, a component of oxidized LDL (and β-VLDL, another atherogenic lipoprotein in the rabbit), have shown that this material can selectively up-regulate VCAM-1 expression in cultured rabbit aortic endothelial cells.[54] Conceivably, this phospholipid could act alone or in combination with cytokines generated locally by activated vessel wall cells or emigrating leukocytes to up-regulate endothelium-leukocyte adhesion molecules, and thus contribute to localized mononuclear leukocyte recruitment.

In addition to a VCAM-1/VLA-4 adhesive interaction, other endothelial-dependent mechanisms are also potentially relevant to mononuclear recruitment in atherogenesis. These include ICAM-1, a widely expressed member of the immunoglobulin superfamily that is also up-regulated in vascular endothelium as a "chronic ELAM" and can interact with various components of the CD11/CD18 integrin complex[44]; E-selectin (ELAM-1), an "acute ELAM" that interacts with sialyl-Lewis and related carbohydrate ligands[55] and an inducible endothelial counterreceptor for L-selectin, a ligand constitutively present on blood leukocyte surfaces.[56] Interestingly, although all of the above counterreceptor pairs have been implicated in monocyte-endothelial adhesion, only VCAM-1/VLA-4 has the potential to mediate mononuclear leukocyte, but not polymorphonuclear leukocyte, interactions. Two other relevant endothelial products that are secreted upon cytokine activation include monocyte chemoattractant protein-1, a monocyte-selected chemoattractant that has been implicated in monocyte-endothelial transmigration,[57] and macrophage colony-stimulating factor, a cytokine that can promote activation and maturation of monocytes and macrophages.[58] Recent immunohistochemical studies have localized the expression of these molecules at various stages of atherosclerotic lesion development in experimental animals and, in some instances, in humans.[59–61] The relative contributions of these mechanisms of leukocyte recruitment to the atherogenic process is an area of ongoing study that has important pathogenetic as well as therapeutic implications.

PATHOPHYSIOLOGICAL IMPLICATIONS AND POTENTIAL CLINICAL APPLICATIONS OF ATHERO-ELAMS

The identification of an inducible mononuclear leukocyte-selective adhesion molecule that is expressed in developing atherosclerotic lesions in a well-defined experimental model has several conceptual as well as practical implications. First, this provides evidence that endothelial activation/dysfunction is occurring early in the atherosclerotic process. It suggests that the net balance of local pathophysiological stimuli has elicited a pattern of response in the endothelium that is manifested by this change in surface phenotype. Second, endothelial VCAM-1 interacting with its leukocyte counterreceptor, VLA-4, is a molecular event in mononuclear leukocyte recruitment that may be susceptible to some form of antiadhesion therapeutic intervention. Third, characterization of the expression of VCAM-1 or other athero-ELAMs in human atherosclerotic lesions may provide novel markers for the early stages of this complex disease process, potentially of use in both diagnosis and treatment. These clinical applications might take the form of (1) noninvasive imaging of early lesions via labeled monoclonal antibodies, (2) differential analysis of the pattern of endothelial activation antigens as an indicator of the stage of underlying vessel wall pathology, or (3) selective targeting to early atherosclerotic lesions of a conventional therapeutic agent or specifically engineered genetic construct for "gene therapy." Clearly, the successful application of such diagnostic and therapeutic strategies will require better understanding of the basic mechanisms of endothelial activation in the context of human atherosclerotic vascular disease.

ATHEROGENESIS: STATE OF THE ART AND FUTURE DIRECTIONS

This brief synopsis of the current concepts of atherogenesis was meant to illustrate the remarkable progress that has been made in our understanding of the pathogenetic mechanisms that underlie this complex disease process. Starting with a hypothesis that is more than a century old, and that traces its origins to the descriptive anatomical pathology of Virchow and Rokitansky, modern experimental pathologists have arrived at a dynamic working concept of the cellular and molecular mechanisms involved in atherosclerotic lesion initiation, progression, and regression. Central to this working concept is the notion that the vascular endothelial lining is a dynamically mutable interface that can exhibit a spectrum of adaptive and nonadaptive changes in response to various pathophysiological stimuli—circulating lipoproteins, locally generated cytokines and growth factors, and even biomechanical forces. As our knowledge of the stimuli and consequences of dysfunctional endothelial phenotypes increases, so will our working concept of the pathogenesis of atherosclerosis. Perhaps, this will provide a rational basis for innovative diagnostic and therapeutic interventions in human coronary artery disease in the near future.

ACKNOWLEDGMENTS

Research in the author's laboratory has been supported primarily by grants from the National Heart, Lung, and Blood Institute, and the American Heart Association and its Massachusetts affiliate. The author wishes to acknowledge his colleagues and collaborators, especially Drs. Ramzi Cotran, Tucker Collins, Myron Cybulsky, Peter Libby, William Luscinskas, and Nitzan Resnick.

REFERENCES

1. World Health Organization. Classification of atherosclerotic lesions. *WHO Tech Rep Serv* 1985;153:1–20.
2. von Rokitansky C. *A manual of pathological anatomy,* vol. 4. Translated by Day GE. London: The Sydenham Society, 1852.
3. Stary HC. Evolution and progression of atherosclerotic lesions in coronary arteries of children and young adults. *Atherosclerosis* 1989;(Suppl)9:119–132.

4. PDAY Research Group. Natural history of aortic and coronary atherosclerotic lesions in youth. *Atherosclerosis Thrombosis* 1993;13:1291–1298.

5. Ross R. The pathogenesis of atherosclerosis: a perspective for the 1990s. *Nature* 1993;362:801–809.

6. Ross R. Atherosclerosis: a defense mechanism gone awry. *Am J Pathol* 1993;143:987–1002.

7. Libby P, Hansson GK. Involvement of the immune system in human atherogenesis: current knowledge and unanswered questions. *Lab Invest* 1991;64:5–15.

8. Majno G, Joris J, Z and T. Atherosclerosis: new horizons. *Hum Pathol* 1985;16:3–5.

9. Schwartz CJ, Valente AJ, Sprague EA, Kelley JL, Nerem RM. The pathogenesis of atherosclerosis: an overview. *Clin Cardiol* 1991;14:1–16.

10. Witztum JL, Steinberg D. Role of oxidized low density lipoprotein in atherogenesis. *J Clin Invest* 1991;88:1785–1792.

11. Fuster V, Badimon L. Badimon JJ, Chesebro JH. The pathogenesis of coronary artery disease and the acute coronary syndromes. *N Engl J Med* 1992;326:242–250.

12. Hajjar DP. Viral pathogenesis of atherosclerosis. Impact of molecular mimicry and viral genes. *Am J Pathol* 1991;139:1195–1211.

13. Munro JM, Cotran RS. The pathogenesis of atherosclerosis: atherogenesis and inflammation. *Lab Invest* 1988;58:249–261.

14. Simionescu M, Simionescu N. Proatherosclerotic events: pathobiochemical changes occurring in the arterial wall before monocyte migration. *FASEB J* 1993;7:1359–1366.

15. Virchow R. *Gesammelte Abhandlungen zur Wissenschaftlichen Medicin. Phlogose unq thrombose im gefassystem.* Berlin: Meidinger Sohn and Co., 1856:458–463.

16. French JE. Atherosclerosis in relation to the structure and function of the arterial intima, with special reference to the endothelium. *Int Rev Exp Pathol* 1966;5:253–353.

17. Ross R, Glomset JA. Atherosclerosis and the arterial smooth muscle cell. *Science* 1973;180:1332–1339.

18. Ross R, Glomset JA. The pathogenesis of atherosclerosis. *N Engl J Med* 1976;295:369–377, 420–425.

19. Ross R. The pathogenesis of atherosclerosis—an update. *N Engl J Med* 1986;314:488–500.

20. Bjorkerud S, Bondjers G. Arterial repair in atherosclerosis after mechanical injury: Part 5. Tissue response after induction of large superficial transverse injury. *Atherosclerosis* 1973;18:253–255.

21. Clowes AW, Reidy MA, Clowes MM. Kinetics of cellular proliferation after arterial injury. I: Smooth muscle growth in the absence of endothelium. *Lab Invest* 1983;49:327–333.

22. Fingerle J, Tina Au VP, Clowes AW, Reidy MA. Intimal lesion formation in rat carotid arteries after endothelial denudation in absence of medial injury. *Atherosclerosis* 1990;10:1082–1087.

23. Stadius ML, Rowan R, Franklin Fleischhauer F, Kernoff R, Billingham M, Gown AM. Time course and cellular characteristics of the iliac artery response to acute balloon injury. *Arteriosclerosis Thrombosis* 1992;12:1267–1273.

24. Jackson CL, Schwartz SM. Pharmacology of smooth muscle cell replication. (Tutorial.) *Hypertension* 1992;20:713–736.

25. Raines EW, Bowen-Pope DF, Ross R. Platelet-derived growth factor. In: Sporn MB, Roberts AB, eds. *Handbook of experimental pharmacology: peptide growth factors and their receptors.* Berlin: Springer-Verlag, 1990:173–262.

26. Klagsbrun M, Edelman ER. Biological and biochemical properties of fibroblast growth factors: implications for the pathogenesis of atherosclerosis. *Arteriosclerosis* 1989;9:269–278.

27. Roberts AB, Sporn MB. The transforming growth factors. In: Sporn MB, Roberts AB, eds. *Handbook of experimental pharmacology: peptide growth factors and their receptors.* Berlin: Springer-Verlag, 1990:419–472.

28. Deuel TF. Polypeptide growth factors: roles in normal and abnormal cell growth. *Annu Rev Cell Biol* 1987;3:443–492.

29. Liu MW, Roubin GS, King SB. Restenosis after coronary angioplasty: potential biologic determinants and role of intimal hyperplasia. *Circulation* 1989;79:1374–1387.

30. Clowes AW, Clowes MM. Kinetics of cellular proliferation after arterial injury. III. Heparin inhibits rat smooth muscle mitogenesis and migration. *Circ Res* 1986;58:839–845.

31. Gimbrone MA Jr. Vascular endothelium in health and disease. In: Haber E, ed. *Molecular cardiovascular medicine*. New York: Scientific American Medicine, 1994, In press.
32. Gimbrone MA Jr, ed. *Vascular endothelium in hemostasis and thrombosis*. Edinburgh: Churchill Livingstone, 1986.
33. Luscher TF, Vanhouette PM, eds. *The endothelium: modulator of cardiovascular function*. Boca Raton, FL: CRC Press, 1990.
34. Cybulsky MI, Gimbrone MA Jr. Endothelial leukocyte adhesion molecules in acute inflammation and atherogenesis. In: Simionescu N, Simionescu M, eds. *Endothelial cell dysfunctions*. New York: Plenum Press, 1992:129–140.
35. Simionescu N, Simionescu M, eds. *Endothelial cell dysfunctions*. New York: Plenum Press, 1992.
36. Pober JS, Cotran RC. Cytokines and endothelial cell biology. *Physiol Rev* 1990;70:427–451.
37. Collins TC. Endothelial nuclear factor-kB and the initiation of the atherosclerotic lesion. *Lab Invest* 1993;68:499.
38. Davies PF, Tripathi SC. Mechanical stress mechanisms and the cell: an endothelial paradigm. *Circ Res* 1993;72:239.
39. Resnick N, Collins T, Atkinson W, Bonthron DT, Dewey CF, Jr., Gimbrone MA, Jr. Platelet-derived growth factor B chain promoter contains a cis-acting fluid shear-stress-responsive element. *Proc Nat Acad Sci U.S.A.* 1993;90:4591–4595.
40. Gerrity RG, Naito HK, Richardson M, Schwartz CJ. Dietary induced atherogenesis in swine. Am J Pathol 1979;95:775–785.
41. Joris I, Nunnari JJ, Krolikowski FJ, Majno G. Studies on the pathogenesis of atherosclerosis. I. Adhesion and emigration of mononuclear cells in the aorta of hypercholesterolemic rats. *Am J Pathol* 1983;113:341–358.
42. Faggiotto A, Ross R, Harker L. Studies of hypercholesterolemia in the nonhuman primates. I. Changes that lead to fatty streak formation. *Arteriosclerosis* 1984;4:323–340.
43. Libby P, Hansson GK. Involvement of the immune system in human atherogenesis: current knowledge and unanswered questions. *Lab Invest* 1991;64:5–15.
44. Springer TA. Adhesion receptors of the immune system. *Nature* 1990;346:425–434.
45. Cybulsky MI, Gimbrone MA, Jr. Endothelial expression of a mononuclear leukocyte adhesion molecule during atherogenesis. *Science* 1991;251:788–791.
46. Rice GE, Munro JM, Bevilacqua MP. Inducible cell adhesion molecule 110(INCAM-110) is an endothelial receptor for lymphocytes: a CD11/CD18-independent adhesion mechanism. *J Exp Med* 1990;171:1369–1374.
47. Osborn L, Hession C, Tizard R, Vassallo C, Lubowskyj S, Chi-Rosso G, Lobb R. Direct expression of cloning of vascular cell adhesion molecule 1, a cytokine-induced endothelial protein that binds to lymphocytes. *Cell* 1989;59:1203–1211.
48. Cybulsky MI, Fries JWU, Williams AJ, Sultan P, Gimbrone MA, Jr, Collins T. Gene structure, chromosomal location, and basis for alternative mRNA splicing of the human VCAM1 gene. *Proc Natl Acad Sci U.S.A.* 1991;88:7859–7863.
49. Elices MJ, Osborn L, Takada Y, Crouse C, Lubowskyj S, Hemler ME, Lobb RR. VCAM-1 on activated endothelium interacts with the leukocyte integrin VLA-4 at a site distinct from the VLA-4/fibronectin binding site. *Cell* 1990;60:577–584.
50. Bochner BS, Luscinskas FW, Gimbrone MA, Jr, *et al*. Adhesion of human basophils, eosinophils, and neutrophils to interleukin-1-activated human vascular endothelial cells: contributions of endothelial cell adhesion molecules. *J Exp Med* 1991;173:1553–1556.
51. Li H, Cybulsky MI, Gimbrone MA, Jr, Libby P. An atherogenic diet rapidly induces VCAM-1, a cytokine-regulated mononuclear leukocyte adhesion molecule, in rabbit aortic endothelium. *Arteriosclerosis Thrombosis* 1993;13:197–204.
52. Schwenke DC, Carew TE. Initiation of atherosclerotic lesions in cholesterol-fed rabbits. II. Selective retention of LDL vs. selective increases in LDL permeability in susceptible sites of arteries. *Atherosclerosis* 1989;9:908–918.
53. Witztum JL, Steinberg D. Role of oxidized low density lipoprotein in atherogenesis. *J Clin Invest* 1991;88:1785–1792.

54. Kume N, Cybulsky MI, Gimbrone MA, Jr. Lysophosphatidylcholine, a component of atherogenic lipoproteins, induces mononuclear leukocyte adhesion molecules in cultured arterial endothelial cells. *J Clin Invest* 1992;90:1138–1144.
55. Bevilacqua MP, Nelson RM. Selectins. *J Clin Invest* 1993;91:379–387.
56. Spertini O, Luscinskas FW, Kansas GS, Munro JM, Griffin JD, Gimbrone MA, Jr, Tedder TF. Leukocyte adhesion molecule-1 (LAM-1, L-selectin) interacts with an inducible endothelial cell ligand to support leukocyte adhesion. *J Immunol* 1991;147:2565–2573.
57. Berliner JA, Territo MC, Sevanian A, *et al.* Minimal modified low density lipoprotein stimulates monocyte endothelial interactions. *J Clin Invest* 1990;85:1260–1266.
58. Clinton SK, Underwood R, Hayes L, Sherman ML, Kufe DW, Libby P. Macrophage colony-stimulating factor gene expression in vascular cells and in experimental and human atherosclerosis. *Am J Pathol* 1992;140:301–316.
59. Poston RN, Haskard DO, Coucher JR, Gall NP, Johnson-Tiedy RR. Expression of intercellular adhesion molecule-1 in atherosclerotic plaques. *Am J Pathol* 1992;140:665–673.
60. Nelken NA, Coughlin SR, Gordon D, Wilcox JN. Monocyte chemoattractant protein-1 in human atheromatous plaques. *J Clin Invest* 1991;88:1121–1127.
61. O'Brien KD, Allen MD, McDonald TO, *et al.* Vascular cell adhesion molecule-1 is expressed in human coronary atherosclerotic plaques. Implications for the mode of progression of advanced coronary atherosclerosis. *J Clin Invest* 1993;92:945–951.

Chapter 2

Atherosclerotic Plaques: Natural and Unnatural History

WILLIAM D. EDWARDS

Atherosclerosis is unquestionably the leading cause of death in Western society. Nearly one-half of all deaths in the United States are due to cardiovascular diseases, and approximately 90% of these are attributable to atherosclerosis. Ischemic heart disease, as a consequence of coronary atherosclerosis, accounts for about one-third of all deaths and two-thirds of all cardiovascular deaths.

Shallow focal atherosclerotic plaques can be identified in the coronary arteries of a substantial number of otherwise healthy young adults.[1,2] Even so, the disease is generally asymptomatic for several decades, until the size or number of plaques is sufficient to produce severe stenosis. When symptoms do develop, they tend to be episodic in nature, with intervening symptom-free periods of varying duration. Over time, atheromatous plaques change in size, shape, and number, and their enlargement is generally the consequence of chronic exposure to risk factors. With control of risk factors, progression of the disease may slow or halt, and in some cases, regression of lesions begins to take place.

Thus, plaques are dynamic lesions that are in a continuous state of flux. Those that are not enlarging are considered to be stable or quiescent, whereas atheromas that *are* expanding represent unstable or vulnerable lesions. Plaque growth, whether slow or abrupt, is usually associated with surface erosion, internal hemorrhage, luminal thrombosis, or a combination of these processes.[3–6] In *population* studies, various risk factors have been identified both for atherosclerosis and for plaque rupture (Tables 2.1 and 2.2). For *individual* patients and *individual* lesions, however, disease progression is a highly unpredictable process.[7]

To prevent, or at least minimize, the development of atherosclerosis, the elimination or control of chronic risk factors is advocated. Once the disease is present and symptomatic, however, therapy is generally directed toward relieving obstruction and preventing plaque rupture, thrombosis, and embolization. In this regard, the goals of current research and treatment are to understand and control the risk factors for acute plaque rupture and to transform unstable plaques into stable and quiescent lesions.[8–10]

TABLE 2.1.   RISK FACTORS FOR DEVELOPING ATHEROSCLEROSIS

Major Risk Factors	Other Risk Factors
Hypertension	Male gender
Hyperlipidemia	Advanced age
Cigarette smoking	Obesity
Diabetes mellitus	Insufficient regular physical activity
Family history	Homocystinuria

TABLE 2.2.   RISK FACTORS FOR SPONTANEOUS PLAQUE RUPTURE

Soft plaque with a necrotic core
Atheroma with a thin fibrous cap
Clusters of foam cells within the fibrous cap
Atherophagocytosis by giant cells
Intimal clusters of leukocytes
Adventitial bands of mononuclear leukocytes

MORPHOLOGY OF STABLE ATHEROSCLEROTIC PLAQUES

DEFINITION OF ATHEROSCLEROSIS

Atherosclerosis is a chronic, progressive, multifocal *intimal* disease, whose basic lesion is the atheroma or plaque. It primarily affects the large elastic arteries and large and medium-sized muscular arteries of the systemic circulation. Venous bypass grafts that are interposed within the arterial system can also develop atherosclerotic obstructions. For inexplicable reasons, the internal thoracic (mammary) artery, which is an elastic artery rather than muscular, is often spared the ravages of this disease.

In children and adolescents in all cultures, intimal fatty streaks form near the branch points of large arteries. These represent an adaptive response of the arterial intimal to chronic injury, usually from oxidized low-density lipoproteins. Their development entails the entry of lipids and monocytes into the subendothelial space (that is, beneath the basement membrane and above the internal elastic membrane). Here, under the direction of numerous chemical mediators, monocytes are transformed into macrophages and then into foam cells, and medial smooth muscle cells migrate and begin to proliferate.

Microscopically, it is foam cell necrosis, due to the toxic effects of excessive oxidized low-density lipoproteins, that heralds the transformation of an adaptive fatty streak into an atherosclerotic plaque.[5] In Western countries, arterial plaque is evident grossly at autopsy in virtually all persons older than 60 years. However, regardless of its prevalence, atherosclerosis clearly represents a *disease state* and not simply a degenerative or adaptive process.

PLAQUE DISTRIBUTION

Although atherosclerosis can occur throughout the systemic arterial circulation, it is often extensive only in certain regions. In the aorta, for example, severe ulcerocalcific disease with aneurysms and mural thrombus primarily affects the descending thoracic and abdominal regions and tends to be particularly prominent in the infrarenal segment. Furthermore, although mural thrombus can cause occlusive distal aortic disease, significant luminal obstruction by plaque is rare in the aorta. In contrast, severe obstruction is the primary consequence of atherosclerosis in muscular arteries and is most commonly observed in the coronary, carotid, cerebral, renal, and mesenteric arteries and in the arteries of the lower extremities (iliofemoral, popliteal, and tibial).

Coronary atherosclerosis is limited to the epicardial vessels and does not involve their intramural branches. Consequently, obstructions in the septal perforating branches of the anterior and posterior descending arteries occur only near their origins. Plaques also tend to be most severely obstructive in the proximal half of the left anterior descending and circumflex arteries (and their diagonal and marginal branches, respectively), whereas they may produce severe narrowing anywhere along the course of the right coronary artery.[11,12] High-grade disease distally in the left coronary system generally occurs only in hearts with severe proximal disease and usually is associated with shorter and more discrete lesions than those observed proximally. Critical obstruction of the left main coronary artery rarely occurs as an isolated lesion but, rather, is typically associated with severe disease in the other three major epicardial coronary arteries.

Among persons exposed similarly to the same risk factors, the extent and distribution of plaques can vary tremendously. Moreover, within the same person, atherosclerosis may be severe in some arteries and yet only mild or moderate in other vessels. Thus, although the term "generalized atherosclerosis" enjoys common usage, it does not adequately convey the variation in severity that often exists between different organ systems in the same subject. For this reason, the extent of atherosclerosis observed at autopsy should be recorded separately for the aorta, coronary arteries, and other major arterial regions.

PLAQUE COMPOSITION

The classic atheroma represents a raised fibrofatty plaque with a necrotic core and a fibrous outer coat. Within the core commonly are found degenerating blood elements, foam cells, cholesterol crystals, granulation tissue, smooth muscle cells, myofibroblasts, capillaries, calcium, iron pigment, giant cells, mononuclear leukocytes, and necrotic debris (Fig. 2.1). Adjacent to the internal elastic membrane, which often exhibits numerous focal disruptions and duplications, the plaque is frequently characterized by a prominent deposition of elastin and collagen in an onionskin pattern.

The overlying fibrous cap varies appreciably in thickness, and its endothelial lining often exhibits focal areas of denudation associated with adherent monocytes and platelets.[13] Whereas fibroblasts and smooth muscles of intimal origin produce nonthrombogenic collagen, those within an atheroma, that have migrated from the media, produce collagen that is very thrombogenic. Calcification appears to be related to the severity of stenosis and the age of the patient.[14]

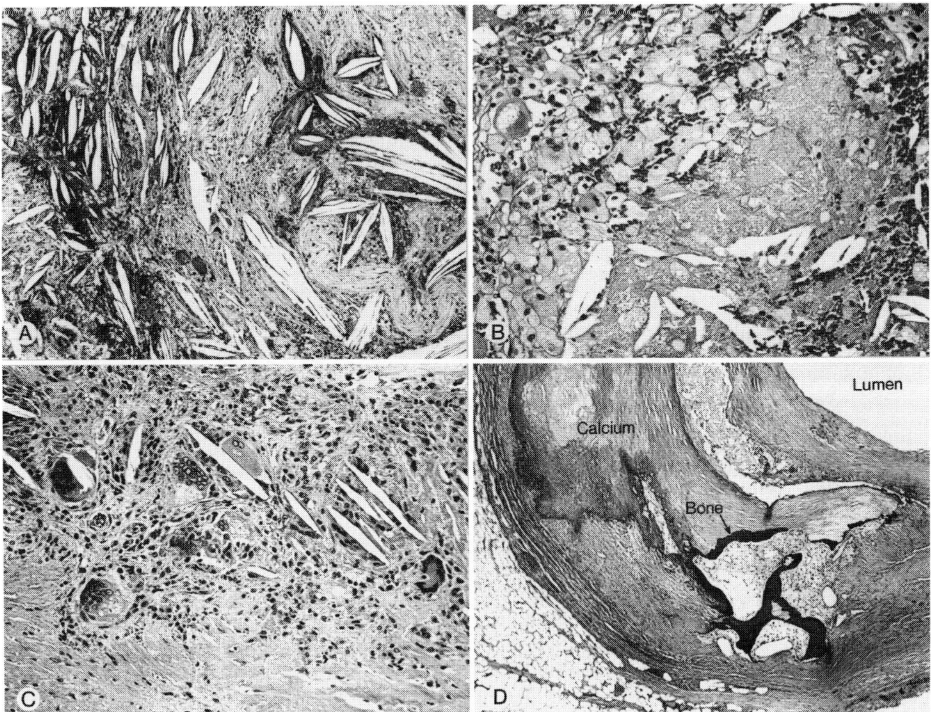

FIG. 2.1.   Plaque composition. *A,* cholesterol clefts. *B,* foam cells (*upper left*) and necrotic debris (*lower right*). *C,* giant cells adjacent to cholesterol crystals (atherophagocytosis). *D,* calcium deposition with focal bone formation (osseous metaplasia). Hematoxylin-eosin stain; *A,* ×90; *B* and *C,* ×180; *D,* ×36).

As with plaque distribution, the composition of atheromas can vary considerably, not only between persons, but also between arteries in the same person, or in the same organ, or even within the same artery itself. Plaque composition also affects vascular compliance.[15] Soft atheromas primarily consist of necrotic debris and are potentially moldable, whereas hard plaques usually represent rigid fibrocalcific structures (Fig. 2.2). Microscopically, many plaques contain both soft and hard elements. Thus, atherosclerotic plaques can be designated as fatty, fibrofatty, or fibrous, based on the relative contribution by soft and firm components. As atheromas age, they become more fibrotic and less cellular.[16] Coronary plaques in men tend to be more densely fibrotic and less cellular than those in women, perhaps indicating the earlier age at which the disease develops in men.[17]

The distinction between soft and hard lesions may be important clinically because plaque compliance can influence the success rate of interventions such as balloon angioplasty. By using invasive intravascular ultrasound, it is possible to determine whether an individual plaque is soft or hard. Moreover, the presence of calcium, indicative of a hard plaque, can be detected noninvasively by ultrafast computed tomography.[18]

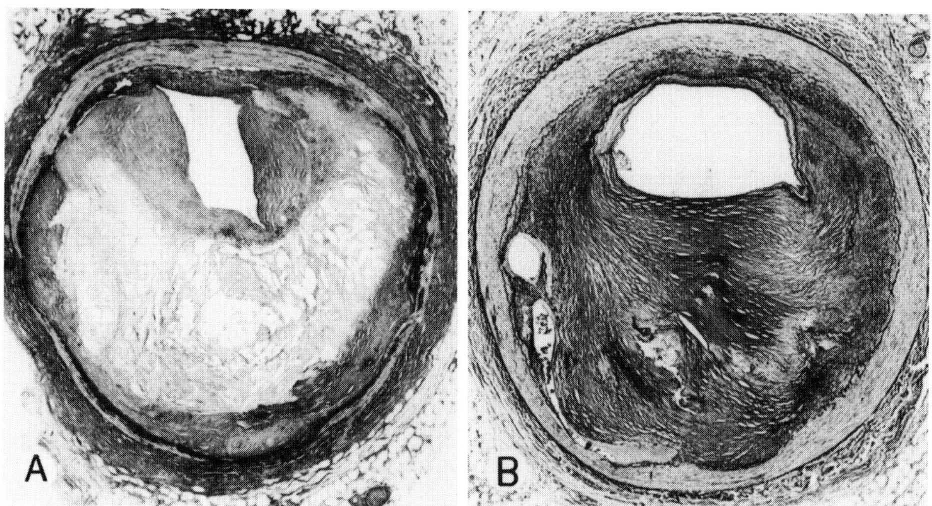

FIG. 2.2.　Plaque composition shown in coronary arteries. A, soft plaque, with necrotic core. B, hard plaque, with fibrocalcific core. Elastic-van Gieson; ×18.

PLAQUE MORPHOLOGY

Atherosclerotic plaques in the aorta are virtually always eccentric in location, such that they do not encircle the entire circumference of the artery. With time, however, adjacent plaques can enlarge and coalesce and eventually line the luminal circumference. By comparison, atheromas in muscular arteries may be either concentric or eccentric in location (Fig. 2.3). In coronary arteries, for example, about 70–75% of plaques are eccentric, and 25–30% are concentric. When viewed in cross-section, eccentric lesions are characterized by a disease-free segment that often exhibits medial hypertrophy.[19,20]

During the early stage of atherogenesis in muscular arteries, plaques are shallow and crescent shaped. As a result of dilation (or remodeling) of the involved arterial segment, the lumen remains relatively circular in shape and normal in diameter.[21] This capacity for dilation is limited, however, and coronary arteries rarely expand beyond twice their expected diameters.[22] Thus, as dilation begins to cease and as atheromas continue to increase in size and number, the result is appreciable luminal narrowing and eventual tissue ischemia.

In general, coronary arteries are considerably larger than necessary to provide adequate myocardial perfusion at rest. Even with vigorous exertion, their flow reserve is more than sufficient to supply the increased metabolic demands of the myocardium. In fact, the luminal cross-sectional area must decrease by more than 75% before coronary blood flow becomes insufficient with exertion, and it must decrease by at least 90% to be considered inadequate at rest.

Consequently, pathologists define critical lesions in muscular arteries as those that produce >75% obstruction of the luminal cross-sectional area. Be-

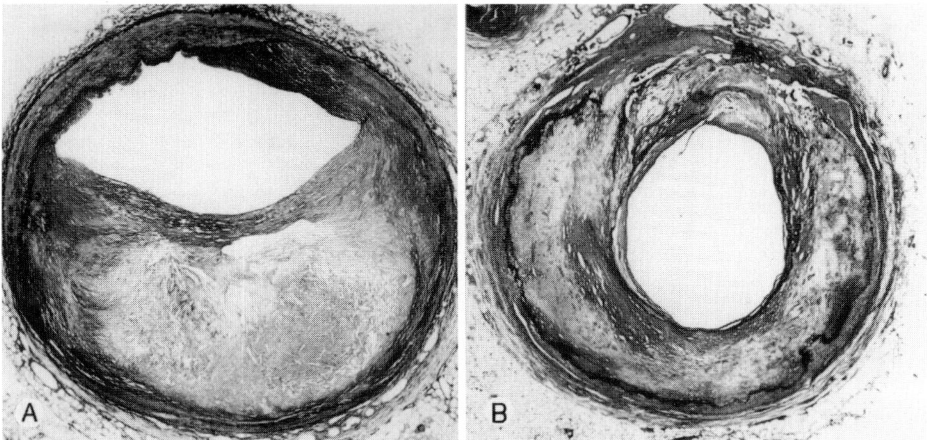

FIG. 2.3. Plaque location, demonstrated in coronary arteries. A, eccentric lesion (bottom) with disease-free segment (top). B, markedly calcified concentric plaque. Elastic-van Gieson; ×18. (From Edwards,22 with permission.)

cause the internal elastic membrane serves as an indicator of the ideal luminal size, its identification is necessary to evaluate the extent of obstruction. Bear in mind, however, that fibroelastic thickening of the intima occurs as an aging change and may achieve a thickness equal to that of the media by the age of 70 years. Age-related intimal thickening and atherosclerosis-related arterial dilatation should be taken into account when attempting to estimate the expected ideal luminal size.

For this purpose, arteries should be decalcified, cut in cross-section, and stained with an elastic-van Gieson or Movat pentachrome stain. Obstructions can then be assessed and graded according to 25% increments of cross-sectional luminal narrowing, such that grade 4 lesions (that is, those >75%) correspond to areas of critical stenosis (Fig. 2.4). A relatively easy method for determining the percent of stenosis is to estimate the number of lumens that can fit within the area bordered by the internal elastic membrane (Table 2.3). Planimetry may be used for studies in which more exact measurements are required. Complications, such as calcification, plaque rupture, or mural thrombosis, should be described in addition to the numerical grade.

For the coronary arteries, it is important to designate the number of epicardial vessels with critical (grade 4) lesions. In this regard, four major vessels are recognized and include the right coronary artery (RCA) and its acute marginal (RCA-AM), posterior descending (RCA-PD), and posterolateral (RCA-PL) branches; the left anterior descending artery (LAD) and its diagonal branches (LAD-D); the left circumflex artery (LCX) and its obtuse marginal branches (LCX-OM); and the left main coronary artery (LMA). The abbreviations shown in parentheses may be used for labeling microscopic slides of the epicardial coronary arteries. Patients can be described angiographically or pathologically as having one-vessel, two-vessel, three-vessel, or four-vessel disease. It is im-

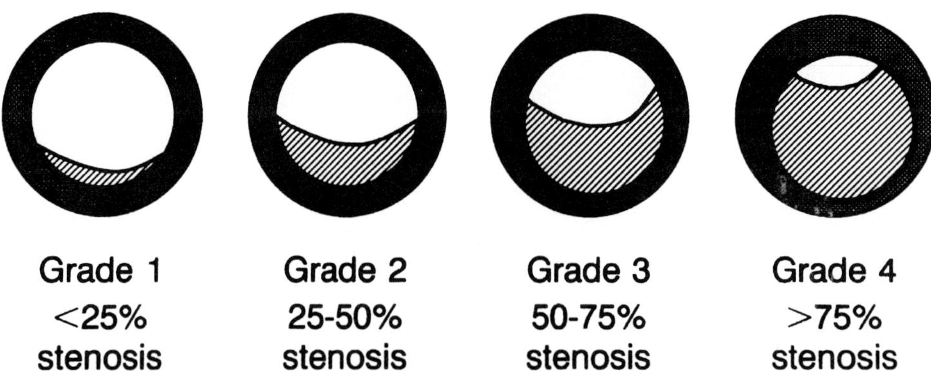

FIG. 2.4.   Plaque size, shown schematically. Using increments of 25%, narrowing of the luminal cross-sectional area can be expressed as a grade from 1 to 4. Grade 0 implies an absence of atherosclerosis, and grade 5 is occasionally used to indicate total (100%) occlusion. (From Edwards,[22] with permission.)

TABLE 2.3.   METHOD FOR RAPID MICROSCOPIC DETERMINATION OF PERCENT DECREASE IN CROSS-SECTIONAL LUMINAL AREA[a]

Actual Lumens per Expected Luminal Size[b]	Percent Obstruction in Luminal Area[c]
1	0 (Grade 0)
1.25	20 (Grade 1)
1.5	33 (Grade 2)
2	50 (Grade 3)
2.5	60
3	67
4	75 (Grade 4)
5	80
6	83
7	86
8	87
9	89
10	90
15	93
20	95
25	96
33	97
50	98
100	99

[a]Requires elastic-van Gieson or Movat pentachrome stain.
[b]Expected luminal size is determined by the area outlined by the internal elastic membrane.
[c]Grade 1, ≤25%; grade 2,>25% but ≤50%; grade 3,>50% but ≤75%; and grade 4,>75%.

portant to emphasize, however, that the other coronary arteries are rarely normal but, rather, contain numerous noncritical plaques.

For the aorta, a grading scale with 25% increments can also be applied, based on the percentage of surface area that is involved, rather than cross-sectional area. Complications of atherosclerosis, including aneurysms, should be designated separately. The extent and complications should be listed for each of the four aortic regions (ascending, arch, descending thoracic, and abdominal). For example, one may describe grade 3 ulcerocalcific disease in the descending thoracic aorta and grade 4 ulcerocalcific disease of the abdominal aorta with a thrombus-filled aneurysm (5.3 cm in diameter and 6.7 cm in length) of the infrarenal segment.

Because the cross-sectional shapes of atheromatous plaques in muscular arteries are so variable, it is not surprising that the corresponding residual lumens also have a variety of possible shapes.[23] Eccentric plaques generally produce lumens that are elliptical, circular, or D-shaped, and concentric lesions are often associated with circular or elliptical lumens (Fig. 2.5). Other shapes are encountered less frequently.

In the cardiac catheterization laboratory, coronary angiography produces a luminogram in which vessels are imaged longitudinally, not in cross-section. Stenosis is described in terms of the percentage of narrowing in luminal diameter, rather than luminal area. Moreover, in contrast to the definition used by pathologists that is based on inadequate blood flow with exertion, cardiologists define critical plaques as those that produce insufficient blood flow at rest. This represents a decrease in luminal area by >90%, which corresponds to a decrease in luminal diameter by >70% (Table 2.4).

In most cases, the degree of obstruction determined angiographically corresponds closely to that which is observed microscopically. Discrepancies, when they occur, are generally attributable to one of two errors.[22] Angiographically, the percent of narrowing is assessed by comparing the diameter at the point of obstruction with that proximally, assuming that the proximal segment is not

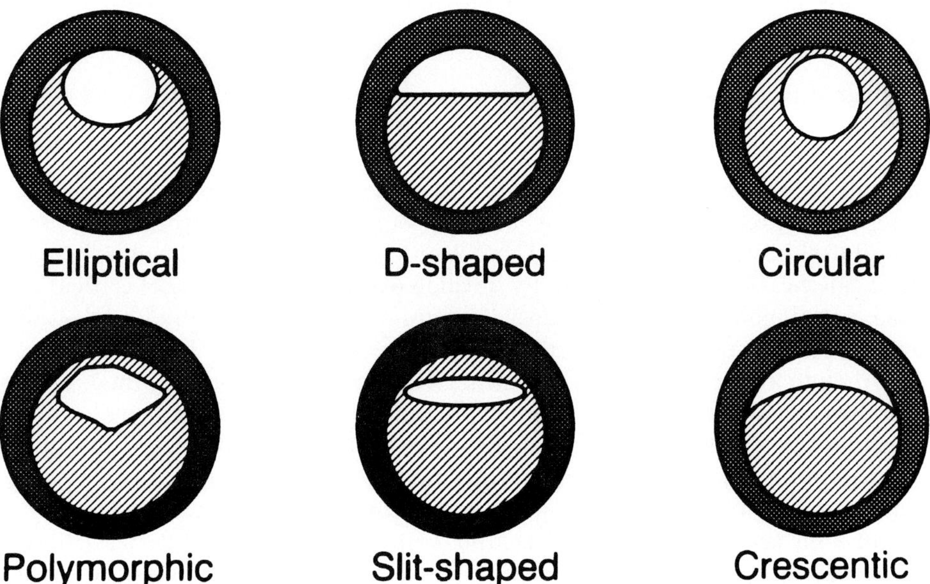

FIG. 2.5. Luminal shapes, shown schematically in cross-section. For atherosclerotic muscular arteries, most lumens are elliptical, D-shaped, or circular. (From Edwards,[22] with permission.)

TABLE 2.4. NARROWING IN LUMINAL DIAMETER COMPARED WITH NARROWING IN LUMINAL CROSS-SECTIONAL AREA

Percent Decrease in Luminal Diameter	Percent Decrease in Luminal Area	
	Actual	Approximate
10	19	20
20	36	35
30	51	50
40	64	65
50	75	75[a]
60	84	85
70[b]	91	90
80	96	95
90	99	99
100	100	100

[a]Critical lesion microscopically (>75% narrowing in luminal cross-sectional area).
[b]Critical lesion angiographically (>70% narrowing in luminal diameter).

diseased. If this assumption is faulty, which it often is, then the severity of obstruction will be *under*estimated (Fig. 2.6).[24,25] In contrast, if pathologists ignore the effect of arterial dilation and do not evaluate absolute luminal sizes in addition to the grade of stenosis, then the degree of obstruction can be overestimated (Figs. 2.7 and 2.8). Another potential source of error is the evaluation of coronary arteries that have not been perfusion fixed, in which collapse of the disease-free portion of the vessel wall produces a luminal area that is appreciably smaller than that which existed during life (see Fig. 2.16*B*).

Secondary Vascular Lesions

Intimal calcification commonly affects atherosclerotic plaques, and its occurence is related to plaque size and patient age. Clinically, even very small amounts of calcium can be detected with ultrafast computed tomography.[18] Although the presence of calcium generally indicates the presence of significant disease, it is recognized that the calcified segment does not necessarily correspond to the site of most severe obstruction. Furthermore, in the elderly, coronary calcification may occasionally develop even in the absence of critical disease, and in subjects younger than 40 years, it may be clinically undetectable even in the presence of critical disease.

Although atherosclerosis is an intimal disease, the underlying media often becomes secondarily affected. Remodeling and dilation (as described above) result in a stretched and thinned media. In general, the more severe the stenosis, the more extensive the underlying medial thinning and atrophy will be. Occasionally, large calcified plaques, particularly in the aorta, can erode into or through the media. For a muscular artery, dilation beyond twice its expected diameter is considered aneurysmal. Furthermore, in muscular vessels with eccentric plaques, the disease-free wall opposite the atheroma is often involved by compensatory medial hypertrophy, a process that may play a role in subsequent spasm at that site.

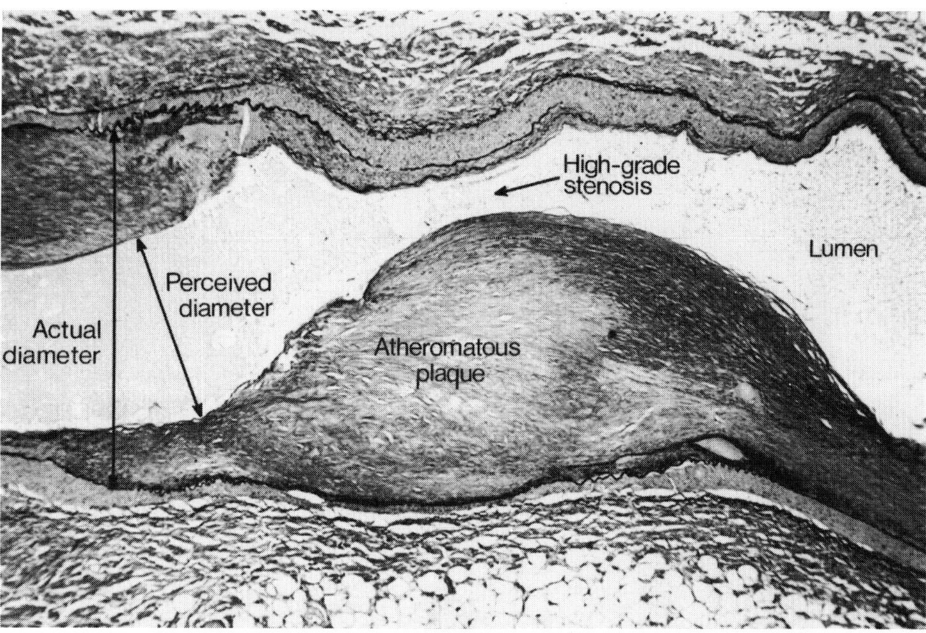

FIG. 2.6.   A clinical source for error in determining the severity of vascular obstruction, shown in a longitudinal section of a coronary artery. If the region proximal to the high-grade obstruction is considered disease-free angiographically, then the calculated degree of stenosis will be underestimated. Elastic-van Gieson; ×36. (From Edwards,[22] with permission.)

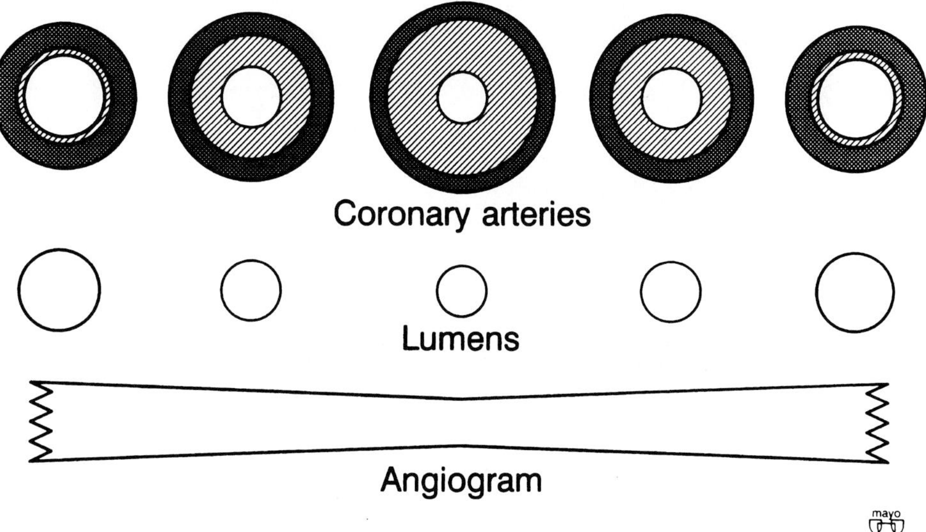

FIG. 2.7.   A microscopic source for error in determining the severity of vascular stenosis, shown schematically. If the effects of arterial dilation are not considered, and if the degree of change in absolute luminal size is also ignored, then the severity of obstruction will be overestimated. (From Edwards,[22] with permission.)

     Cardiovascular Pathology

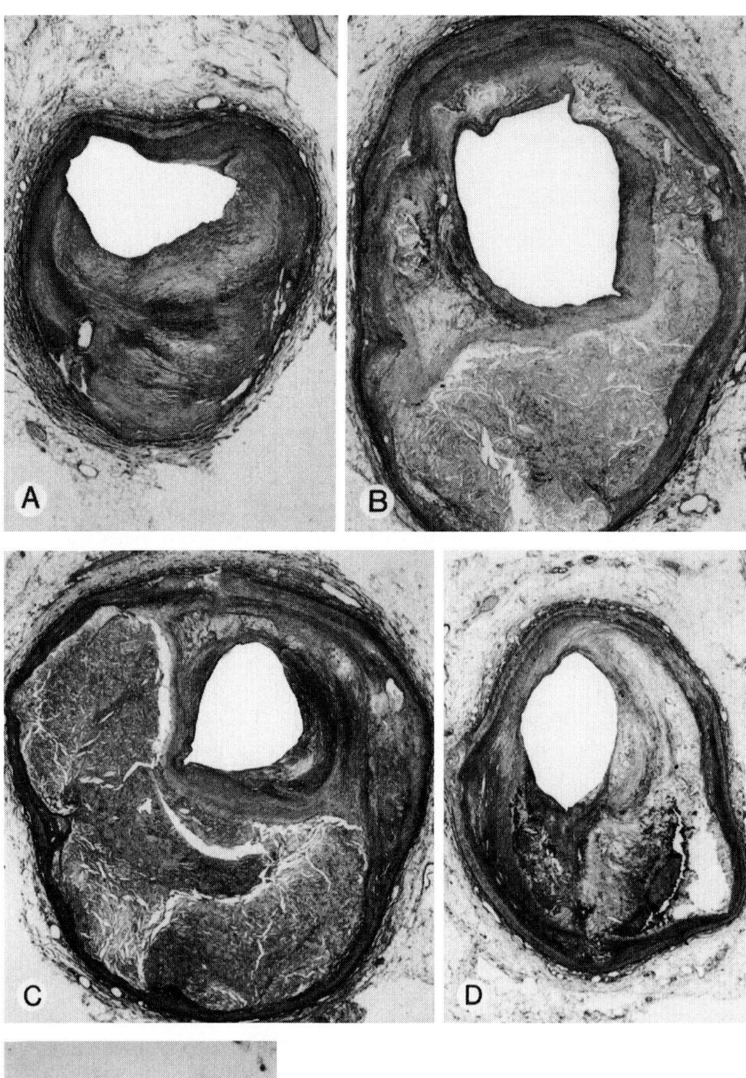

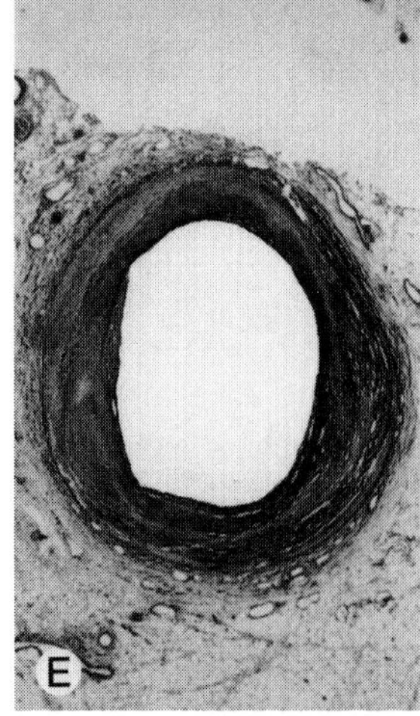

FIG. 2.8. Serial cross-sections from a coronary artery (*A–E*), showing the microscopic source of error described in Fig. 7. *C* appears to represent a grade 4 lesion, with 85–90% obstruction. However, note the degree of dilation (compared with *A* and *E*), and note the small difference in absolute luminal area (compared with *E*). In reality, the lumen in *C* is narrowed by only about 50–60%. Elastic-van Gieson; ×12). (From Edwards,[22] with permission.)

Beneath a region of medial dilation and atrophy, fibroelastic thickening of the adventitia may occur. This phenomenon helps to explain why interventionally related transmural lacerations of the coronary arteries rarely produce a hemopericardium. The adventitia can also become the site of a dense lymphoplasmacytic infiltrate, with a propensity for perineural involvement.[26] Similar infiltrates are commonly observed in the media and intima. Although this process does not represent vasculitis, it does indicate an unstable plaque that is prone to rupture.[27]

MORPHOLOGY OF UNSTABLE ATHEROSCLEROTIC PLAQUES

DEFINITION OF UNSTABLE PLAQUES

Stable plaques become unstable lesions when dynamic alterations occur that lead, either directly or indirectly, to abrupt luminal narrowing. The four most frequently encountered alterations are plaque rupture, plaque hemorrhage, thrombosis, and medial spasm.[26–30] Although each of these four processes is discussed separately below, it is important to recognize that they generally act in concert. Plaque rupture often results in thrombosis and, through various chemical mediators, thrombosis can promote vasospasm. Spasm, in turn, may cause mechanical stresses that extend the site of plaque rupture, and so the cycle continues.

The response-to-injury model of atherogenesis implies a dynamic, ongoing process that is driven by repetitive injury over time.[3–9] Obstructive lesions may develop slowly and insidiously, as atheromas coalesce or develop atop one another, or they can grow in spurts, as a period of quiescence or slow progression is punctuated by an acute, and often catastrophic, occlusion. Clinical studies have increased our understanding of the dynamic nature of atherosclerosis in living patients and have demonstrated not only the transformation of stable plaques into unstable ones but also the rapid, minute-by-minute changes that take place during acute coronary thrombosis.[28–31] Angiographically, the appearance of unstable plaques differs substantially from that of chronic stable plaques (Fig. 2.9).

Although the following discussion is based primarily on observations in the coronary circulation, these findings also apply to other muscular arteries. In contrast, aortic plaques are more often associated with aneurysm formation and atheroembolization than with acute obstruction.

PLAQUE RUPTURE

Numerous clinicopathologic investigations have demonstrated that surface injury is the most common feature of unstable plaques.[3–6,8,9,32–36] Microscopically, the observed sites of injury span a broad morphologic range, from minimal surface erosions, at one extreme, to lacerations that extend deep within the plaque, at the other extreme. Because of these different appearances, various authors have coined several terms for the site of injury, including erosion, ulceration, fissure, laceration, tear, and rupture. Regardless of the extent of injury, however, the result is exposure of the luminal blood to a thrombogenic

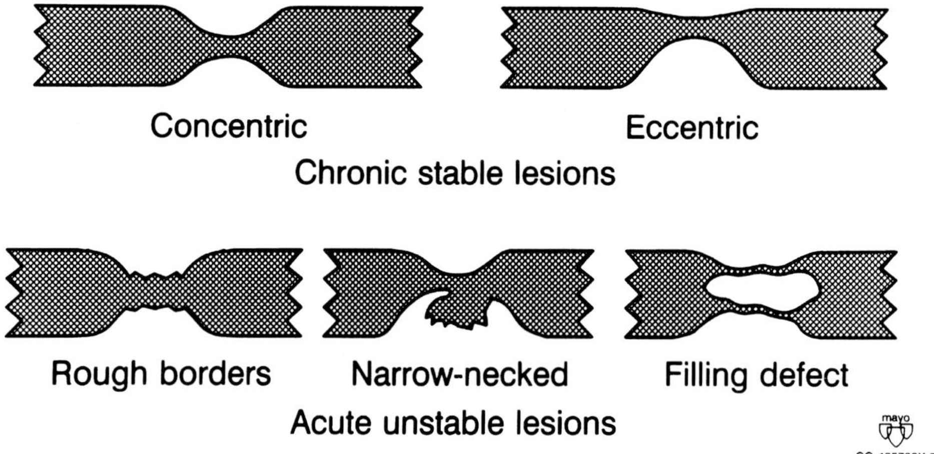

FIG. 2.9. Angiographic appearance of stable and unstable coronary atherosclerotic lesions, shown schematically. (From Edwards,[22] with permission.)

surface (collagen or necrotic debris), thereby setting the stage for acute thrombotic obstruction.

The causes of plaque rupture are complex and poorly understood, and they encompass both functional disturbances at the biochemical level and structural alterations at the microscopic level.[3] Surface erosions and fissures are more likely to involve soft and eccentric plaques than hard and concentric lesions.[37] Based on postmortem studies, various risk factors for plaque rupture have been identified (Table 2.2) and include atheromas that are soft or contain areas of atherophagocytosis by giant cells, fibrous caps that are thin or contain focal clusters of foam cells or inflammatory cells, and adventitial regions that harbor clusters of mononuclear leukocytes.[33,38,39] Mechanical stress points for eccentric lesions have been identified at the junction of the plaque with the more normal-appearing arterial wall and along the center of the plaque.[40,41] These points correspond precisely to the actual sites of rupture most commonly encountered at autopsy.

Currently, the only risk factor for rupture that can be detected clinically in living patients is plaque compliance.[15] Even so, one cannot accurately predict if or when a particular soft plaque will undergo surface ulceration. None of the other factors can be assessed clinically. Furthermore, among those features that can be evaluated, such as calcification and critical stenoses, none are risk factors for plaque rupture. The implication is that plaque erosion and secondary thrombosis are just as likely to occur on noncritical lesions as critical ones, and this has been demonstrated in various clinical studies.[42,43]

Once plaque rupture has occurred, several different outcomes are possible in muscular arteries (Figs. 2.10 and 2.11).[22] In some cases, thrombosis is minimal, and the fissure or erosion is simply filled in by fibrous tissue. For soft plaques, atheroembolization to small distal arterial branches also may occur,

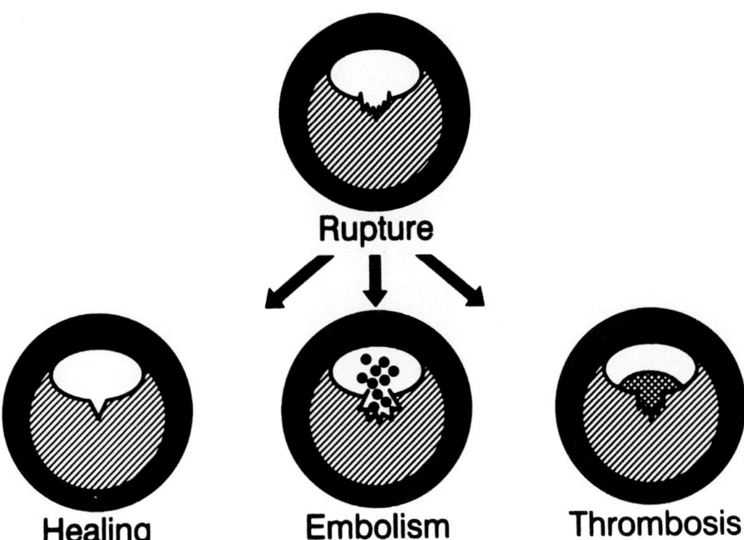

FIG. 2.10. Possible fates of ruptured atherosclerotic plaques in muscular arteries, shown schematically in cross-section. (From Edwards,[22] with permission.)

and in the heart, this phenomenon can cause various arrhythmias, including ventricular tachycardia. Although the formation of a platelet-fibrin thrombus over an area of surface erosion is probably the most common scenario, it is important to emphasize that the early thrombus is generally shallow and may undergo numerous cycles of enlargement, only to be washed away by the continual flow of luminal blood.

In the aorta, the possible consequences of plaque ulceration are somewhat different than those discussed for the coronary and other muscular arteries. Areas of ulceration often produce showers of atheroemboli to the spleen, kidneys, and lower extremities. In some cases, the ulcer site remains open but endothelialized, and in other cases, it becomes coated with mural thrombus. Less commonly, the ulceration burrows beyond the confines of the intima and into the media and even the adventitia. These so-called penetrating ulcers of the aorta may be associated with medial hematomas, intramedial dissections, thrombus-filled false aneurysms, or transmural ruptures (Fig. 2.12).[44–46] Such lesions are most frequently found in the distal portion of the descending thoracic aorta, although any region of the aorta can be involved.

PLAQUE HEMORRHAGE

Plaque rupture may lead not only to thrombosis but also to hemorrhage within the atheroma. Although the region of hemorrhage consists primarily of red blood cells, the surfaces along the rupture tract are often lined by aggregates of platelets.[34] With deep intimal lacerations, luminal blood under systemic pressure gains entry into the core of the plaque. This, in turn, causes a

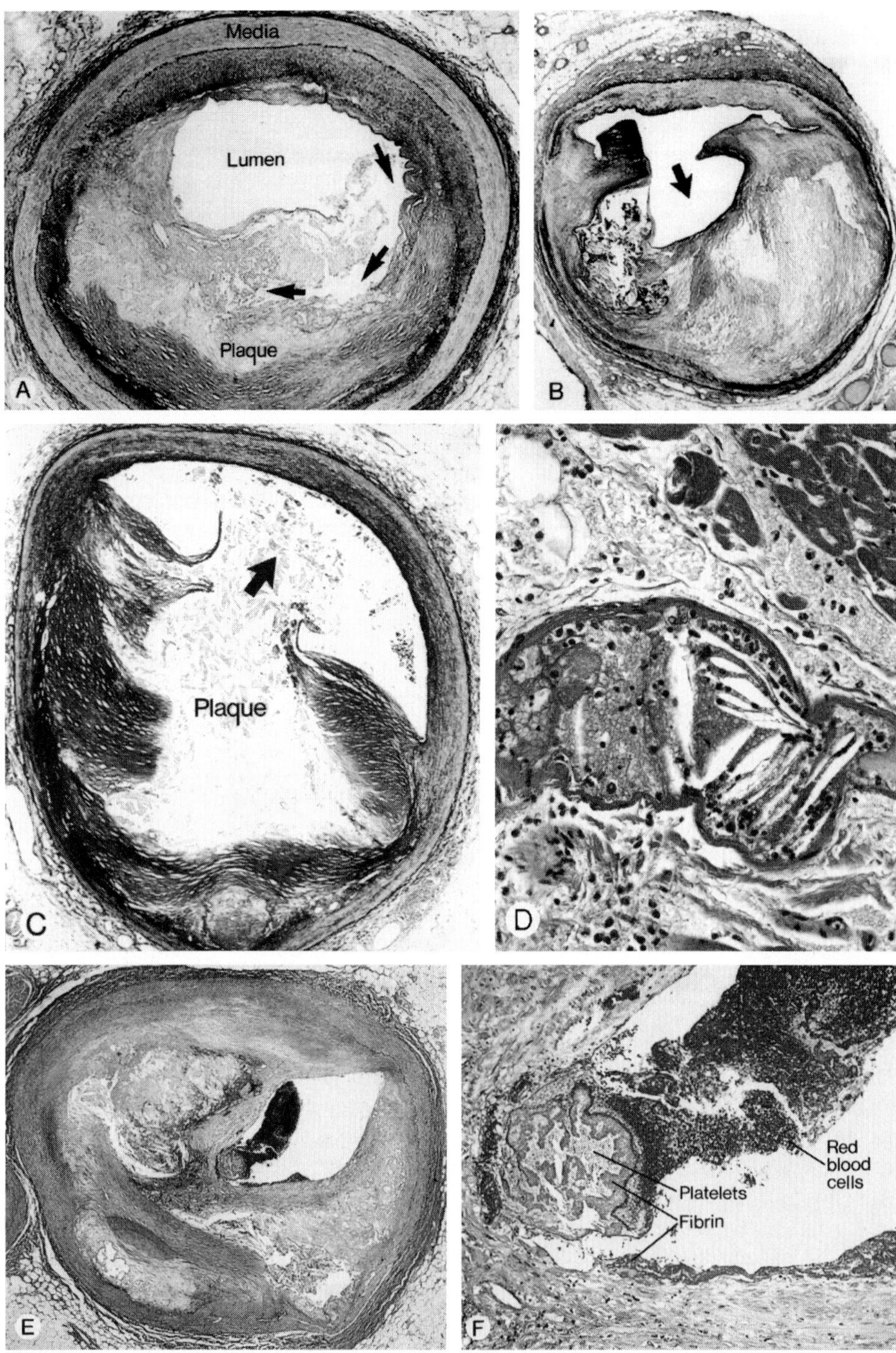

FIG. 2.11. Spontaneous plaque rupture and its consequences, demonstrated in coronary arteries. *A,* deep intimal fissure tract (*arrows*) at a vulnerable junction between the plaque and disease-free wall. *B,* old healed rupture site (*arrow*) without evidence of thrombus. *C,* erosion of thin fibrous cap, with expulsion of atheromatous debris into the lumen (*arrow*). *D,* atheroembolus in a small intramural coronary artery branch. *E, F,* shallow ulceration associated with early thrombosis, shown in overview (*E*) and close-up (*F*) to emphasize the variable composition of a thrombus. *A–C,* elastic-van Gieson; ×24, ×18, ×18, respectively. *D–F,* hematoxylin-eosin; ×180, ×18, ×90, respectively. (From Edwards,[22] with permission.)

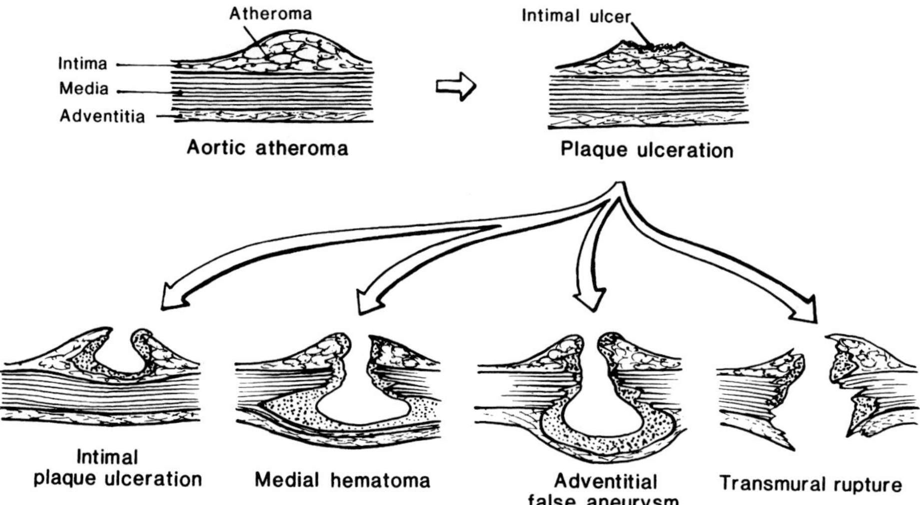

FIG. 2.12. Possible fates of ulcerated atherosclerotic plaques in the aorta, shown schematically. (From Stanson et al.,[46] with permission.)

rapid expansion in plaque volume and a rapid diminution in luminal area.[34] Expulsion and embolization of necrotic atheromatous debris may occur in the aftermath.

Plaque hemorrhage can also develop by an entirely different mechanism, one that does not involve plaque rupture. Within the core of a soft atheroma, primary disruption of capillary channels, derived from the vasa vasorum, may occur and lead to rapid plaque enlargement.[47,48] Because small hemorrhages are observed so frequently in nonruptured plaques, this mechanism presumably occurs with some regularity, particularly in large soft atheromas, and is important in the progressive enlargement of plaques over time. However, among patients with acute myocardial infarction, plaque rupture is a more common cause of intimal hemorrhage than disruption of intraatheromatous vasa vasorum.[49]

Microscopically, acute intimal hemorrhage generally is characterized by focal collections of intact red blood cells within the pultaceous core of an atheroma.[50] The core, in turn, often contains evidence of older hemorrhagic or thrombotic events, including degenerating red blood cells, compact fibrin, and hemosiderin pigment, in addition to the usual macrophages, foam cells, giant cells, and cholesterol crystals.

THROMBOSIS

Autopsy studies indicate that plaque erosions underlie coronary thrombosis in at least 90% of the cases.[51] From a clinical perspective, thrombosis represents the most important complication of plaque rupture because of its relationship to sudden and often catastrophic tissue infarction. Nevertheless, it is important to emphasize that infarction is *not* the most common consequence of arterial thrombosis. Whether thrombus remains shallow and nonocclusive or progresses to form an occlusive mass depends on several factors, including exposure to thrombogenic material, the balance between thrombosis and thrombolysis, and local flow disturbances caused by the underlying plaque.[52] Current dogma suggests that a deep plaque rupture is more likely than a shallow surface erosion to produce an occlusive thrombus.[9]

However, the prevalent notions that deep injury involves the arterial media and that medial tissue is substantially more thrombogenic than an intimal plaque represent erroneous concepts. First, spontaneous plaque ruptures, regardless of their depth, are virtually always confined to the intimal layer and do not extend into the media (with the exception of penetrating ulcerations of the aorta). Second, plaque collagen, produced by medially derived smooth muscle cells, is quite thrombogenic, and necrotic core debris is even more so.[53] Third, injury produced in animals by balloon dilation of normal arteries is not directly comparable with that which occurs spontaneously in atherosclerotic arteries from humans.

Just as plaque rupture has several potential outcomes, so also does luminal thrombosis (Fig. 2.13).[34] Following endothelial disruption (whether functional or structural), shallow thrombus covers the site of injury and initially primarily consists of platelets with little fibrin. The opposing effects of thrombosis and intrinsic thrombolysis, coupled with the hemodynamic effects of pulsatile luminal blood flow, lead to rapid alterations in thrombus size. Within the coronary arteries of living patients, angioscopy has demonstrated that dramatic changes occur rapidly, over the course of minutes, as thrombus is formed and then washed away, only to form again.[28–31]

With time, as the fibrin content increases, the thrombus begins to stabilize

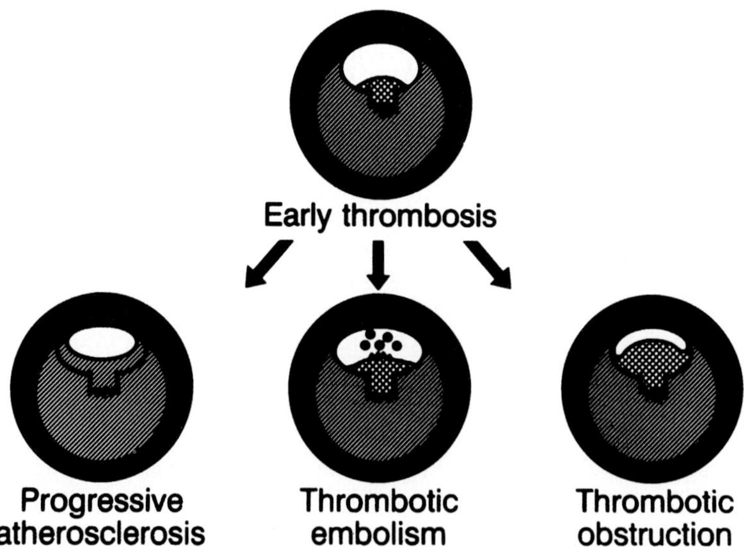

FIG. 2.13.   Possible fates of arterial thrombus, shown schematically in cross-section. (From Edwards,[22] with permission.)

and form a relatively shallow nonocclusive mass. Eventually, degeneration and organization lead to incorporation into the underlying atheroma. This and plaque hemorrhage represent the two most common mechanisms for chronic plaque progression. Although these processes are acute, their extent is generally mild, such that luminal narrowing most often progresses by numerous small steps, rather than by one catastrophic step. In the coronary circulation, this is borne out both pathologically by the large number of stable plaques that exist compared with the smaller number of unstable lesions and clinically by the results of sequential angiograms in individual patients.[7,54] Less commonly, the process becomes occlusive, or nearly so, and stagnant blood flow leads to the propagation of a red thrombus both proximally and distally to the site of plaque rupture. Thromboembolization represents another possible consequence of coronary thrombosis.

For pathologists, the microscopic evaluation of atherosclerosis entails playing the role of a medical archeologist and interpreting both recent lesions and the fibrotic aftermath of lesions that may have occurred months to years earlier. For this challenge, an elastic-van Gieson or Movat pentachrome stain is not only recommended, it is considered a necessity. Tissues should be decalcified, arteries should be cut in cross-section, and slides should be prepared with as few wrinkles as possible. With practice and experience, one will readily begin to identify evidence of plaque progression due to previous cycles of rupture and thrombosis (Fig. 2.14).

Old arterial thrombus has a wide range of microscopic appearances that depend in part on the size and age of the lesion. Some become densely fibrotic, whereas others remain loose and myxoid. Many contain small capillary channels, and a few develop multiple large recanalization channels. In this regard, even so-called chronic total coronary occlusions often exhibit several prominent vascular channels, into which a guidewire might be inserted during an interventional procedure in the cardiac catheterization laboratory.

The microscopic appearance of acute thrombotic lesions is also somewhat variable. Classically, the initial thrombus over a site of plaque erosion consists of platelets and fibrin. As the thrombus enlarges, generally it is characterized by a loose mesh of fibrin in which large numbers of red blood cells become trapped. In some patients, however, the thrombus consists entirely of platelets and fibrin regardless of its size, and in others, it represents primarily a mass of red blood cells almost from its inception.

MEDIAL SPASM

Coronary spasm represents a medial phenomenon. As such, the severity of acute luminal narrowing is greater for arteries harboring eccentric plaques, with medial hypertrophy of the disease-free portion of the arterial wall, than for those with concentric lesions with diffuse medial atrophy.[55] Even among eccentric plaques, luminal size and shape affect the extent to which medial spasm can produce acute luminal obstruction (Figs. 2.15 and 2.16). Vasospasm may also occur in arteries without appreciable atherosclerosis. Although one generally associates acute vasoconstriction with coronary arteries, spasm is

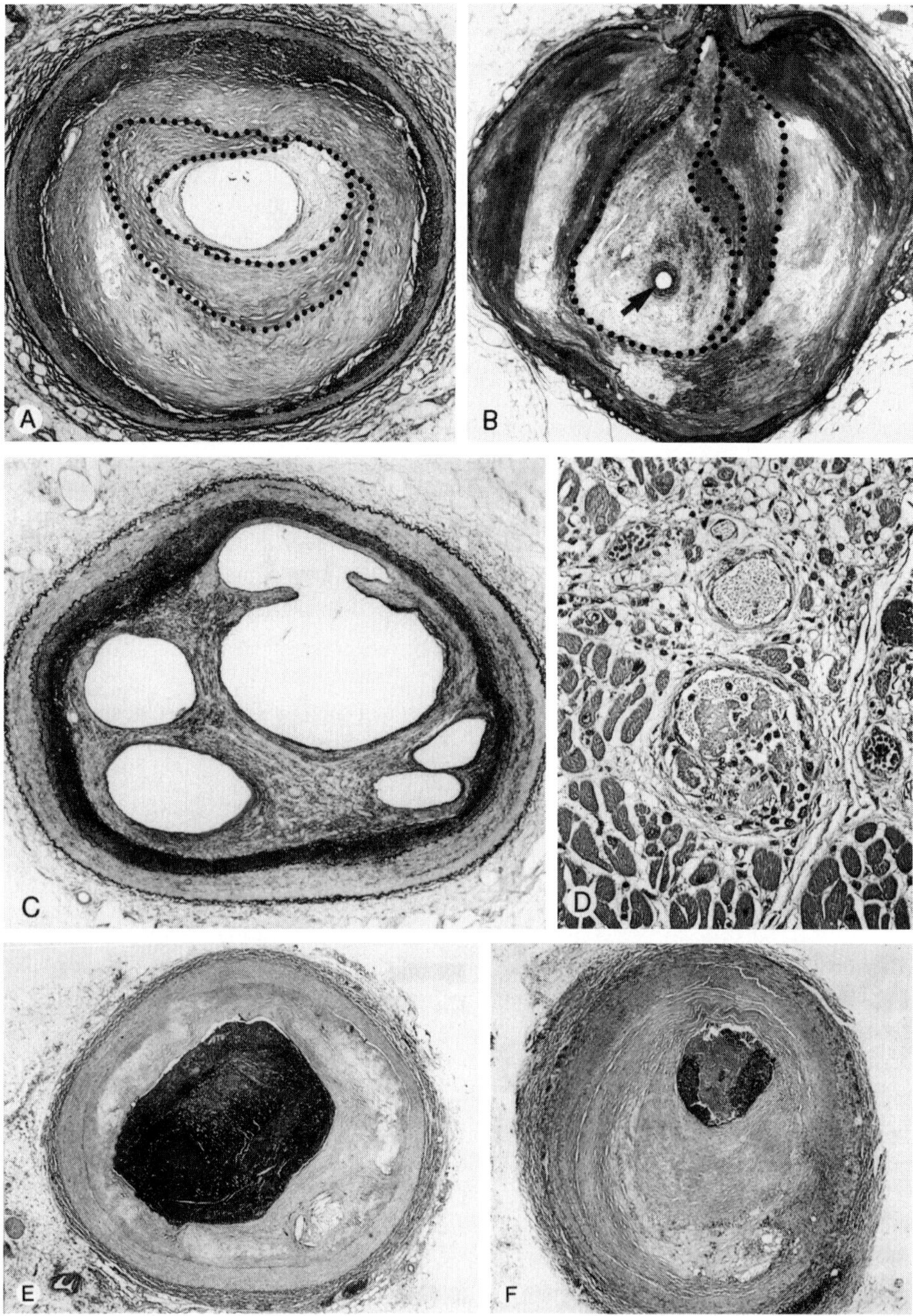

FIG. 2.14.　Thrombosis and its consequences, shown in coronary arteries. *A,* healing by fibrosis (twice), with progression of atherosclerotic narrowing (black dotted lines indicate previous luminal borders). *B,* organization of occlusive thrombus, with extremely small residual lumen (*arrow*) (black dotted line indicates previous luminal borders). *C,* organization of an occlusive thrombus, with apparent endogenous thrombolysis and formation of large recanalization channels. *D,* embolization of platelet-fibrin thrombus to an intramural coronary artery branch. *E, F,* enlargement of an acute thrombus, with luminal occlusion, occuring on noncritical (*E*) and critical (*F*) plaques. *A–C,* elastic-van Gieson; ×36, ×18, ×36, respectively. *D–F,* hematoxylin-eosin, ×360, ×36, ×24, respectively. (From Edwards,[22] with permission.)

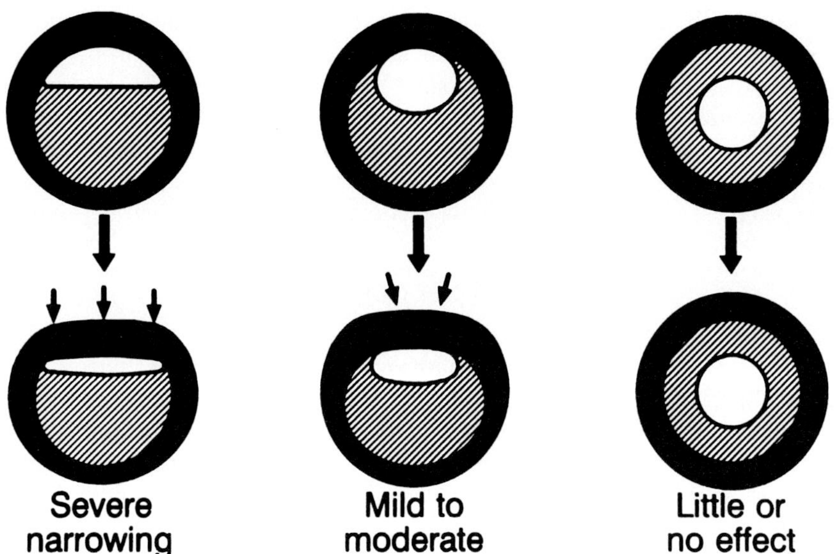

FIG. 2.15. Effect of coronary artery spasm on lumens of varying size, shape, and location, shown schematically. (From Edwards,[22] with permission.)

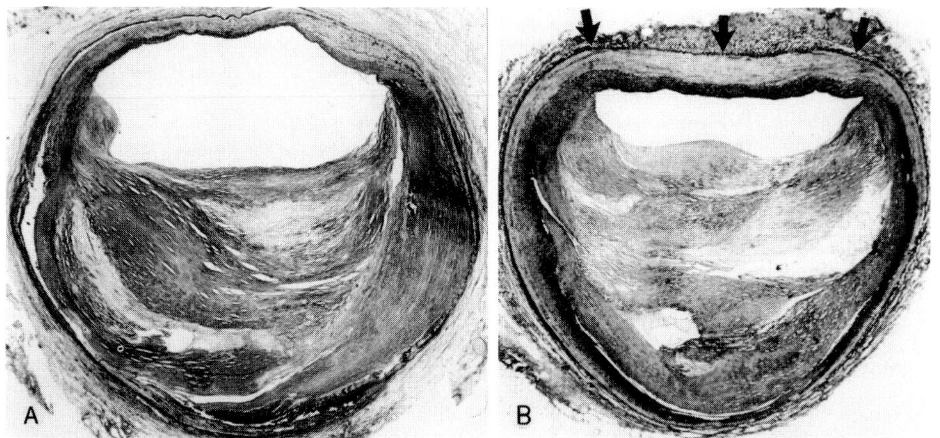

FIG. 2.16. Simulation of the effect of coronary vasospasm on luminal dimensions. *A,* perfusion-fixed vessel has a large elliptical lumen. *B,* nonperfusion-fixed specimen exhibits collapse of disease-free segment (*arrows*), simulating spasm-related luminal narrowing. Elastic-van Gieson; ×18. (*A,* from Edwards,[22] with permission.)

also clinically important in other muscular arteries, including mesenteric, renal, cerebral, digital, and pulmonary. In addition, it may affect internal thoracic (mammary) arteries used as coronary bypass grafts, as well as aortocoronary saphenous vein bypass grafts.

In some cases, medial spasm alone causes sufficient acute stenosis to produce myocardial ischemia and chest pain, even in patients who otherwise have angiographically normal coronary arteries. Spasm may also produce sufficient wall stress and buckling to result in surface disruption, thereby initiating plaque rupture and mural thrombosis.[56] For other patients, spasm follows, rather than precedes, an episode of plaque erosion and thrombosis, due to the release of vasoconstrictive substances. Depending on the extent of thrombosis (that is, either mural or occlusive), spasm can be associated with chronic plaque progression or with the acute ischemic syndromes such as myocardial infarction.[57]

FATE OF UNSTABLE PLAQUES

Plaque instability is characterized microscopically by rupture or hemorrhage of the atheroma, with or without overlying thrombosis. Thrombus may be nonocclusive (mural) or occlusive. As a functional rather than structural disorder, medial spasm can be observed during angiography or angioscopy but not microscopically. In the cardiac catheterization laboratory, vasospasm is usually induced by the intracoronary administration of ergonovine. However, it is recognized that other agents, such as cocaine, may also cause coronary vasospasm in susceptible persons, presumably by acting on receptors other than those operative for ergonovine.

Potential outcomes for unstable lesions include healing at the site of plaque erosion, atheroembolization, nonocclusive thrombosis, thromboembolization, organization of mural thrombus (plaque progression), acute thrombotic occlusion, and organization of the occlusive mass, with varying degrees of recanalization.[34] Among these outcomes, the most common fate is plaque progression, due to either resealing of the plaque fissure or organization of a nonocclusive mural thrombus.

CLINICAL CORRELATIONS WITH STABLE AND UNSTABLE PLAQUES

GENERAL FEATURES

Discussion in this section is limited primarily to the coronary arteries. However, the observations in these vessels are also generally applicable to other muscular arteries that become involved by atherosclerosis.

Patients with coronary artery disease may be categorized into one of five clinical groups, including asymptomatic disease and four symptomatic categories—angina pectoris, myocardial infarction, chronic heart failure, and sudden death. Within these five groups, several important clinical subgroups are recognized. Angina pectoris may be stable, variant, microvascular, or unstable, and myocardial infarctions can be acute or old and either subendocardial or transmural. Unstable angina, acute myocardial infarction, and sudden death are known collectively as the acute coronary syndromes. Some microscopic lesions, such as plaque hemorrhage, occur with similar frequency in each of the four major symptomatic categories.[50] Others, such as plaque rupture and luminal thrombosis, occur predominantly with the acute coronary syndromes.

With progression of atherosclerosis, the clinical state often shifts from one major group to another (Fig. 2.17). Whereas the shift from asymptomatic to

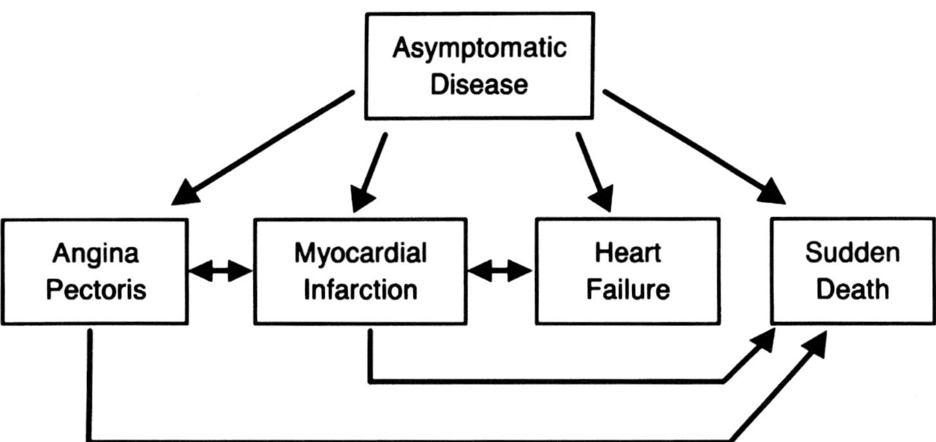

FIG. 2.17. Clinical coronary syndromes, showing transitions that can occur as the disease progresses. Because a fatal outcome is expected in unoperated patients with ischemic heart disease and severe congestive heart failure, death is usually neither sudden nor unexpected, hence the absence of an arrow between heart failure and sudden death.

symptomatic disease generally occurs over the course of decades, the transition from unstable angina to acute myocardial infarction can occur over weeks or days. In general, non-Q wave infarctions involve only the subendocardial region, and Q wave lesions correspond to transmural necrosis. Clinically, there is a continuous spectrum from unstable angina to subendocardial infarction to transmural infarction.[58]

ASYMPTOMATIC CORONARY ARTERY DISEASE

Asymptomatic coronary atherosclerosis is generally characterized by stable noncritical plaques or by single-vessel disease. Occasionally, however, a previously asymptomatic patient is found at autopsy to have critical two-vessel or three-vessel disease. In this setting, death may be attributed to an ischemia-related arrhythmia or to nonischemic causes, depending on the other autopsy findings. Similarly, a hypotension-related perioperative myocardial infarction can be the first clinical manifestation of severe coronary artery disease. Unstable atheromas also can be asymptomatic and usually are characterized either by simple resealing of a plaque fissure or by a very shallow mural thrombus along an area of surface erosion.

Clearly, then, absence of symptoms does not necessarily imply an absence of disease. This is an important concept. In living patients, assurance that there is no critical coronary stenosis is based on actual visualization of the arterial lumens and not solely on a negative history for chest pain or myocardial infarction. This also pertains to symptomatic patients with heart failure, among whom some, particularly diabetics, will be misdiagnosed as having idiopathic dilated cardiomyopathy if their coronary arteries are not properly evaluated.

ANGINA PECTORIS

In subjects at rest, stable atheromatous plaques in the coronary circulation are usually asymptomatic. With exercise, however, blood flow through segments with critical (grade 4) lesions may be inadequate to meet the increased myocardial oxygen demand. Ischemic chest pain can result and is referred to as chronic stable angina pectoris. Synonyms include exertional and classic angina. Most patients with stable angina have either two-vessel or three-vessel critical coronary atherosclerosis (Table 2.5).[59,60]

Vasotonic angina occurs as a result of medial spasm and can affect either the epicardial coronary arteries, as variant or Prinzmetal's angina, or the smaller transmural branches, as microvascular angina.[61] Variant angina is generally nonexertional in nature and, in the cardiac catheterization laboratory, can be induced with ergonovine. Microscopically, stable plaques of either noncritical or critical severity usually characterize the site of angiographically proven spasm.[34,62] Because vasospasm can produce surface buckling and erosions, intimal hyperplasia and plaque progression also may be identified in autopsy specimens.[63]

Microvascular angina, also known as syndrome X, is defined clinically as anginal chest pain (often exertional) that is associated with a positive exercise stress test but angiographically normal coronary arteries, with a negative ergonovin challenge.[64] It is thought to be due to diffuse narrowing of the small intramural coronary arteries and microcirculation, with a reduced vasodilator reserve. Although the number of microscopic studies is small, the available findings substantiate the clinical hypothesis and include medial hypertrophy and intimal proliferation of the intramural coronary arteries.[64,65] Capillaries also may be thickened and exhibit swollen and obstructive endothelial cells. Similar microvascular disease is also a feature of intramural arteries in patients with left venticular hypertrophy in hypertension and in hypertrophic cardiomyopathy and may be responsible for angina in these patients as well.[66] Among patients with angiographically normal coronary arteries, it is important to emphasize that chest pain may also be noncardiac in origin, as can occur with esophageal dysfunction, for example.

Unstable angina refers to episodic ischemic myocardial pain that has increased in frequency or severity or persists at rest. Synonyms include not only preinfarction, accelerated, and crescendo angina but also acute coronary insufficiency and the intermediate coronary syndrome. Among the acute coronary syndromes, the epicardial arteries in patients with unstable angina more closely resemble those reported for sudden death than for acute myocardial infarction. Most patients have critical three-vessel disease, and 30–50% of the lengths of their coronary vessels are obstructed by critical lesions, compared with 30–35% for the other acute coronary syndromes.[26,67] Grade 4 stenosis of the left main coronary artery is also observed relatively frequently in autopsied cases. Plaques are more often fibrous than fatty and eccentric than concentric, and virtually all hearts harbor at least one old organized and recanalized thrombus. Clusters of adventitial lymphocytes are observed in about 35%

TABLE 2.5. CORRELATION BETWEEN CLINICAL MANIFESTATION OF CORONARY ARTERY DISEASE AND PATHOLOGIC FEATURES OF ATHEROSCLEROTIC PLAQUES[a]

Clinical State	Microscopic Features of Coronary Atherosclerosis
Asymptomatic	Stable noncritical plaques; occasionally, critical stable plaques (generally one-vessel disease)
Angina pectoris	
Chronic stable (exertional)	Stable critical plaques (usually two-vessel or three-vessel disease)
Variant (Prinzmetal's)	Stable noncritical or critical plaques; evidence of plaque progression; occasionally an unstable atheroma
Microvascular (syndrome X)	No significant disease of epicardial coronary arteries; medial and intimal thickening of intramural arteries; swollen capillary endothelial cells
Unstable (preinfarction)	Unstable plaque, either critical or noncritical, with rupture and acute nonocclusive platelet-rich thrombus; also stable critical plaques (usually three-vessel disease)
Myocardial infarction (MI)	
Acute myocardial ischemia[b]	Unstable plaque, either critical or noncritical, with rupture and acute thrombus, either nonocclusive or occlusive; often associated with other stable critical plaques
Acute subendocardial MI	Same as for unstable angina
Acute transmural MI	Unstable plaque, either critical or noncritical, with rupture and acute occlusive fibrin-rich thrombus; also stable critical plaques (usually two-vessel or three-vessel disease)
Chronic myocardial ischemia[c]	Stable critical plaques (usually two-vessel or three-vessel disease)
Old healed MI (scars >1 cm)	Stable critical plaques (usually two-vessel or three-vessel disease); old organized thrombus, especially with transmural infarcts
Chronic heart failure	Stable critical plaques (usually two-vessel or three-vessel disease; old organized thrombus; evidence of plaque progression
Sudden death	Unstable plaque, either critical or noncritical, with rupture and acute thrombus, either nonocclusive or occlusive; associated with other stable critical plaques (two-vessel or three-vessel disease in 80%, one-vessel disease in 15%, and four-vessel disease in 5%)

[a]Represents autopsied cases only (a source of bias). See text for detailed descriptions.

[b]Characterized microscopically by contraction band necrosis or by nuclear pyknosis and intense sarcoplasmic staining with eosin, occurring in the *absence* of an infiltrate of neutrophils or, with reperfusion, macrophages. These features generally represent preinfarction changes in which the patient died before leukocytic infiltration occurred. It is possible that at least some clinical cases of stunned myocardium harbor similar microscopic changes.

[c]Characterized microscopically by patchy subendocardial collections of vacuolated myocytes or by small (<1 cm) subendocardial patches of fibrosis or granulation tissue. Vacuolated myocytes may possibly correspond clinically to hibernating myocardium.

of the microscopic coronary sections, half of which also show vascular nerve involvement that may lead to vasospasm.[26]

Acute lesions, indicative of an unstable plaque, are also commonly encountered in patients with unstable angina. Plaque hemorrhage is found in about

65% of the patients, and plaque rupture and acute thrombosis are each present in 35% of the cases.[68] Thrombus tends to be platelet rich and nonocclusive in nature, and its frequent layered appearance indicates episodic growth.[68,69] Within the small arterial branches of the downstream myocardium, micro-emboli commonly are encountered and may be the cause not only of unstable angina, but also of subsequent ventricular arrhythmias and sudden death.[70,71]

Myocardial Infarction

Although acute myocardial infarction can occur among patients with critical one-vessel disease or even noncritical disease, it most commonly is associated with underlying two-vessel or three-vessel critical (grade 4) coronary athero-sclerosis (Table 2.5). Only infrequently does thrombus-related myocardial in-farction develop in the setting of critical left main artery disease. Patients with acute left ventricular infarctions also tend to have a preponderance of fatty plaques and fewer fibrous lesions.[67] In 90% of the cases, at least one coronary artery contains an obstructive old organized and recanalized thrombus.

Acute coronary lesions include intimal hemorrhage in 90% of the patients, plaque rupture in 75% (usually involving fatty atheromas), and luminal thrombosis in 70–90%.[68] In most cases, the thrombus is occlusive and fibrin rich, as documented by angiography, angioscopy, and microscopy.[68,72] Al-though thrombotic occlusion is as likely to occur on a noncritical plaque as on a critical lesion, it is more likely to be associated with a fatal outcome if it oc-curs on a critical lesion.[42] This is difficult to explain in light of the observations that thrombosis on a noncritical plaque is often associated with a Q-wave (transmural) infarction, whereas thrombosis on a critical atheroma generally produces a non-Q-wave (subendocardial) infarction, presumably due to the myocardial protection afforded by chronically dilated collateral vessels.[58]

It is important to emphasize that, in certain circumstances, acute myocar-dial infarction can occur among patients with stable coronary atherosclerosis. Two such situations include prolonged hypotension, usually associated with anesthesia induction or inadequate myocardial protection during open heart surgery, and hypoxemia, often due to an acute exacerbation of chronic pul-monary disease. In these settings, global myocardial infarction may result, with circumferential and subendocardial involvement of the entire left ventri-cle. The right ventricular free wall and anterior tricuspid papillary muscle can also be affected, particularly if they are hypertrophied. In addition, among pa-tients with stable coronary artery disease and coexistent aortic stenosis, aor-tic regurgitation, or hypertrophic cardiomyopathy, old infarctions in their hy-pertrophied left ventricles are frequently observed at autopsy.

Finally, in patients with old healed myocardial infarctions, the coronary ar-teries most commonly exhibit critical two-vessel or three-vessel disease.[67] Moreover, for old transmural scars, the infarct-related artery is usually the site of a chronic total occlusion, either with or without recanalization channels. In contrast, old subendocardial infarcts are more often associated with critical but nonocclusive atheromas with microscopic features of plaque progression. If thrombolysis has occurred, either intrinsically or following thrombolytic therapy, then the infarct-related artery may in fact harbor no critical lesions.

Similar clinical scenarios also can pertain to arteries other than the coronaries. For example, in patients with severe aortoiliac disease or severe atherosclerosis in the more distal arteries of the legs (arteriosclerosis obliterans, or ASO), exertional leg pain may occur and is referred to as intermittent claudication. Moreover, following a period of hypotension, acute infarction of the bowel can result in patients with either ostial stenosis of the superior or inferior mesenteric arteries or atherosclerotic obstructions within the mesenteric arterial branches. Less commonly, renal infarctions develop under similar circumstances.

CONGESTIVE HEART FAILURE

End-stage ischemic heart disease (so-called ischemic cardiomyopathy) is characterized by intractable congestive heart failure. Most patients have a clinical history of either numerous myocardial infarctions or one massive event. Less commonly, and primarily in diabetics, heart failure represents the initial manifestation of chronic severe coronary atherosclerosis. Autopsy studies indicate that about 90% of the cases have critical two-vessel or three-vessel disease, and 10% have single-vessel disease.[73] Critical left main artery disease is virtually nonexistent in this group of patients, and a history of exertional angina pectoris is also uncommon.

SUDDEN CORONARY DEATH

Sudden coronary death is generally defined as unexpected death that occurs within 6 hours, and usually within 1 hour, of the onset of symptoms. Clinical follow-ups in successfully resuscitated victims have confirmed that cardiac arrest is more often the result of an ischemia-related arrhythmic event than acute myocardial infarction. Autopsy studies of fatal cases document critical two-vessel or three-vessel coronary atherosclerosis in 85–90%, single-vessel disease in 10–15%, and critical left main artery lesions in fewer than 5%. Fibrous plaques generally outnumber fatty atheromas, and old organized thrombi are identified in about 80% of the patients.[68,74] Features of unstable lesions include intimal hemorrhage in about 40%, plaque rupture in 20%, and platelet-rich nonocclusive thrombi in 30–75% of the cases.[68,75] Showers of microemboli also occur frequently and are thought to be important in the pathogenesis of fatal cardiac arrhythmias.

UNNATURAL HISTORY OF ATHEROSCLEROTIC PLAQUES

DEFINITION OF UNNATURAL HISTORY

Compared with the natural history of atherosclerosis, its *unnatural* history refers to vascular responses to interventional procedures that are associated with iatrogenic injury. Interventions include surgical resections, such as endarterectomy, and nonsurgical procedures, such as balloon angioplasty, directional or rotational atherectomy, laser angioplasty, or stent placement. The resulting arterial injuries share many features in common with spontaneous plaque rupture, but there are important differences as well. Regardless of the type of interventional procedure, an unstable region is produced that is prone to develop thrombosis or intimal hyperplasia. With time, the healed area of injury may begin to resemble a fibrotic or fibrofatty atheroma.

MECHANISMS OF BALLOON ANGIOPLASTY

The mechanisms responsible for successful balloon dilation of an obstructed artery are variable, but most entail plaque rupture.[76,77] Like spontaneous fissures, these most commonly occur ether at the junction between the plaque and the disease-free wall or along a thin point in the fibrous cap, where mechanical stress is the greatest (Fig. 2.18).[40] However, in contrast to plaque ruptures that are spontaneous, those associated with balloon angioplasty are most

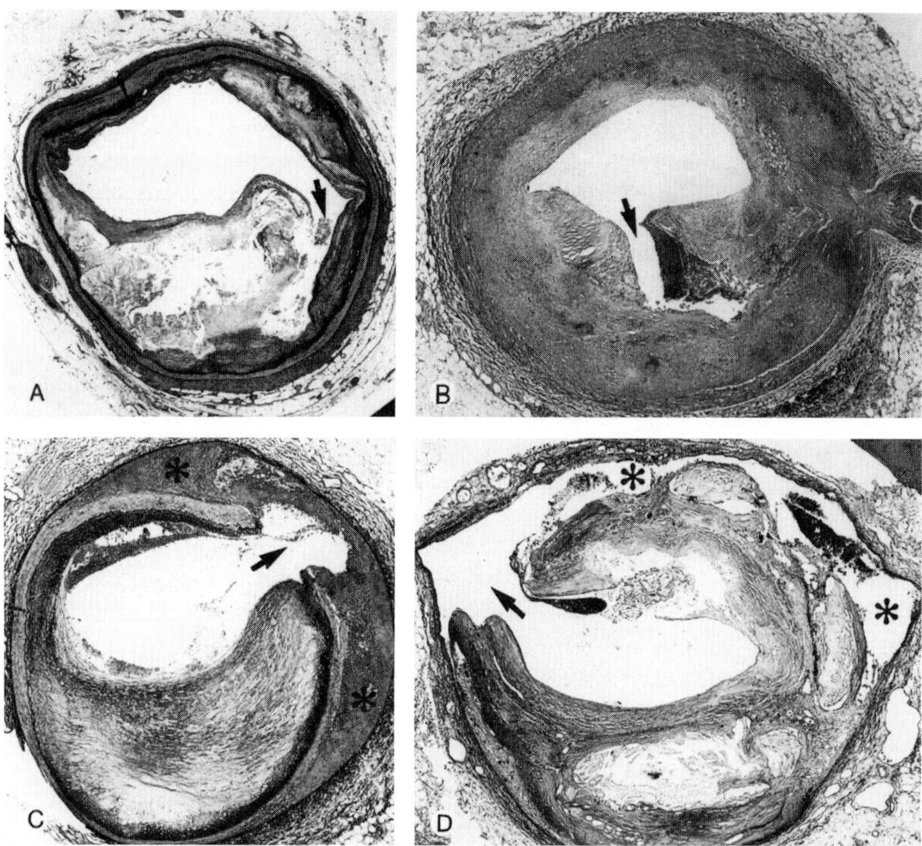

FIG. 2.18. Iatrogenic plaque rupture during clinically successful percutaneous transluminal coronary angioplasty. *A*, a fracture (*arrow*) has occurred at the junction between the lipid-rich plaque and the relatively disease-free wall. *B*, a deep intimal laceration (*arrow*) involves the midportion of a fibrous plaque and is partially lined by fresh thrombus. *C*, a deep tear (*arrow*) at the plaque border extends through the media to the external elastic membrane and is associated with a localized intramedial dissection and hematoma formation (*). *D*, fracture (*arrow*) of a concentric fibrofatty atheroma has occurred at its thinnest point and has led to a prominent intramedial dissection (*). *A, C, D*, elastic-van Gieson; *B*, hematoxylin-eosin; *A*, ×12; *B–D*, ×24. (From Edwards,[22] with permission.)

commonly associated with extension not only into the intima but also well into the media, often to the level of the external elastic membrane. Such deep lacerations may result in formation of an intimal flap or an intramedial dissection. For balloon angioplasty of arteries with unstable plaques, the procedure usually causes extension along the original rupture tract, although new sites of intimal disruption can also occur.

However, despite the prevalence of iatrogenic arterial disruption, it is only by substantial stretching of medial and adventitial tissues that luminal enlargement is achieved.[76] This generally involves laceration of medial elements, slippage of parallel layers of medial smooth muscle cells, and disruption and slippage of adventitial collagen and elastin. The result is focal dilation and remodeling of the arterial wall, often associated with formation of an aneurysm or even a pseudoaneurysm (that is, a contained rupture). Predictably, balloon angioplasty is more likely to be successful for eccentric plaques that are fatty or fibrofatty than for concentric plaques that are primarily fibrous or calcific.

From a practical perspective, for arterial segments being evaluated microscopically at autopsy, distinction must be made between lacerations that have occurred as a result of balloon dilation and clefts that represent artifacts of tissue processing. Although such clefts may resemble either spontaneous or iatrogenic rupture sites, an absence along the rupture tract of red blood cells, fibrin, or platelets in young lesions or a reparative response in older lesions usually allows their identification to be made readily. To minimize the likelihood of artifactual clefts, an artery that has been subjected to an interventional procedure should be perfusion fixed, carefully dissected from the surrounding tissues, decalcified for at least 24 hours, and then step sectioned at 2–3-mm intervals, using a new scalpel blade and a gentle slicing motion rather than a back-and-forth sawing action or a downward guillotinelike crushing method.

HEALING AND RESTENOSIS

Plaque ruptures produced by balloon angioplasty represent sites of vascular injury that are prone to the same complications and types of healing described for spontaneous ruptures, even though the patients are anticoagulated and the lacerations often extend into the media. Autopsy studies of coronary arteries from patients who have undergone balloon dilation procedures, coupled with information derived from various animal models, indicate that postinterventional healing shares numerous features in common with the response-to-injury model for atherogenesis.[22,76–82]

After an angioplasty procedure, the area of injury becomes lined by platelets and later by a fibrin meshwork in which platelets and red blood cells become entrapped. Thrombosis at this time is dynamic and may be accompanied by rapid changes in size and shape. In the setting of anticoagulation, the thrombus begins to stabilize over the course of minutes to hours, rather than hours to days, and it generally becomes endothelialized within the first several days.

At this time, blood-borne monocytes line the new endothelium and migrate into the underlying thrombus. There, monocytes are transformed into tissue macrophages and begin to phagocytose the mass of compact fibrin, agglutinated platelets, and degenerating red cells. Simultaneously, smooth muscle cells, apparently derived primarily from the media, enter the intimal subendothelial space and undergo a phenotypic transformation from the usual spindle-shaped contractile cells, which are strongly immunoreactive for α-actin, into polygonal or stellate synthetic cells, which stain weakly. The extracellular matrix is abundant, appears myxoid by light microscopy, and is rich in glycosaminoglycans (acid mucopolysaccharides).

Over weeks to months, the neointima becomes less cellular, and smooth muscle cells revert from a haphazardly arranged synthetic type to the parallel contractile form. Concurrently, the extracellular matrix becomes less myxoid and more collagenous. As a result, the site of healing begins to resemble a fibrous plaque. If the red cell component of the initial thrombus is prominent, or if the patient is hyperlipidemic after the procedure, then the site of healing may also contain foam cells and cholesterol crystals, similar to a fibrofatty atheroma.

In most patients, the lumen-enlarging effect of balloon dilation outweighs the lumen-narrowing effect of neointimal hyperplasia, such that significant relief of stenosis represents both the early and late result of balloon dilation. However, in about 40% of the patients undergoing nonsurgical interventions for obstructive coronary atherosclerosis, neointimal hyperplasia is excessive and results in clinically symptomatic restenosis within 3–6 months (Fig. 2.19).

Obstructive neointimal tissue can be removed from living patients by coronary atherectomy and has been the source of numerous investigations[83–88]. In clinically young lesions, it is characterized by a loose myxoid matrix in which numerous stellate smooth muscle cells are haphazardly arranged, reminiscent of their appearance in tissue cultures. Older lesions, in contrast, feature a densely collagenous matrix in which scattered, spindle-shaped cells exhibit a parallel arrangement. Thus, the microscopic appearance of restenosis tissue obtained by atherectomy is virtually identical to that described at autopsy and in experimental animals.

Moreover, young lesions are indistinguishable from the intimal proliferation associated with such diverse forms of vascular injury as cardiac transplant vasculopathy, mediastinal irradiation, and chronic exposure to cocaine, as well as injury to saphenous vein bypass grafts (Fig. 2.20).[22,89,90] Old restenosis lesions are identical to those associated with plaque progression. These examples serve to emphasize that the vascular wall has a relatively limited response to injury. Thus, it is not surprising that arterial healing after an interventional procedure resembles many aspects of atherosclerosis.

SUMMARY OF NATURAL AND UNNATURAL HISTORY OF ATHEROSCLEROSIS

Atherosclerosis is a chronic but dynamic intimal disease whose progression is characterized by alternating episodes of stability and instability. Chronic plaque progression appears to be the result of surface erosions or fissures, secondary nonocclusive mural thrombosis, healing intimal fibrosis, and eventual

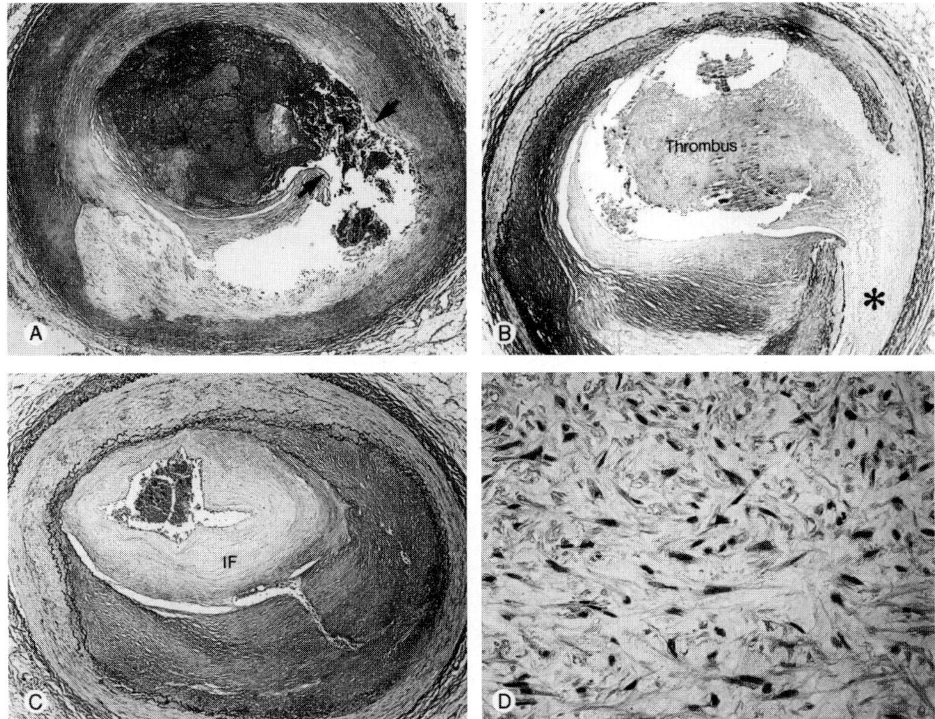

FIG. 2.19. Obstructive consequences of iatrogenic plaque rupture related to percutaneous transluminal coronary angioplasty. *A,* rupture at the plaque border (between the *arrows*) is associated with acute luminal thrombotic occlusion. *B,* healing is characterized by loose fibroplasia within the rupture site and intramedial dissection channel (*) and by ongoing luminal thrombosis. *C,* chronic restenosis is the result of intimal fibroplasia (*IF*). *D,* restenosis in a younger lesion is associated with smooth muscle hyperplasia and myxoid extracellular matrix, as shown at high power. *A, D,* hematoxylin-eosin; *C, D,* elastic-van Gieson; *A,* ×18; *B, C,* ×36; *D,* ×360. (From Edwards,[22] with permission.)

incorporation into the underlying atheroma. Such episodes usually are asymptomatic but may be associated with unstable angina, subendocardial myocardial infarction, or sudden death. Occlusive thrombosis usually is acutely symptomatic and accompanied by transmural myocardial infarction, unless coronary blood flow is rapidly reestablished by thrombolytic therapy or an interventional procedure. Thrombosis is as likely to involve a noncritical plaque as a critical lesion. Currently, there are no means available to predict accurately on an individual basis, who is at high risk for an acute symptomatic coronary event.

Interventional therapies cause vascular injury that shares several features in common with unstable atherosclerosis. For example, both are associated with plaque rupture, both involve platelet-fibrin thrombosis, and both initially heal by intimal hyperplasia that represents a stereotypical response to injury.

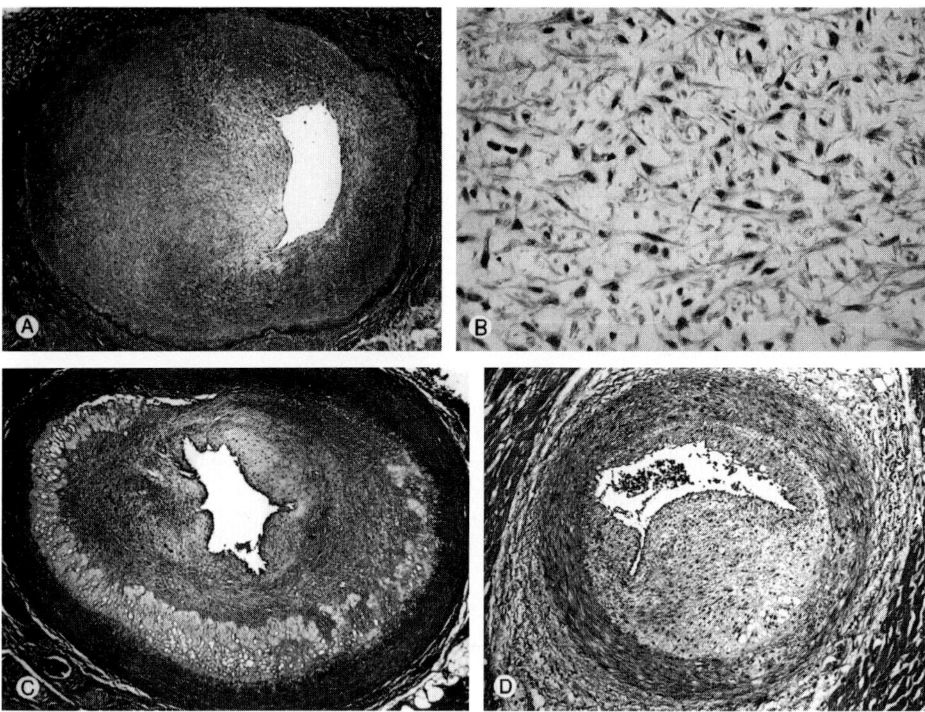

FIG. 2.20.　Intimal hyperplasia unrelated to coronary balloon angioplasty. *A, B,* severe obstruction of an aortocoronary saphenous vein bypass graft is the result of excessive intimal proliferation, as shown at low power (*A*) and high power (*B*). *C, D,* chronic cardiac transplant vasculopathy is responsible for the intimal hyperplasia and critical luminal stenosis in epicardial (*C*) and intramural (*D*) coronary arteries. *A,* elastic-van Gieson; *B–D,* hematoxylin-eosin; *A, C,* ×36; *B,* ×360; *D,* ×90.

Plaque rupture due to interventional procedures, however, is generally more extensive than that which occurs spontaneously and characteristically involves the media or adventitia as well. Nonetheless, the results of functional and structural studies (at the cell biology and microscopic levels, respectively) indicate more similarities than differences. Thus, new strategies directed toward the control of postinterventional restenosis may have applicability in the treatment of atherosclerosis, and vice versa.

REFERENCES

1. Mizgala HF, Gray LH, Ferris JA, Bociek V, Allard P, Davies C. Coronary artery luminal narrowing in the young with sudden unexpected death: a coroner's autopsy study in 350 subjects age 40 years and under. *Can J Cardiol* 1993;9:33–40.
2. Joseph A, Ackermann D, Talley JD, Johnstone J, Kupersmith J. Manifestations of coronary atherosclerosis in young trauma victims: an autopsy study. *J Am Coll Cardiol* 1993;22:459–467.

3. Ross R. The pathogenesis of atherosclerosis: a perspective for the 1990s. *Nature* 1993;362: 801–809.
4. Loscalzo J. The relation between atherosclerosis and thrombosis. *Circulation* 1992;86(Suppl III):95–99.
5. Schwartz CJ, Valente AJ, Sprague EA, Kelley JL, Nerem RM. The pathogenesis of atherosclerosis: an overview. *Clin Cardiol* 1991;14(Suppl I):1–16.
6. Munro JM, Cotran RS. The pathogenesis of atherosclerosis: atherogenesis and inflammation. *Lab Invest* 1988;58:249–261.
7. Bruschke AVG, Kramer JR, Jr, Bal ET, Haque IU, Detrano RC, Goormastic M. The dynamics of progression of coronary atherosclerosis studied in 168 medically treated patients who underwent coronary arteriography three times. *Am Heart J* 1989;117:296–305.
8. Muller JE, Abela GS, Nesto RW, Tofler GH. Triggers, acute risk factors and vulnerable plaques: the lexicon of a new frontier. *J Am Coll Cardiol* 1994;23:809–813.
9. MacIsaac AI, Thomas JD, Topol EJ. Toward the quiescent plaque. *J Am Coll Cardiol* 1993; 22:1228–1241.
10. Sytkowski P, Kannel W, D'Agostino R. Changes in risk factors and the decline in mortality from cardiovascular disease: the Framingham heart study. *N Engl J Med* 1990;322:1635–1641.
11. Jost S, Deckers JW, Nikutta P, et al. Progression of coronary artery disease is dependent on anatomic location and diameter. *J Am Coll Cardiol* 1993;21:1339–1346.
12. Hochman JS, Phillips WJ, Ruggieri D, Ryan SF. The distribution of atherosclerotic lesions in the coronary arterial tree: relation to cardiac risk factors. *Am Heart J* 1988;116:1217–1222.
13. Davies MJ, Woolf N, Rowles PM, Pepper J. Morphology of the endothelium over atherosclerotic plaques in human coronary arteries. *Br Heart J* 1988;60:459–464.
14. Kragel AH, Reddy SG, Wittes JT, Roberts WC. Morphometric analysis of the composition of atherosclerotic plaques in the four major epicardial coronary arteries in acute myocardial infarction and in sudden coronary death. *Circulation* 1989;80:1747–1756.
15. Alfonso F, Macaya C, Goicolea J, et al. Determinants of coronary compliance in patients with coronary artery disease: an intravascular ultrasound study. *J Am Coll Cardiol* 1994;23: 879–884.
16. Stary HC. The sequence of cell and matrix changes in atherosclerotic lesions of coronary arteries in the first forty years of life. *Eur Heart J* 1990;11(Suppl E):3–19.
17. Mautner SL, Lin F, Mautner GC, Roberts WC. Comparison of women versus men of composition of atherosclerotic plaques in native coronary arteries and in saphenous veins used as aortocoronary conduits. *J Am Coll Cardiol* 1993;21:1312–1318.
18. Simons DB, Schwartz RS, Edwards WD, Sheedy PF, Breen JF, Rumberger JA. Noninvasive definition of anatomic coronary artery disease by ultrafast computed tomographic scanning: a quantitative pathologic comparison study. *J Am Coll Cardiol* 1992;20:1118–1126.
19. Waller BF. The eccentric coronary atherosclerotic plaque: morphologic observations and clinical relevance. *Clin Cardiol* 1989;12:14–20.
20. Saner HE, Gobel FL, Salomonowitz E, Erlien DA, Edwards JE. The disease-free wall in coronary atherosclerosis: its relation to degree of obstruction. *J Am Coll Cardiol* 1985;6: 1096–1099.
21. Clarkson TB, Prichard RW, Morgan TM, Petrick GS, Klein KP. Remodeling of coronary arteries in human and nonhuman primates. *JAMA* 1994;271:289–294.
22. Edwards WD. Pathology of myocardial infarction and reperfusion. In: Gersh BJ, Rahimtoola SH, eds. *Acute myocardial infarction.* New York: Elsevier, 1991:14–48.
23. McPherson DD, Johnson MR, Alvarez NM, et al. Variable morphology of coronary atherosclerosis: characterization of atherosclerotic plaque and residual arterial lumen size and shape by epicardial echocardiography. *J Am Coll Cardiol* 1992;19:593–599.
24. Stone PH, Gibson M, Pasternak RC, et al. Natural history of coronary atherosclerosis using quantitative angiography in men, and implications for clinical trials of coronary regression. *Am J Cardiol* 1993;71:766–772.
25. Stiel GM, Stiel LSG, Schofer J, Donath K, Mathey DG. Impact of compensatory enlargement of atherosclerotic coronary arteries on angiographic assessment of coronary artery disease. *Circulation* 1989;80:1603–1609.

26. Kohchi K, Takebayashi S, Hiroki T, Nobuyoshi M. Significance of adventitial inflammation of the coronary artery in patients with unstable angina: results at autopsy. *Circulation* 1985;71:709–716.

27. Baroldi G, Silver MD, Mariani F, Giuliano G. Correlation of morphological variables in the coronary atherosclerotic plaque with clinical patterns of ischemic heart disease. *Am J Cardiovasc Pathol* 1988;2;159–172.

28. Reddy KG, Nair RN, Sheehan HM, Hodgson JMcB. Evidence that selective endothelial dysfunction may occur in the absence of angiographic or ultrasound atherosclerosis in patients with risk factors for atherosclerosis. *J Am Coll Cardiol* 1994;23:833–843.

29. Yamagishi M, Miyatake K, Tamai J, Nakatani S, Koyma J, Nissen SE. Intravascular ultrasound detection of atherosclerosis at the site of focal vasospasm in angiographically normal or minimally narrowed coronary segments. *J Am Coll Cardiol* 1994;23:352–357.

30. Porter TR, Sears T, Xie F, Michels A, Mata J, Welsh D, Shurmur S. Intravascular ultrasound study of angiographically mildly diseased coronary arteries. *J Am Coll Cardiol* 1993;22: 1858–1865.

31. Mizuno K, Satomura K, Miyamota A, et al. Angioscopic evaluation of coronary artery thrombi in acute coronary syndromes. *N Engl J Med* 1992;326:287–291.

32. Fuster V, Badimon L, Badimon JJ, Chesebro JH. The pathogenesis of coronary artery disease and the acute coronary syndromes. *N Engl J Med* 1992;326;242–250.

33. Buja LM, Willerson JT. The role of coronary artery lesions in ischemic heart disease: insights from recent clinicopathologic, coronary angiographic, and experimental studies. *Major Probl Pathol* 1991;23:42–60.

34. Davies MJ. A macro and micro view of coronary vascular insult in ischemic heart disease. *Circulation* 1990;82(Suppl II):38–46.

35. Fuster V, Stein B, Ambrose JA, Badimon L, Badimon JJ, Chesebro JH. Atherosclerotic plaque rupture and thrombosis: evolving concepts. *Circulation* 1990;82(Suppl II):47–59.

36. Dinerman JL, Mehta JL. Endothelial, platelet and leukocyte interactions in ischemic heart disease: insights into potential mechanisms and their clinical relevance. *J Am Coll Cardiol* 1990;16:207–222.

37. Arbustini E, Maurizia G, Diegoli M, et al. Coronary atherosclerotic plaques with and without thrombus in ischemic heart syndromes: a morphologic, immunohistochemical, and biochemical study. *Am J Cardiol* 1991;68:36B–50B.

38. van der Wal AC, Becker AE, van der Loos CM, Das PK. Site of intimal rupture or erosion of thrombosed coronary atherosclerotic plaques is characterized by an inflammatory process irrespective of the dominant plaque morphology. *Circulation* 1994;89:36–44.

39. Tracy RE, Devaney K, Kissling G. Characteristic of the plaque under a coronary thrombus. *Virchows Arch [A]* 1985;405:411–427.

40. Loree HM, Kamm RD, Stringfellow RG, Lee RT. Effects of fibrous cap thickness on peak circumferential stress in model atherosclerotic vessels. *Circ Res* 1992;71:850–858.

41. Richardson PD, Davies MJ, Born GVR. Influence of plaque configuration and stress distribution on fissuring of coronary atherosclerotic plaques. *Lancet* 1989;21:941–944.

42. Qiao J-H, Fishbein MC. The severity of coronary atherosclerosis at sites of plaque rupture with occlusive thrombosis. *J Am Coll Cardiol* 1991;17:1138–1142.

43. Marshall JC, Waxman HL, Sauerwein A, et al. Frequency of low-grade residual stenosis after thrombolytic therapy during acute myocardial infarction. *Am J Cardiol* 1990;66:773–778.

44. Kazerooni EA, Bree RL, Williams DM. Penetrating atherosclerotic ulcers of the descending thoracic aorta: evaluation with CT and distinction from aortic dissection. *Radiology* 1992;183:759–765.

45. Hussain S, Glover JL, Bree R, Bendick PJ. Penetrating atherosclerotic ulcers of the thoracic aorta. *J Vasc Surg* 1989;9:710–717.

46. Stanson AW, Kazmier FJ, Hollier LH, et al. Penetraing atherosclerotic ulcers of the thoracic aorta: natural history and clinicopathologic correlations. *Ann Vasc Surg* 1986;1:15–23.

47. Zamir M, Silver MD. "Hemorrhagic" and microvascular phenomena within the arterial wall. *Can J Cardiol* 1992;8:981–984.

48. Barger AC, Beeuwkes R. Rupture of coronary vasa vasorum as a trigger of acute myocardial infarction. *Am J Cardiol* 1990;66:41G–43G.
49. Constantinides P. Causes of thrombosis in human atherosclerotic arteries. *Am J Cardiol* 1990;66:37G–40G.
50. Virmani R, Roberts WC. Extravasated erythrocytes, iron, and fibrin in atherosclerotic plaques of coronary arteries in fatal coronary heart disease and their relation to luminal thrombus: frequency and significance in 57 necropsy patients and in 2958 five mm segments of 224 major epicardial coronary arteries. *Am Heart J* 1983;105:788–797.
51. Forrester J. Intimal disruption and coronary thrombosis: its role in the pathogenesis of human coronary disease. *Am J Cardiol* 1991;68:69B–77B.
52. Falk E. Coronary thrombosis: pathogenesis and clinical manifestations. *Am J Cardiol* 1991;68:28B–35B.
53. Fernandez-Ortiz A, Badimon JJ, Falk E, et al. Characterization of the relative thrombogenicity of atherosclerotic plaque components: implications for consequences of plaque rupture. *J Am Coll Cardiol* 1994;23:1562–1569.
54. Haft JI, Haik BJ, Goldstein JE, Brodyn NE. Development of significant coronary artery lesions in areas of minimal disease: a common mechanism for coronary disease progression. *Chest* 1988;94:731–736.
55. Kaski J, Tousoulis D, Haider A, Gavrielides S, Crea F, Maseri A. Reactivity of eccentric and concentric coronary stenosis in patients with chronic stable angina. *J Am Coll Cardiol* 1991;17:627–633.
56. Lin C-S, Penha PG, Zak FG, et al. Morphodynamic interpretation of acute coronary thrombosis with special reference to volcano-like eruption of atheromatous plaque caused by coronary artery spasm. *Angiology* 1988;88:535–547.
57. Nobuyshi M, Tanaka M, Nosaka H, et al. Progression of coronary atherosclerosis: Is coronary spasm related to progression? *J Am Coll Cardiol* 1991;18:904–910.
58. Ambrose JA, Hjemdahl-Monsen CE, Borrico S, et al. Angiographic demonstration of a common link between unstable angina pectoris and non-Q wave acute myocardial infarction. *Am J Cardiol* 1988;61:244–247.
59. Hangartner JRW, Charleston AJ, Davies MJ, Thomas AC. Morphological characteristics of clinically significant coronary artery stenosis in stable angina. *Br Heart J* 1986;56:501–508.
60. Roberts WC. The coronary arteries and left ventricle in clinically isolated angina pectoris: a necropsy analysis. *Circulation* 1976;54:388–390.
61. Bugiardini R, Pozzati A, Ottani F, Morgagni GL, Puddu P. Vasotonic angina: a spectrum of ischemic syndromes involving functional abnormalities of the epicardial and microvascular coronary circulation. *J Am Coll Cardiol* 1993;22:417–425.
62. Rizzon P, Rossi L, Calabrese P, et al. Angiographic and pathologic correlations in Prinzmetal variant angina. *Angiology* 1978;29:486–490.
63. Corrado D, Thiene G, Buja GF, et al. The relationship between growth of atherosclerotic plaques, variant angina and sudden death. *Int J Cardiol* 1990;26:361–367.
64. Cannon RO III, Epstein SE. "Microvascular angina" as a cause of chest pain with angiographically normal coronary arteries. (Editorial.) *Am J Cardiol* 1988;61:1338–1343.
65. Moseri M, Yarom R, Gotsman MS, Hasin Y. Histologic evidence for small-vessel coronary artery disease in patients with angina pectoris and patent large coronary arteries. *Circulation* 1986;74:964–972.
66. Tanaka M, Fujiwara H, Onodera T, et al. Quantitative analysis of narrowing of intramyocardial small arteries in normal hearts, hypertensive hearts, and hearts with hypertrophic cardiomyopathy. *Circulation* 1987;75:1130–1139.
67. Roberts WC. Qualitative and quantitative comparison of amounts of narrowing by atherosclerotic plaques in the major epicardial coronary arteries at necropsy in sudden coronary death, transmural healed myocardial infarction and unstable angina pectoris. *Am J Cardiol* 1989;64:324–328.
68. Kragel AH, Gertz SD, Roberts WC. Morphologic comparison of frequency and types of acute lesions in the major epicardial coronary arteries in unstable angina pectoris, sudden coronary death and acute myocardial infarction. *J Am Coll Cardiol* 1991;18:801–808.

69. Falk E. Morphologic features of unstable atherothrombotic plaques underlying acute coronary syndromes. *Am J Cardiol* 1989;63:114E–120E.
70. Davies MJ, Thomas AC, Knapman PA, Hangartner JR. Intramyocardial platelet aggregation in patients with unstable angina suffering sudden ischemic cardiac death. *Circulation* 1986;73:418–427.
71. Gotlieb AI, Freeman MR, Salerno TA, et al. Ultrastructural studies of unstable angina in living man. *Mod Pathol* 1991;4:75–80.
72. Ambrose JA. Plaque disruption and the acute coronary syndromes of unstable angina and myocardial infarction: if the substrate is similar, why is the clinical presentation different? *J Am Coll Cardiol* 1992;19:1653–1658.
73. Virmani R, Roberts WC. Quantification of coronary arterial narrowing and of left ventricular myocardial scarring in healed myocardial infarction with chronic, eventually fatal congestive heart failure. *Am J Med* 1980;68:831–838.
74. Roberts WC, Kragel AH, Gertz SD, et al. The heart in fatal unstable angina pectoris. *Am J Cardiol* 1991;68:22B–27B.
75. Davies MJ. Anatomic features in victims of sudden coronary death: Coronary artery pathology. *Circulation* 1992;85(Suppl I):19–24.
76. Virmani R, Farb A, Burke AP. Coronary angiplasty from the perspective of atherosclerotic plaque: morphologic predictors of immediate success and restenosis. *Am Heart J* 1994;127:163–179.
77. Waller BF. Morphology of percutaneous transluminal coronary angioplasty used in the treatment of coronary heart disease. *Major Probl Pathol* 1991;23:100–133.
78. Schoen FJ. *Interventional and surgical cardiovascular pathology: clinical correlations and basic principles.* Philadelphia: WB Saunders, 1989:59–107.
79. Reidy MA, Fingerle J, Lindner V. Factors controlling the development of arterial lesions after injury. *Circulation* 1992;87(Suppl III):43–46.
80. Anderson PG. Restenosis: animal models and morphometric techniques in studies of the vascular response to injury. *Cardiovasc Pathol* 1992;1:263–278.
81. Muller DWM, Ellis SG, Topol EJ. Experimental models of coronary artery restenosis. *J Am Coll Cardiol* 1992;19:418–432.
82. Schwartz RS, Huber KC, Murphy JG, et al. Restenosis and the proportional neointimal response to coronary artery injury: results in a porcine model. *J Am Coll Cardiol* 1992;19:267–274.
83. Casscells W, Engler D, Willerson JT. Mechanisms of restenosis. *Texas Heart Inst J* 1994;21:68–77.
84. MacLeod DC, Strauss BH, de Jong M, et al. Proliferation and extracellular matrix synthesis of smooth muscle cells cultured from human coronary atherosclerotic and restenotic lesions. *J Am Coll Cardiol* 1994;23:59–65.
85. Simons M, Leclerc G, Safian RD, et al. Relation between activated smooth-muscle cells in coronary artery lesions and restenosis after atherectomy. *N Engl J Med* 1993;328:608–613.
86. Miller MJ, Kuntz RE, Friedrich SP, et al. Frequency and consequences of intimal hyperplasia in specimens retrieved by directional atherectomy of native primary coronary artery stenoses and subsequent restenoses. *Am J Cardiol* 1993;71:652–658.
87. Bauriedel G, Windstetter U, DeMaio SJ, Jr, et al. Migratory activity of human smooth muscle cells cultivated from coronary and peripheral primary and restenotic lesions removed by percutaneous atherectomy. *Circulation* 1992;85:554–564.
88. Garratt KN, Edwards WD, Kaufmann UP, et al. Differential histopathology of primary atherosclerotic and restenotic lesions in coronary arteries and saphenous vein bypass grafts: analysis of tissue obtained from 73 patients by directional atherectomy. *J Am Coll Cardiol* 1991;17:442–448.
89. Johnson DE, Alderman EL, Schroeder JS, et al. Transplant coronary artery disease: Histopathologic correlations with angiographic morphology. *J Am Coll Cardiol* 1991;17:449–457.
90. de Lorgeril M, Loire R, Guidollet J, et al. Accelerated coronary artery disease after heart transplantation: the role of enhanced platelet aggregation and thrombosis. *J Intern Med* 1993;233:343–350.

Chapter 3

Myocardial Ischemia and Reperfusion

ROBERT B. JENNINGS, CHARLES STEENBERGEN, JR.,
AND KEITH A. REIMER

Most of our knowledge of the pathobiology of acute myocardial ischemia has been derived from studies of acute ischemia in experimental animals. The results of these studies show that the general effects of acute ischemia are similar in the hearts of all mammalian species tested, including humans. The differences between species are minor and are accounted for by circumstances such as differences in (1) enzyme distribution, (2) cardiac rate, and (3) the volume of collateral circulation reaching the ischemic myocardium. Thus, the timing of various changes such as myocyte death often differs between species, but the changes leading to myocyte death and the process of repair are generally similar in all mammalian hearts.

Most of the information presented in this chapter has been derived from studies of the ischemic canine heart.[1] Wherever possible, we shall relate the changes observed in the canine heart to those seen in human heart disease. In this process, it is important to remember that extrapolation of data from animals to patients requires appropriate caution.

Myocardial infarction is defined as the death (necrosis) of myocardium caused by the development of *ischemia,* i.e., the reduction of arterial blood flow to levels at which oxygen delivery is inadequate to meet the metabolic needs of the myocardium. Although the clinical features associated with the onset of severe and persistent myocardial ischemia often are equated with the onset of myocardial infarction, the distinction between ischemia and infarction is crucial. The recognition that ischemia initially causes reversible cellular injury, which becomes irreversible sometime later,[2] provides the basis for the concept that appropriate interventions might salvage ischemic myocardium and thereby limit ultimate infarct size by, for example, treating evolving acute myocardial infarction with thrombolysis. This concept has sparked widespread research efforts to establish the early subcellular events associated with myocardial ischemia, the pathogenesis of the transition to irreversible injury, and the biologic determinants of ultimate infarct size. This chapter will provide a brief overview of the biology of acute myocardial ischemia and infarction.

BIOLOGY OF MYOCARDIAL ISCHEMIA AND INFARCTION

Myocardial infarction is a dynamic process that is initiated by ischemia of sufficient duration and severity to cause irreversible cell injury. The development of ischemic necrosis elicits an acute inflammatory reaction, phagocytosis, and repair. The culmination of this process is the removal of the dead myocytes, followed by their replacement by a fibrous scar.

ETIOLOGY OF INFARCTION IN HUMANS

Most myocardial infarcts occur in hearts supplied by arteries exhibiting severe and generally long-standing coronary atherosclerosis. However, atherosclerosis alone does not lead to the clinical syndrome of acute infarction. Infarction arises when flow to the myocardium through a diseased vessel is obstructed acutely. Although a subject of debate in the past, angiographic studies of the coronary arteries of patients with evolving acute myocardial infarction have shown that more than 85% of cases are due to thrombi totally or partially obstructing the coronary artery supplying the area of acute ischemia.[3] These thrombi usually are attached to an ulcerated, often eccentric atherosclerotic plaque.[4,5] Careful postmortem studies of the relationship between an occluding thrombus and the underlying plaque in transmural infarcts have shown that the fibrous cap of the atherosclerotic plaque usually is ruptured at the site of the thrombus, a finding that suggests that the thrombosis occurs because of the rupture. Eccentric plaques with abundant lipid appear to be especially prone to rupture.[5] In addition to the overlying thrombus, the underlying plaques often exhibit hemorrhage and clotting within their grumous contents. This hemorrhage may expand the plaque to the point that it narrows the vessel enough to induce ischemia.

The thrombi that cause acute infarction can be lysed by the intravenous or intracoronary injection of thrombolytic agents such as tissue plasminogen activator, streptokinase, or other fibrinolytic enzymes, so-called thrombolytic therapy.[6] A fresh intracoronary clot usually lyses a few minutes after initiation of therapy; as soon as the clot dissolves, arterial flow is restored to the damaged myocardium. The ischemic tissue also can be reperfused successfully by coronary bypass surgery as long as the site of obstruction has been identified by coronary angiography.

Coronary spasm of sufficient degree to induce symptomatic ischemia has been demonstrated in some patients, especially those with variant angina; in addition, spasm clearly can cause acute myocardial infarction.[7] In such hearts, no thrombi are noted in the involved coronary artery. However, spasm of sufficient duration to induce infarction appears to be uncommon. On the other hand, minor degrees of spasm may be common, especially in unstable angina. In any event, the true incidence of spasm is very difficult to determine. Another potential cause of coronary occlusion is platelet aggregation, especially the embolization of platelet aggregates. Platelet embolism of adequate size to induce infarction has not been shown to occur experimentally and seems an unlikely cause of clinical infarction in humans. On the other hand, both spasm and platelet aggregration could cause small foci of ischemia that might lead to sudden death from a ventricular arrhythmia like ventricular fibrillation.

Variations in Severity of Acute Ischemia

The onset of ischemia is accompanied by rapid changes in myocardial metabolism (Fig. 3.1).[1] Sudden occlusion of a major coronary artery reduces or eliminates the flow of oxygenated arterial blood to the myocardium supplied by the occluded vessel. This produces almost instant deleterious effects because the myocardium is so dependent on aerobic respiration to make enough energy to support contractile function. After only 8–10 seconds of ischemia, the supply of oxygen trapped in the tissue as oxygenated hemoglobin or myoglobin is exhausted. Simultaneously, the myocardium ceases contracting efficiently and electrocardiographic changes appear (Fig. 3.1).

To produce symptoms and signs, the degree of reduction in arterial flow has to be sufficiently marked to cause cessation of aerobic metabolism. However, the severity of the ischemia found after sudden complete occlusion of a major coronary artery varies among species. In humans with coronary artery disease, collaterals enlarge after significant narrowing develops. These collaterals can supply arterial flow adequate to maintain the viability of some myocytes when the diseased vessel is suddenly occluded. In many dog hearts, native collateral connections between the arterial beds are present in the subepicardial myocardium. These are 20–200 μm in diameter and provide arterial flow to the ischemic bed during diastole.[8–10] Figure 3.2 shows the distribution of collateral flow after sudden occlusion of the circumflex artery in the open-chest anesthetized dog heart.[11] Local flow in different layers of the left ventricle was measured 20 minutes into the occlusion in 31 consecutive dogs by left atrial injection of 10 − μm plastic microspheres labeled with a γ emitter. Note the subendocarial myocardium received the least and the subepicar-

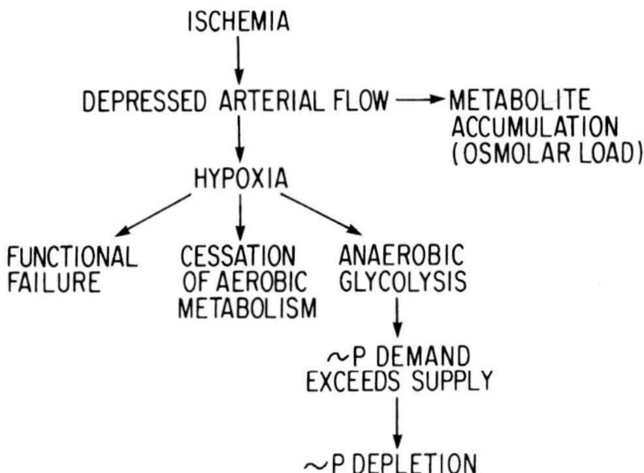

FIG. 3.1. Principal consequences of ischemia are shown in this diagram. Metabolites are produced intracellularly by hypoxic metabolism where they accumulate and equilibrate to a variable extent with extracellular fluid. Because tissue demand for high-energy phosphate (~P) exceeds supply, the net level of adenosine triphosphate decreases until it is virtually zero in zones of low-flow ischemia. Reproduced with permission of the authors and publishers of Ref. 17.

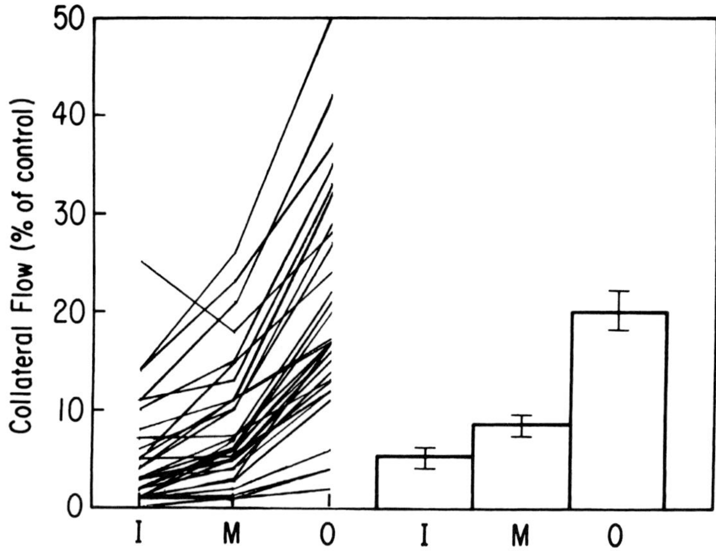

FIG. 3.2. Transmural distribution of collateral flow 20 minutes after proximal circumflex artery occlusion in 31 dogs. Flow was measured with 9 ± 1 μm microspheres before and after coronary artery occlusion. Collateral flow is expressed as percent of preocclusion flow to the same samples. Individual dogs are illustrated on the left, and the group mean $\pm$ SEM are shown on the right. *I, M,* and *O* are inner, middle, and outer thirds, respectively, of the transmural wall in the circumflex bed. In 90% of hearts, there was a transmural flow gradient such that flow to the outer wall was greater than flow to the inner wall. Subendocardial flow was almost always severely depressed (<10%) and averaged 4.5% of control. Subepicardial flow was greater (averaged 20% of control) and much more variable than subendocardial flow. Reproduced with permission of the authors and publishers of Ref. 11.

dial myocardium the most flow in virtually all of the hearts in Fig. 3.2. This gradient of blood flow is characteristic of hearts containing significant collateral connections. However, three hearts exhibited transmural severe ischemia, *i.e.,* virtually no collateral flow, and therefore a negligible transmural gradient of blood flow in the distribution of the occluded major coronary artery. This variation in flow induces a number of biologic consequences that will be discussed subsequently.

Canine myocardium receiving very low (0–5% of control) or no flow, generally termed *severe* or *total ischemia,* respectively, dies quite quickly, whereas *moderately ischemic* myocardium receiving 0.15–0.30 mL of arterial blood per gram wet weight, per minute dies more slowly. *High-flow ischemia* is associated with defective function but generally is not associated with myocyte death.[12] Assessment of the metabolic and ultrastructural changes of ischemia in the remainder of this chapter was performed only on severely ischemic subendocardial myocardium of the canine heart.

EFFECTS OF LOW-FLOW ISCHEMIA ON MYOCARDIUM

The two chief consequences of the reduction in arterial flow are the *depletion of ~P* in the involved myocardium and the accumulation of the products of myocyte metabolism within the area of ischemia (Fig. 3.1). Note that moderate and high-flow ischemia differ from low-flow ischemia because the collateral flow washes products of ischemic metabolism, such as H+ and lactate, to the general circulation. Also, the flow provides some substrate and probably provides small quantities of O_2 to support the aerobic oxidation of lactate or other substrates present in the myocyte. The reduction of the level of substances inhibiting glycolysis by either of these processes, as well as the benefit of small amounts of aerobic metabolism, permit generation of larger quantities of ~P in tissue receiving significant collateral flow. The aphorism that *"a little collateral flow goes a long way"* succinctly summarizes the benefit of collateral flow with respect to its capacity to reduce the severity of the deleterious effects of ischemia.

ENERGY METABOLISM IN ACUTE ISCHEMIA

As soon as the O_2 supplies become limiting, aerobic or mitochondrial respiration ceases. The myocardium then becomes dependent on reserves of ~P, which are small, and anaerobic glycolysis (AG) for its ~P. Creatine phosphate (CP) is the chief readily available reserve of ~P; it is utilized almost completely by a few contractions after aerobic respiration ceases.[13] Myocardial ATP supplies then begin to decline.[14–16] From this point on, AG, utilizing glucose 1-phosphate from glycogen, provides most of the ~P utilized by the ischemic myocytes. Three micromoles of ~P are released per micromole of glucose 1-phosphate converted to 2 μmol of lactate; note that this is less than 10% of the ~P released when glucose is metabolized to CO_2 and H_2O by aerobic metabolism.[1,17] Even though AG is relatively inefficient, it is the most important source of ~P in severe ischemia; at least 80% of the ~P utilized by totally ischemic myocardium is derived from AG.[18]

Rates of AG are high initially but, within 60–90 seconds, slow markedly because of the acidosis that develops secondary to lactate accumulation and the fact that some of the products of glycolysis accumulating in the tissue (osmotic load) inhibit AG.[19–21] Sufficient high-energy phosphate is generated by the high initial rate of AG to maintain the viability of the affected myocytes for many minutes. However, the slowed rate that soon appears is inadequate to maintain ATP. Also contributing to the slowing of glycolysis is a reduction in the rate of ~P utilization.

Net myocardial ATP decreases quickly during the first 10 minutes of low-flow ischemia (Fig. 3.3). Then the rate of decrease slows. However, virtually no ATP remains in the tissue by the time 40 minutes of ischemia have passed. The contribution of AG to ~P release is shown by the rise in tissue lactate. After 40 minutes of ischemia, tissue lactate ranges between 200 and 250 μmol per gram, dry weight. This inverse relationship between ATP depletion and lactate accumulation is a characteristic feature of low-flow or total ischemia but is noted only when ischemia is sufficiently severe to prevent both washout of lactate and metabolism of lactate to CO_2 and H_2O. Although not shown in Fig. 3.3, AG, judging by the rate of lactate production, ceases at about 40 minutes of severe *in vivo* ischemia.[18] It probably ceases because there is insuffi-

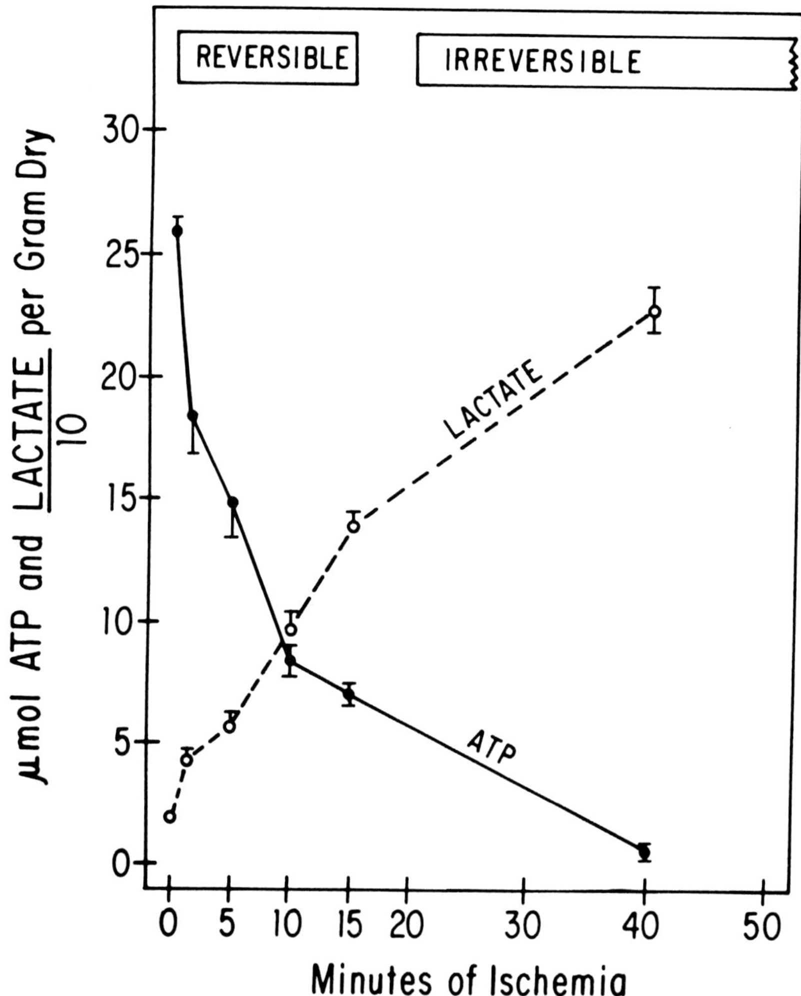

FIG. 3.3. Adenosine triphosphate (ATP) depletion (●) versus lactate production (○) in low-flow regional ischemia. Results were obtained from ischemic posterior papillary muscle tissue of groups of 4–6 hearts of anesthetized open-chest dogs subjected to occlusion of the circumflex branch of the left coronary artery. The tissue was frozen, dried, and analyzed after estimating arterial collateral flow with microspheres. In no case was collateral arterial flow >0.07 ml/min/g. Brackets indicate SEM. The injury is considered to be reversible during the first 15 minutes and irreversible after 20 or more minutes of ischemia. Reproduced with permission of the authors and publishers of Ref. 78.

cient ATP to phosphorylate fructose 6-phosphate to fructose 1,6-diphosphate early in the glycolytic scheme (Fig. 3.4).

Energy supply-and-demand relationships in ischemia are presented in diagrammatic fashion in Fig. 3.5.[22,23] The top half of the diagram presents reactions providing ~P and the bottom half shows reactions utilizing ~P. As indi-

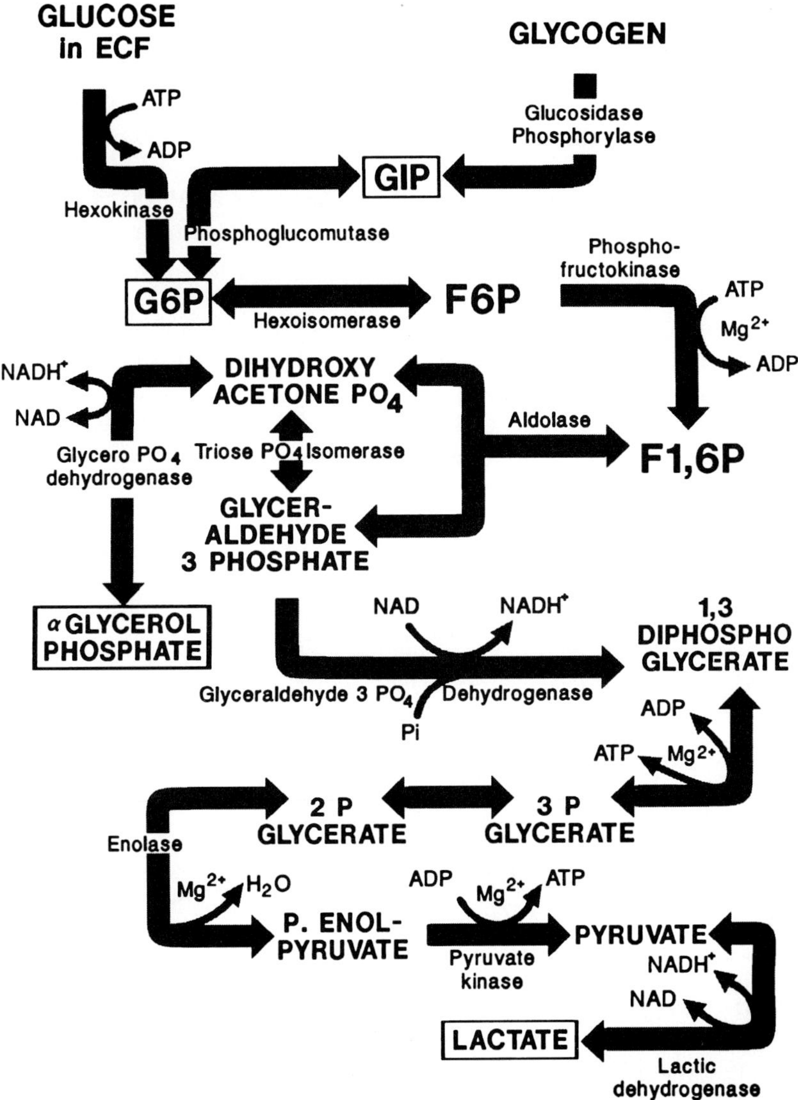

FIG. 3.4. Pathways of anaerobic glycolysis. In severe myocardial ischemia, most of the glucose used is derived from glycogen. Three micromoles of high-energy phosphate (~P) are produced per micromole of glucose 1-phosphate (*G1P*) converted to 2 μmol of lactate. Glyceraldehyde phosphate dehydrogenase is inhibited in ischemia; this inhibition results in accumulation of glucose 6-phosphate (*G6P*), small amounts of glucose 1-phosphate, and in the diversion of some three carbon units to α-glycerol phosphate (*αGP*). This diversion is favored by the high reduced nicotinamide adenine dinucleotide-to-nicotinamide adenine dinucleotide (NADH/NAD) ratio in tissue and provides some of the NAD required to support the activity of glyceraldehyde phosphate dehydrogenase. In low-flow or total ischemia, one can account for virtually all the glycogen used in ischemic tissue as G1P, G6P, αGP, and lactate. Thus, other intermediates do not accumulate to a significant extent. ATP (adenosine triphosphate); ADP (adenosine diphosphate); *F6P,* fructose 6-phosphate; *F1,6P,* fructose diphosphate; *Pi,* inorganic phosphate. Reproduced with permission of the authors and publishers of Ref. 1.

cated earlier, most energy utilized in the ischemic tissue is derived from AG[17], the remainder is derived from reserve ~P. Other reactions, such as substrate level phosphorylation, provide negligible quantities of ~P.

The reactions that consume ~P, *i.e.,* that provide the demand for energy while the tissue is ischemic, are shown on the bottom half of Fig. 3.5. A significant amount of the demand is provided by transport ATPases responding to the continuous electrical stimuli from the AV node and by attempts of the myofibrils to contract. The exact contribution of this source is unknown.[17] On the other hand, it is clear that 35–50% of the energy expended during ischemia is wasted by the mitochondrial ATPase.[24,25] This ATPase is mitochondrial synthase working in reverse. Instead of phosphorylating ADP to ATP, it catabolizes ATP to ADP and P_i. This reaction begins to occur as soon as the mitochondrial proton gradient is lost; it wastes much of the ATP consumed in the ischemic myocardium. It is of interest that ATP depletion and lactate accumulation can be slowed greatly[24,25] if this ATPase is inhibited with oligomycin (Fig. 3.6). Other reactions that consume ATP, such as adenylyl cyclase, fatty acid-coenzyme A synthetase, and phosphorylation reactions involving protein kinases, also contribute to the demand for ATP.[22]

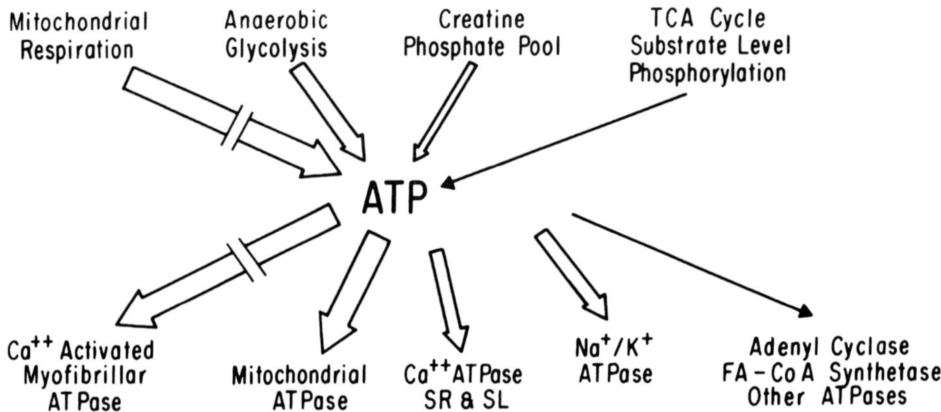

FIG. 3.5. The principal reactions producing and using high-energy phosphate in ischemic tissue are illustrated. The width of the arrows indicates the estimated quantitative importance of the various reactions. In severe ischemia, aerobic respiration is abolished. Preexisting stores of high-energy phosphate, in the form of creatine phosphate or ATP, are relatively small. Thus, anaerobic glycolysis becomes the principal source of energy, producing roughly 80% of the high-energy phosphate bonds that can be used by severely ischemic tissue. Substrate level phosphoryltion of α-ketoglutarate in the mitochondria does not require oxygen, but the tissue content of substrates that can be shuttled to α-ketoglutarate is small. Energy use also is reduced markedly during ischemia. Cardiac contraction, which is mediated by the Ca^{2+} activted myofibrillar ATPase, consumes much of the ATP produced in aerobic myocardium. However, contraction is abolished or depressed markedly in areas of severe ischemia. Some ATP still is required to remove Na+ from the cell, to keep Ca^{2+} sequestered in the sarcoplasmic reticulum, and for a variety of other cellular processes. Studies indicate that a major cause of ATP degradation in ischemia is the squandering of ATP by the mitochondrial ATPase (reverse function of the ATP synthetase). Reproduced with permission of the authors and publishers of Ref. 23.

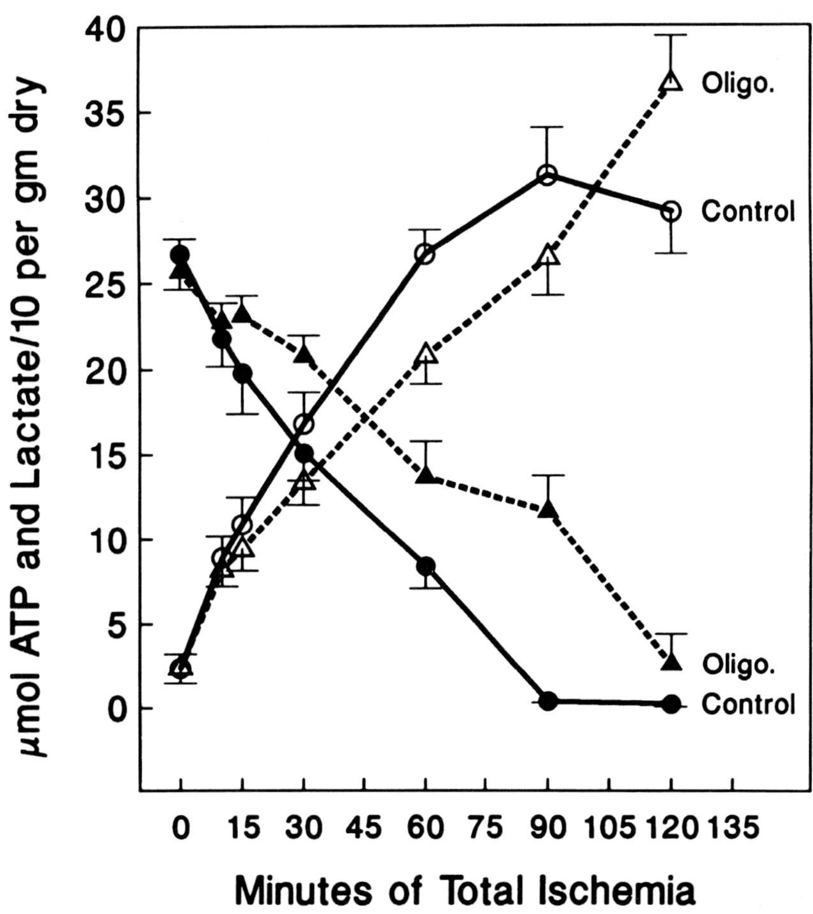

FIG. 3.6.   The effect of oligomycin (*oligo*) on the rate of ATP depletion (▲,●) and lactate accumulation (△,○) is shown in control and treated heart tissue. Note that oligomycin slowed both the rise in lactate (p<.05) and the fall in ATP (P<.01). The rate of ATP depletion from 15 minutes to the time at which ATP was depleted to <1.0 μmol/g dry was significantly different in the control and treated hearts (P<.03). ATP was depleted at a mean rate of 0.316 μmol ATP/g, dry weight/min in control *versus* 0.206 μmol/g, dry weight/min in oligomycin-treated hearts. Thus, inhibition of the mitochondrial ATPase between the 15th and 90th minute of total ischemia reduced the rate of ATP depletion by about 65%. Reproduced with permission of the authors and publishers of Ref. 24.

The conversion of ATP to ADP and then to AMP is followed by catabolism of the adenine nucleotide pool (Fig. 3.7). ADP is in excess in the tissue early in ischemia because glycolytic rephosphorylation cannot meet the rate of production of ADP. Adenylate kinase (myokinase) acts to recover the ~P bond of ADP (2ADP ⇆ATP + AMP). The first step in degradation of the pool involves AMP, which is dephosphorylated by intracellular 5′-nucleotidase to the nucleoside adenosine (Ado). Ado is converted intracellularly or extracellularly to inosine (Ino) by adenosine deaminase. In contrast to ATP, ADP, and AMP, all of which cannot diffuse from the myocyte, both Ado and Ino can and do pass from the myocyte to

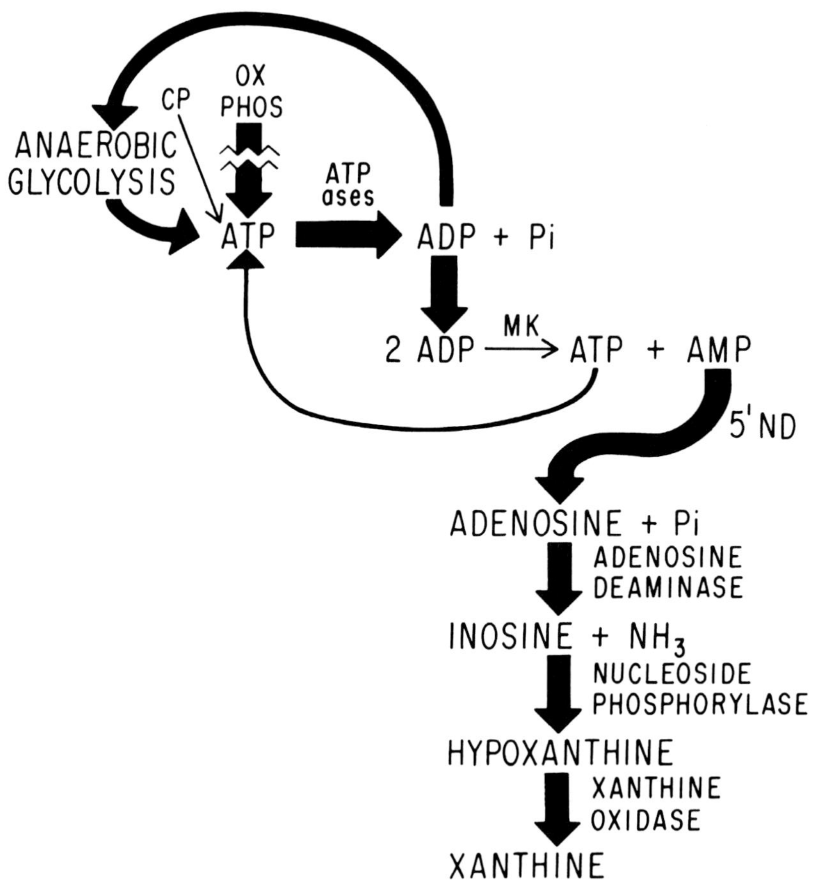

FIG. 3.7.   Major pathways of adenine nucleotide catabolism during myocardial ischemia. The most important routes of ATP and adenine nucleotide degradation are indicated by the heavier arrows. *CP*, creatine phosphate; *MK*, adenylate kinase (myokinase); 5'ND, 5'-nucleotidase. See text for explanation. Reproduced with permission of the authors and publishers of Ref. 79.

the extracellular space via a transporter. In the extracellular space, they are further degraded to hypoxanthine (Hyp) and xanthine (Xan). In those species with significant xanthine oxidase in the heart, Xan is degraded to uric acid. In many species, however, the degradation of the pool essentially stops at Hyp.

As a consequence of the reactions shown in Fig. 3.7, the total adenine nucleotide pool (ΣAd), which is the sum of the nucleotides ATP, ADP, and AMP, decrease rapidly. After 5 minutes of severe ischemia *in vivo,* 34% of it is gone (Fig. 3.8). These changes occur quickly; after only 5 minutes of ischemia, ADP and AMP are increased and significant amounts of Ado, Ino, Hyp, and Xan already are present in the heart. It is of interest that the total purine pool, including nucleotides, nucleosides, and bases, does not decrease over 40 minutes of ischemia even though many of the metabolites are extracellular. This is a reflection of the low collateral flow in the zone of severe ischemia.

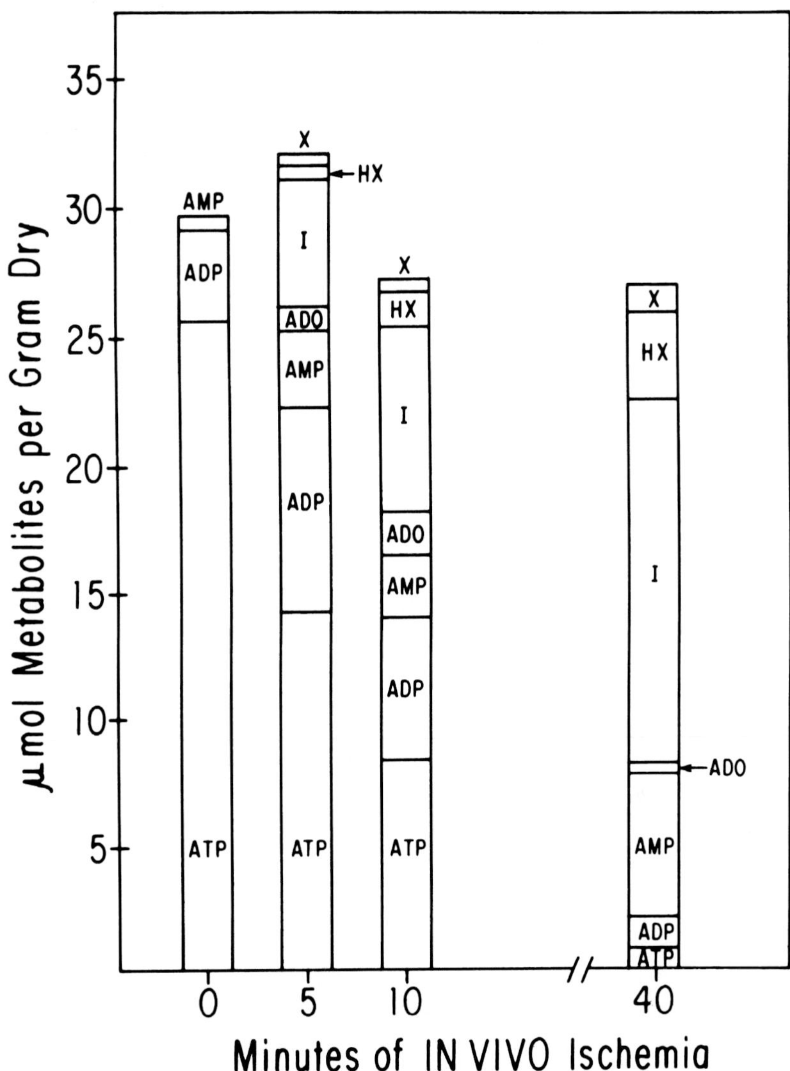

FIG. 3.8. Effect of severe ischemia on myocardial adenine nucleotides, nucleosides, and bases during circumflex artery occlusion in dogs. Measurements were made in nonischemic myocardium (0 min) and in the posterior papillary muscle (representative of the severely ischemic subendocardial zone of the occluded circumflex vascular region). *ADO,* adenosine; *I,* inosine; *HX,* hypoxanthine; *X,* xanthine. Note the transient increase in ADP at 5 and 10 minutes, the progressive decrease in total adenine nucleotides (ΣATP + ADP + AMP), and the stoichiometric recovery of the degraded nucleotides as nucleosides and bases. In more moderately ischemic myocardium, nucleotide catabolites are lost to the circulation.[80]

REVERSIBLE AND IRREVERSIBLE INJURY

Metabolism of the ischemic tissue continues until ATP is essentially gone and anaerobic glycolysis has ceased. About 40–60 minutes are required for completion of this process in zones of severe ischemia (Fig. 3.3). At this point, the tissue is pale because of contracture-rigor development. The tissue compression that results from myofibrillar shortening forces enough erythrocytes from the tissue to change its color from red to pale pink. Shortly after complete development of contracture-rigor, the myocytes cannot be salvaged even if successfully reperfused with arterial blood. Thus, the injury is *irreversible.*[2,26]

Severely ischemic myocytes survive if reperfused within 15 minutes.[22,27,28] Thus, by definition, during a 15-minute period of ischemia, the tissue is *reversibly injured.* The levels of various metabolites in the tissue during the reversible and irreversible phases are shown in Fig. 3.3 and 3.8.

ULTRASTRUCTURAL CHANGES

The ultrastructure of reversibly injured myocardium reflects the underlying metabolic changes. The myocytes are mildly edematous because of the osmotic load and the declining levels of $\sim$P; the sarcoplasmic space is increased and contains less glycogen because of glycogen utilization via AG. Also, the myofibrils of the myocytes are relaxed; *I*-bands appear secondary to the stretching of the acontractile myofibrils that elongate rather than shorten with each contraction of the adjacent viable myocardium. The nucleus shows mild peripheral aggregation of the nuclear chromatin and the sarcolemma is intact. The supporting structure of the tissue is indistinguishable from control.[27,29]

Irreversibly injured myocytes exhibit all of the changes seen during the reversible phase plus two striking additional features (Fig. 3.9). First, all of the mitochondria are swollen, exhibit disorganized cristae, and contain small osmiophilic amorphous densities.[29–31] These densities are composed of lipid and perhaps denatured protein[32,33] and reach their maximal size after about 120 minutes of ischemia. All myocytes in the zone of irreversible injury exhibit these characteristic changes in mitochondrial morphology. The second feature of note is disruption of the plasmalemma of the sarcolemma.[34,35] These breaks are small; they are widely scattered initially, but eventually become extensive (Fig. 3.9C). Also, subsarcolemmal blebs of edema fluid are prominent. These are areas in which the sarcolemma is lifted off the sarcomeres by cellular edema. Sarcolemmal disruption usually is most marked in areas of blebbing. Remnants of plasmalemma appear as circular profiles in the blebs, where they are especially prominent, but the basal lamina tends to remain intact over the bleb (Fig. 3.9D).

The ultrastructural features characteristic of fully developed myocyte coagulation necrosis are found after 90–120 minutes of severe ischemia *in vivo* (Fig. 3.10). Mitochondrial disarray, sarcolemmal disruption, and superstretched myofibrils are the most prominent features. Although the electron microscopic changes are prominent at 2 hours, the necrotic myocytes are difficult to identify objectively by light microscopy because eosin primarily stains myofibrils and myofibrils are not altered significantly, except for stretching,

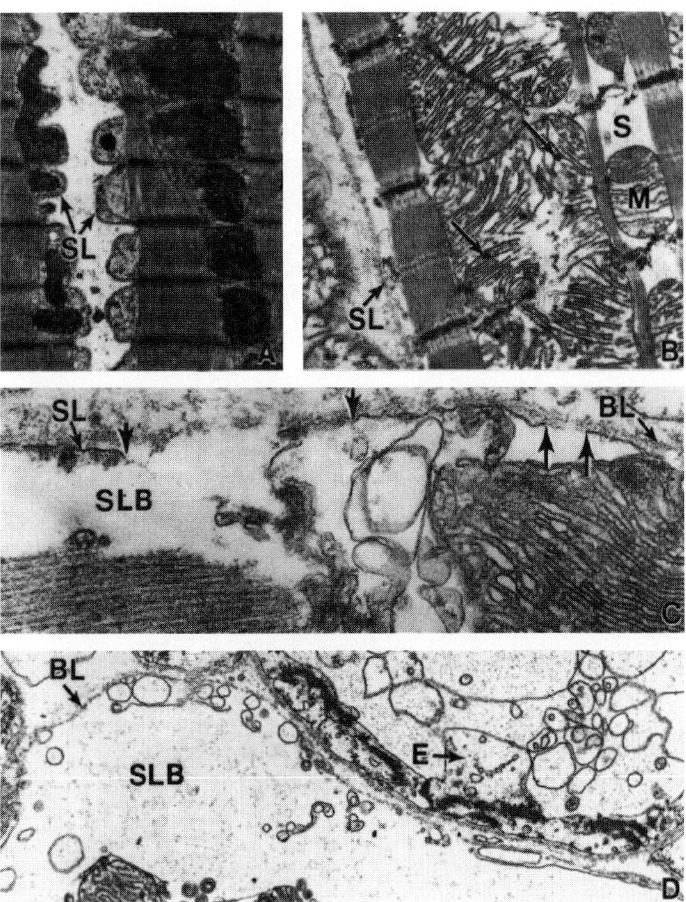

FIG. 3.9.   Control and damaged sarcolemma from canine left ventricle damaged by *in vivo* ischemia and fixed in glutaraldehyde buffered with 0.1 M cacodylate (approximately 600 to 650 millisomolar) followed by postosmication. *Panel A* is representative of control nonischemic myocardium. Note that the sarcolemma (*SL*) is anchored to the underlying myofibrils at the Z-bands. The sarcoplasm is compact and contains granular glycogen and mitochondria. *Panel B* is a representative myocyte irreversibly injured by 40 minutes of permanent ischemia. The myocyte is swollen; note that the SL has detached from the markedly relaxed myofibrils and covers a bleb of edema fluid. Note the swollen mitochondria (*M*) containing amorphous matrix densities (*arrows*). The sarcoplasm (*S*) is clear and is increased in volume. Few glycogen granules are present. *Panel C* is a high-power view of plasmalemmal disruption after 40 minutes of *in vivo* ischemia. The plasmalemma is designated sarcolemma and the point of disruption is shown between the thick arrows where there is persistent basal lamina (*BL*) but no unit membrane. A subsarcolemmal bleb (*SLB*) is present where the SL is lifted off the myofibril. This tissue was fixed by glutaraldehyde perfusion fixation *in vivo* before sectioning. *Panel D* shows a typical well-developed subsarcolemmal bleb after 180 minutes of ischemia. The plasmalemma is fragmented and persists as circular profiles beneath the basal lamina. A capillary lined by swollen endothelial cells (*E*) is in the field. Swollen mitochondria (*M*) of the underlying myocyte are also present. Magnification: *A*, 8,750 ×; *B*, 15,000×; *C*, 62,500×; *D*, 1,900×. Reproduced with permission of the authors and publishers of Ref. 35.

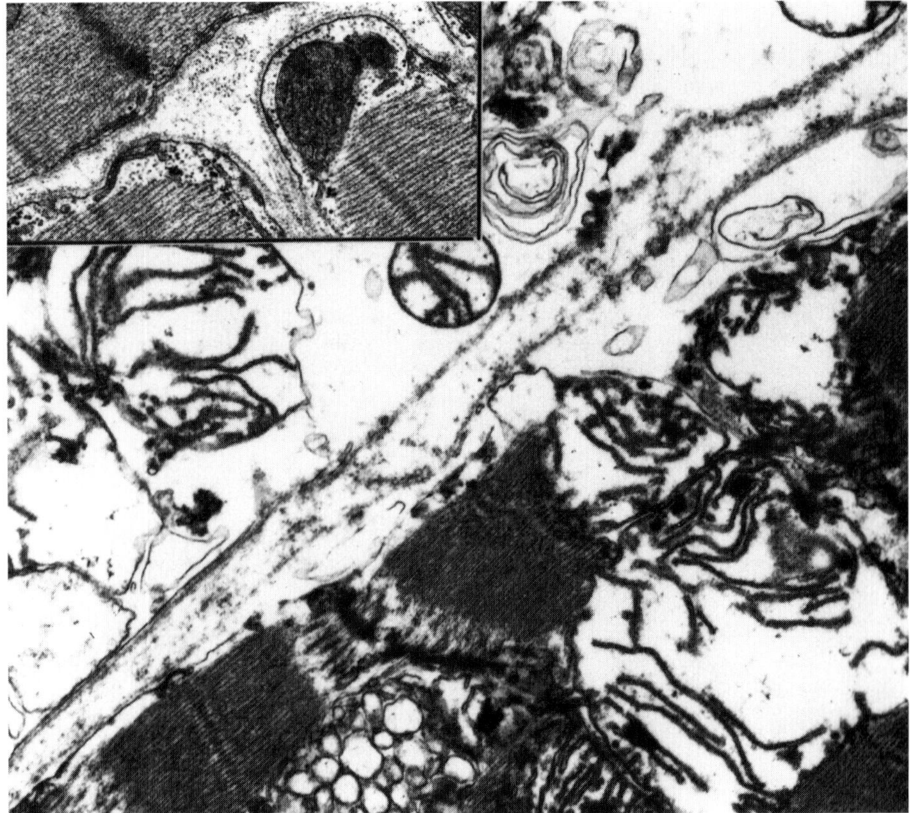

FIG. 3.10.   This micrograph shows the ultrastructure of advanced irreversible injury induced by 2 hours of severe ischemia in the canine heart. The ultrastructure does not change to any significant extent for the next 24–48 hours. The plasmalemma of the sarcolemma is markedly disrupted; the mitochondria are swollen and contain disorganized cristae and amorphous matrix densities. A section showing the sarcolemma of nonischemic control left ventricle of the same heart is shown in the *inset.*

during the initial phase of ischemic injury. Thus, routine techniques of light microscopy reveal little change in the architecture of the dead myocytes until late in ischemia.

The relationship of the striking electron microscopic changes in the mitochondria and sarcolemma during the irreversible phase of ischemic injury to cell death is not clearly established. The sarcolemmal disruption is considered to be the lethal event in ischemic injury.[1] The mitochondrial changes, although important and characteristic, probably do not contribute to myocyte death while the tissue is ischemic because the mitochondria are not functioning when oxygen is unavailable. Thus, alterations in mitochondrial function occurring late in ischemia should not contribute to irreversibility.[36] On the other hand, mitochondrial function must be restored if the myocytes are to survive at the time ischemic tissue is reoxygenated by reperfusion.[12] In this sense, mitochondrial function is critical for survival.

COMPARISON OF *IN VIVO* SEVERE ISCHEMIA WITH TOTAL ISCHEMIA POSTMORTEM

When the heart stops beating, all coronary flow ceases and the myocardium becomes totally ischemic. All of the changes that develop in severe or total ischemia *in vivo* develop *in vitro* in the totally ischemic heart. Thus, after postmortem intervals of several hours have elapsed, the characteristic electron microscopic features of ischemic cell death appear throughout the heart and cannot be used to diagnose early acute myocardial infarction.

Because all of the changes that develop in severe ischemia *in vivo* develop in total ischemia *in vitro,* the total ischemia model has been a very useful and efficient way to study changes in metabolism, ultrastructure, cytoskeletal architecture in ischemia, *etc.* (see data plotted in Fig. 3.6).[18,24,37]

CYTOSKELETAL CHANGES

The disruption of the sarcolemma shown in Figs. 3.9 and 3.10 is believed to be due to disaggregation of the attachment complexes that hold the sarcolemma to the underlying myofibrils.[35,38,39] These attachment complexes are located at each Z-band and consist of a series of cytoskeletal proteins. Talin, actin, α-actinin, integrin, and vinculin all are involved.[40] Vinculin is a distinctive marker protein of the attachment complex because it is found only in the attachment complexes and in the intercalated disk.[41] At or about the time that sarcolemmal disruption is noted by transmission electron microscopy, vinculin staining is much diminished in the attachment complexes (Fig. 3.11). Thus, cytoskeletal disorganization is associated closely with sarcolemmal disruption. It is not clear whether or not this association is causal.

CAUSE OF CELL DEATH IN ISCHEMIA

The molecular event or series of events that cause cell death in low-flow ischemia remains to be established. It is clear that 40–60 minutes of severe ischemia *in vivo* produces changes in the myocytes that make them unsalvageable by reperfusion with arterial blood. These changes include (1) very low tissue ATP (<10% of control); (2) cessation of AG; (3) greatly increased osmotic load composed of lactate, glucose 1-phosphate, glucose 6-phosphate, α-glycerol phosphate, Ado, Ino, inorganic phosphate, ammonia, H+; (4) ion shifts with increased intracellular Na+, Ca^{2+}, Cl-, and H+ along with decreased intracellular K+ and Mg^{2+}; (5) mitochondrial swelling with amorphous matrix densities and functional failure, and (6) sarcolemmal disruption. The development of breaks in the plasmalemma of the sarcolemma is the most likely explanation currently available to explain the demise of the myocytes. These defects allow small molecular weight enzymes and cofactors to leak from the myocyte to the extracellular space. Moreover, the breaks allow massive Ca^{2+} entry to occur when the myocytes are reperfused with arterial blood. This Ca^{2+} overload is very deleterious in that it induces massive contraction of the myofibrils of the myocytes. Contraction-band necrosis appears (Fig. 3.12) rapidly (within 2 minutes) after reperfusion of irreversibly injured tissue.[42,43]

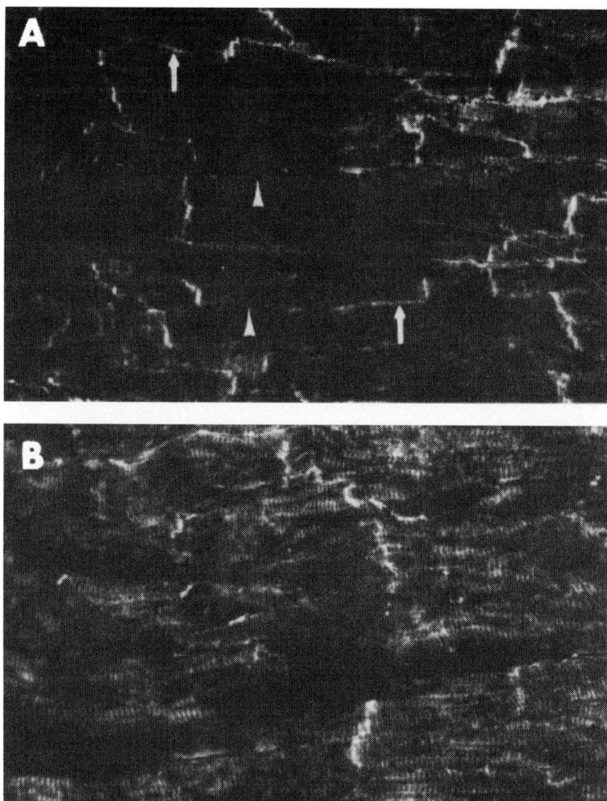

FIG. 3.11.   Vinculin immunofluorescence after 120 minutes of total ischemia (*Panel A*) and after 120 minutes of ischemia and 60 minutes of incubation in oxygenated media (*Panel B*). Representative longitudinal sections labeled with polyclonal antivinculin antibody are shown. In *Panel
A*, portions of the sarcolemma with costameric vinculin staining are indicated by *arrows*, and portions of the sarcolemma lacking vinculin staining are indicated by *arrowheads*. In *Panel B*, there
is no costameric staining. The persistent, faint Z-line and intercalated disk staining can be attributed to nonspecific staining. (Magnification: 500×). Reproduced with permission of the authors and publishers of Ref. 39.

Our current working hypothesis with respect to the cause of myocyte disruption in ischemia is shown in Figure 3.13. It seems likely that disruption is
a two-stage phenomenon. First, the attachment complexes of the sarcolemma
have to be altered in such a way that they lose their capacity to restrain the
sarcolemma at each sarcomere. Our initial hypothesis regarding the mechanism of this phase was that it was mediated by proteolysis induced by a Ca^{2+}-
activated protease specific for vinculin or other components of the attachment
complex. However, no digestion products of appropriate target proteins of the
attachment complex occurs on the time scale associated with disruption.[44] Our
current working hypothesis is that the complex disaggregates, perhaps as a
function of dephosphorylation or secondary to acidosis. Once the sarcolemma

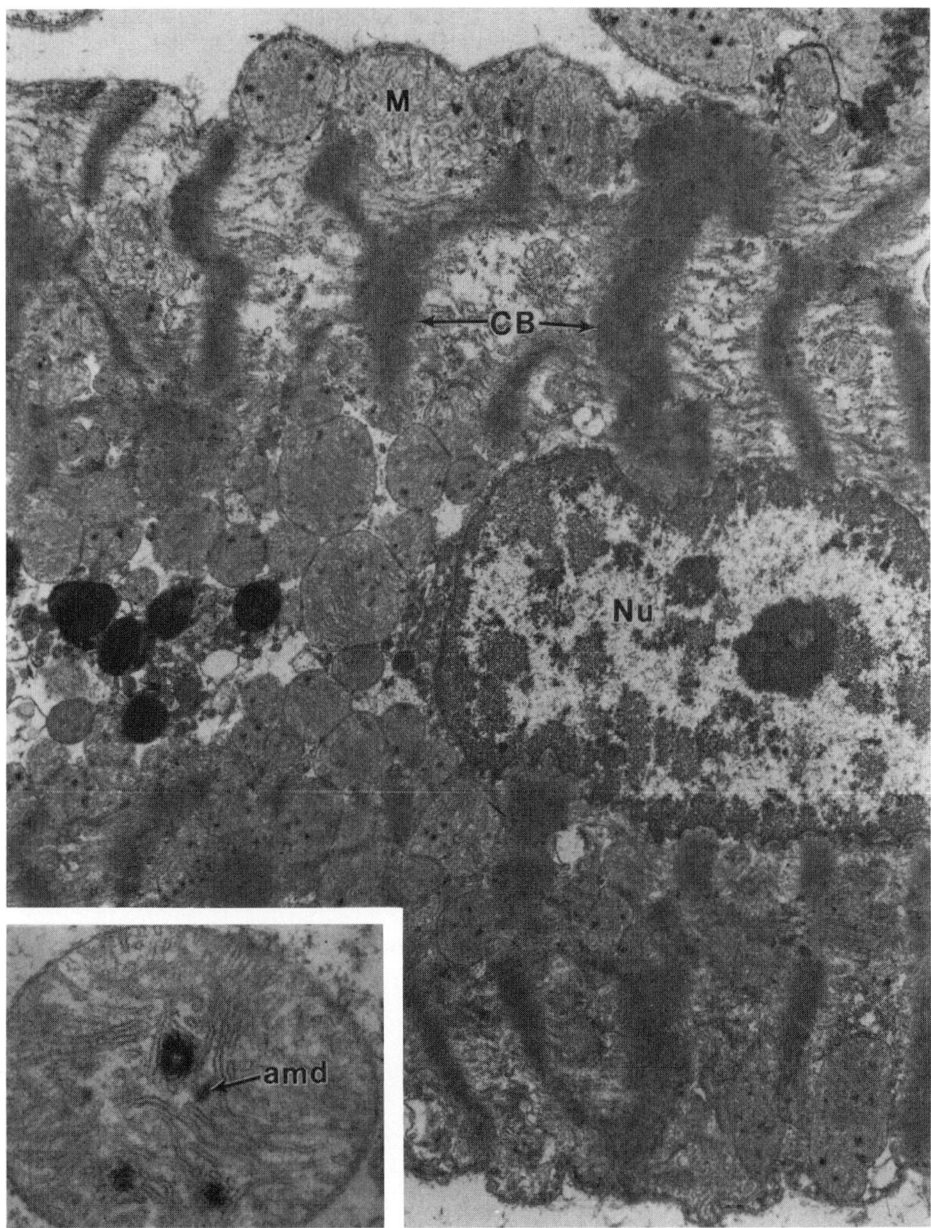

FIG. 3.12. Ultrastructural features of contraction-band necrosis induced by 40 minutes of severe *in vivo* ischemia and 20 minutes of reperfusion in the canine heart. Numerous dense contraction bands (*CB*) are obvious. Peripheral condensation of nuclear chromatin (*Nu*) also is apparent, and the mitochondria (*M*) appear swollen and contain both amorphous and granular matrix densities. The *inset* at lower left shows a higher power view of characteristic granular densities of calcium phosphate in mitochondria of these cells. Both amorphous (*amd*) and granular densities are present. Osmium fixation. Magnification: 14,000×; *inset,* 45,000×. Reproduced with permission of the authors and publishers of Ref. 23.

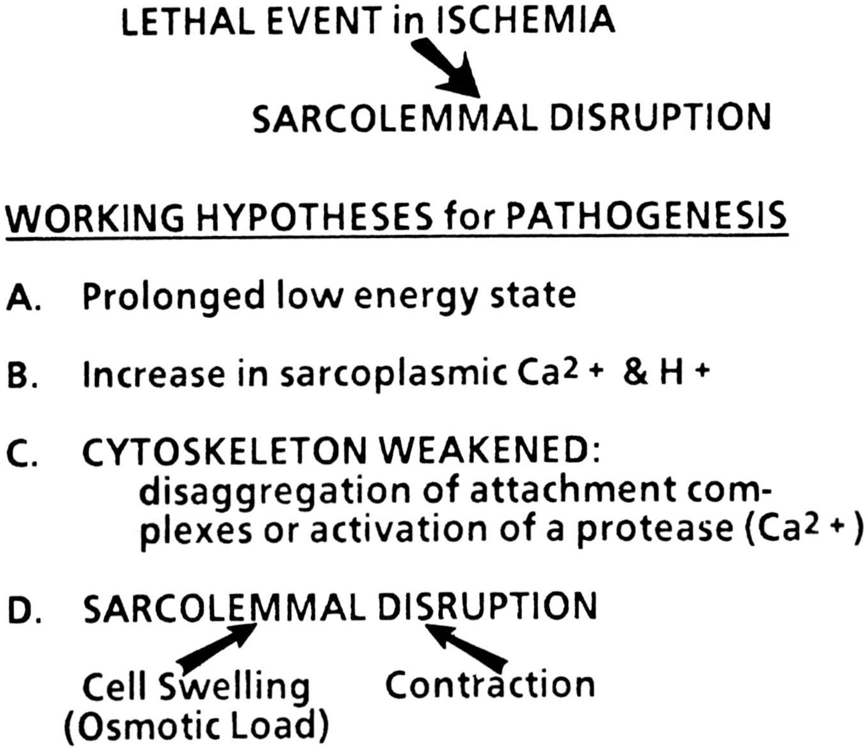

LETHAL EVENT in ISCHEMIA

SARCOLEMMAL DISRUPTION

WORKING HYPOTHESES for PATHOGENESIS

A.   Prolonged low energy state

B.   Increase in sarcoplasmic Ca^{2+} & H^+

C.   CYTOSKELETON WEAKENED:
disaggregation of attachment complexes or activation of a protease (Ca^{2+})

D.   SARCOLEMMAL DISRUPTION

Cell Swelling   Contraction
(Osmotic Load)

FIG. 3.13.   Diagram of the steps involved in a proposed working hypothesis of the cause of sarcolemmal disruption in low-flow ischemia.

or its attachment complexes are altered, the second stage occurs if a force is available to cause the unsupported sarcolemma to disrupt. In severe ischemia, we believe that cell edema developing secondary to the osmotic load and/or contraction of adjacent intact myocytes provides the disruptive force. The subsarcolemmal blebs of edema fluid (Figs. 3.9*C*, 3.9*D*, 3.10) are a reflection of the cell swelling.

High-Energy Phosphate and Cell Death

Because ATP is involved in numerous cell processes critical to the viability of myocytes such as marcomolecular synthesis, ion transport, synthesis of RNA and DNA, etc., ~P depletion has many deleterious effects in the myocyte. Moreover, low ATP is associated with irreversible injury in myocardium, and interventions that maintain cardiac ATP in the range of 5–10 μmol of ATP/g, dry weight, are associated closely with reversible injury as well as salvage of the ischemic myocardium when the tissue is reperfused with arterial blood. We know that not only must ATP be depleted for cell death to occur, but that the depletion must exist for a period of time before the myocytes enter the irreversible phase of injury. For example, a very low ATP develops quickly in iodoacetate poisoning.[37] However, membrane disruption does not occur any faster in iodoacetate treated than in control myocardium. Presumably, ATP depletion results in loss of a reaction or reactions required to maintain viability and does not develop until a system involving ATP becomes defective.

To establish the relationship of ~P depletion (ATP depletion) to cell death, the enzymatic reaction or series of reactions associated with the death of the myocytes must be identified. Until this identification has been made, ATP depletion remains an event that is associated closely with myocyte death. Causality has not been established.

Finally, in severe ischemia, many processes, often interrelated, are occurring simultaneously. It is difficult to pick from this array of phenomena those that are causally associated with the death of the myocyte. At the present time, the cause of membrane disruption is unknown. If the working hypothesis shown in Figure 3.13 is correct, both ATP depletion and the osmotic load may be involved.

MICROVASCULAR INJURY

Myocardial ischemia also results in microvascular damage.[45–47] This is characterized in its early stages by marked endothelial cell swelling and loss of pinocytotic vesicles. The capillaries eventually become obstructed by blebs of swollen endothelial cytoplasm (Fig. 3.9*D*). Fibrin thrombi, erythrocyte rouleaux, and leukocyte entrapment also contribute to obstruction. Eventually, overt microvascular necrosis occurs. Although the role of microvascular injury in the evolution of an acute myocardial infarct still is being debated, available evidence indicates that vascular injury lags behind and does not contribute to the irreversible injury of the ischemic myocytes.

NECROSIS, INFLAMMATION, AND REPAIR

Although the ultrastructural characteristics of irreversible damaged myocytes can be detected as early as 30–40 minutes after the onset of ischemia,[22] acute myocardial infarction often is not detectable by either gross or histologic analysis for 4 hours or longer. After this time, histologic features of necrosis such as hypereosinophilia and nuclear pyknosis are detectable and become more pronounced with time. Other changes, such as loss of myofibrillar cross-striations, develop more slowly. Scattered polymorphonuclear leukocytes may be seen as early as 4 hours at the junction of irreversibly injured and normal myocytes; this junction is identifiable by a tiny zone of myocytes exhibiting contraction-band necrosis at the boundary between irreversibly injured and control myocytes.[48] The number of granulocytes increases during the next 3 days. They degenerate and disappear gradually thereafter (Fig. 3.14). Macrophages are first seen in large numbers on day 4 or 5; they progressively remove the necrotic debris.

Because microvascular necrosis absolishes perfusion of the infarct center, the early inflammatory response often is confined to the periphery of the infarct. Repair of the center of an infarct depends on the ingrowth of new capillaries. A clear-cut rim of granulation tissue often surrounds the infarct by 7–10 days, but complete removal of necrotic muscle and replacement by granulation

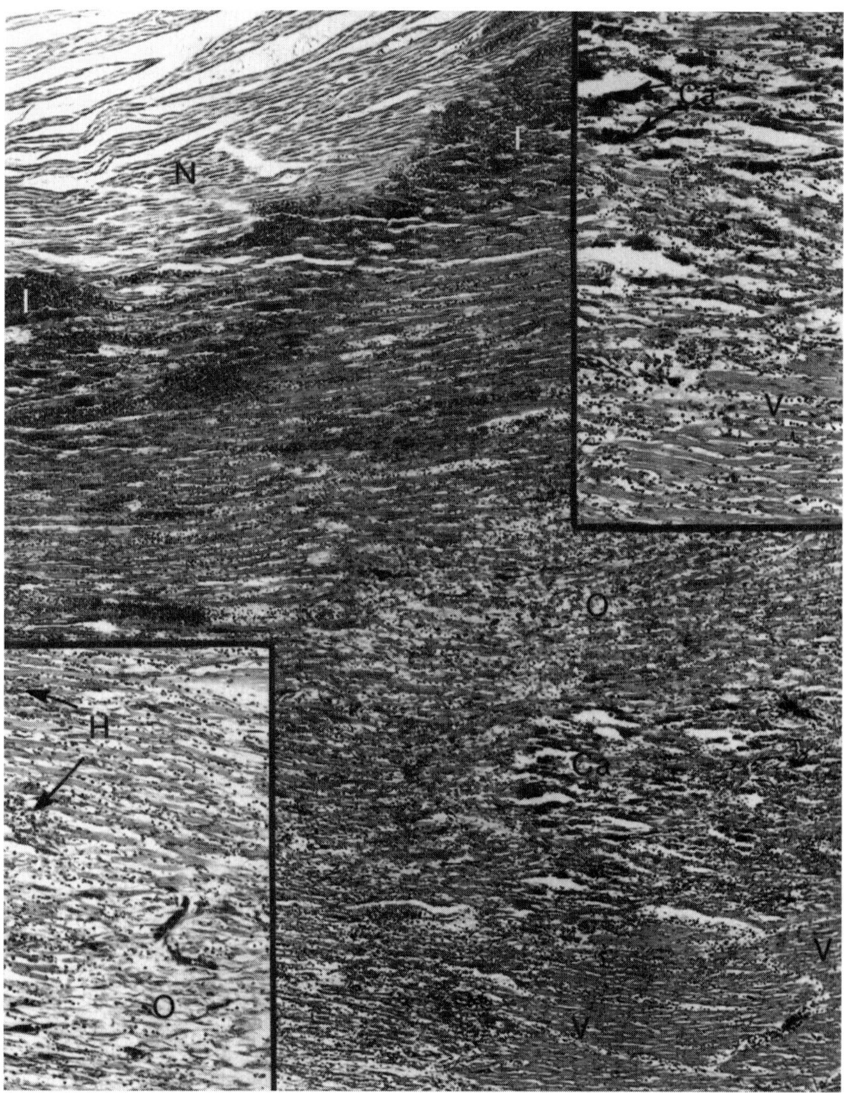

FIG. 3.14. Characteristic histologic zones of inflammation and repair in a 4-day-old myocardial infarct in the dog heart. This view is from the center of the circumflex bed and incorporates much of the transmural wall from the subendocardial region (*top*) to the subepicardial region (*bottom*). There is a subendocardial central core of coagulation necrosis (*N*), with separation of fibers due to interstitial and cellular edema but with relatively little cellular infiltration. This zone is surrounded by a zone with hemorrhage (*H*) and an intense acute inflammatory response (*I*). In the peripheral zone, organization (*O*) has begun and is characterized by macrophages, which have removed some of the necrotic cells, and ingrowth of fibroblasts and capillaries. This is better seen in the lower *inset*. Some heavily calcified cells (*CA*) also are present in the peripheral zone. These cells exhibit contraction-band necrosis and much calcium phosphate in the mitochondria. Some viable muscle (*V*) survived in the subpicardial region seen at the *lower right*. This region between the organizing zone of the infarct and viable myocardium is shown at higher power in the *upper inset*. Hematoxylin and eosin. Magnification: 55×; *insets,* 120×. Reproduced with permission of the authors and publishers of Ref. 72.

tissue requires 2–8 weeks, depending on initial infarct size. Progressive deposition of collagen occurs and the scar may not reach maximum density and strength until 3–6 months have elapsed.

TEMPORAL AND SPATIAL EVOLUTION OF AN ACUTE MYOCARDIAL INFARCT

Not all myocytes die simultaneoulsy in a region of acute myocardial ischemia. The time course of ischemic cell death is of considerable importance inasmuch as the possibility for successful intervention to limit infarct size depends on the persistence of viable myocytes destined to die if untreated.

TRANSMURAL "WAVEFRONT" OF ISCHEMIC CELL DEATH

The time course of ischemic cell death cannot be measured directly in patients and must be inferred from animal studies. The time course of infarction is known in dogs with proximal occlusions of the circumflex artery.[26] In these experiments, reperfusion at 6 hours had no effect on myocardial infarct size. In contrast, infarcts reperfused at 3 hours were significantly smaller compared with nonreperfused infarcts, whereas reperfusion at 40 minutes limited infarct size by 60–70%. The reduction in infarct size was due to salvage of myocardium in the subepicardial region of ischemia. Lateral salvage is unimportant because infarcts extended to within 1–2 mm of the lateral boundaries of the occluded vascular bed in all hearts, regardless of treatment. Thus, limitation of infarct size by reperfusion is primarily due to prevention of subepicardial necrosis. These results are the basis of the transmural "wavefront" phenomenon characteristic of ischemic cell death (Fig. 3.15).

The explanation for the more rapid death of subendocardial region and later transmural extension is complex. Part of the transmural progression of injury is related clearly to the transmural gradient of collateral blood flow. Collateral blood flow following coronary occlusion, although variable in overall amount, always is limited most severely in the subendocardial region and is shunted preferentially to the subepicardial zone. Myocytes only survive in the subepicardial zone if there is collateral flow; thus, collateral flow is the final critical determinant of infarct size.[12] In addition, however, there is a transmural gradient of wall tension, such that tension and, hence, metabolic demands are greatest in the subendocardial region. Moreover, subendocardial myocardium has an intrinsically higher metabolic rate compared with the subepicardial zone.[49] Thus, even in pig hearts, which exhibit no collateral flow, necrosis develops first in the subendocardial layer; note, however, that necrosis becomes transmural very quickly in this species.[50]

Although a transmural progression of myocardial ischemic cell death has not been demonstrated directly in humans, the frequent occurrence of subendocardial infarcts or of transmural infarcts that have variable amounts of viable myocardium in the subepicardial zone clearly indicates that in humans, as in dogs, the subendocardial myocardium is the zone most vulnerable to ischemic injury. The 3–6-hour time period during which ischemic cell death develops after coronary occlusion in anesthetized dogs has been confirmed in closed-chest awake dogs and in nonhuman primates. Results of thrombolysis trials in man indicate that a similar time course applies to patients with severe myocardial

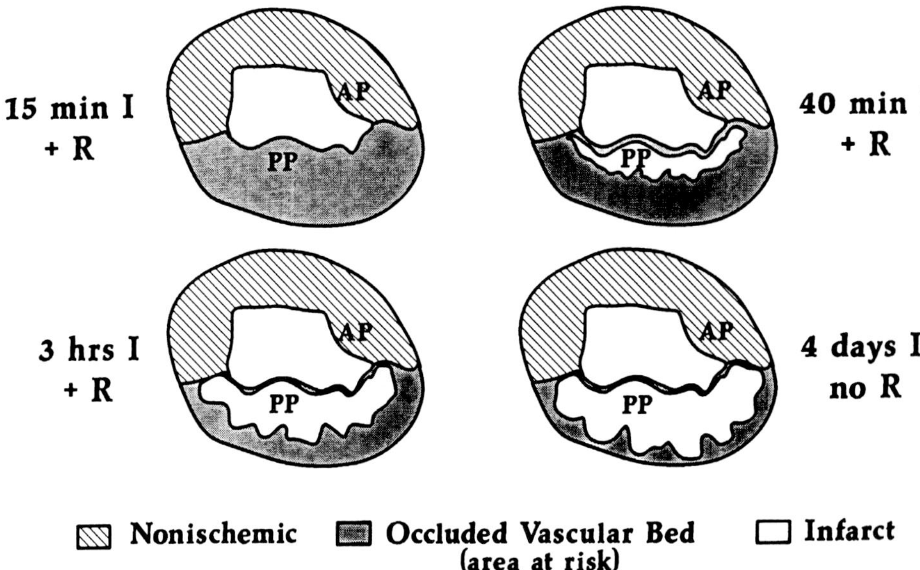

FIG. 3.15.   Progression of cell death *versus* time after circumflex coronary occlusion in dogs. The location of infarcts induced by different periods of ischemia and followed by reperfusion is illustrated. Necrosis occurs first in the subendocardial myocardium. With longer occlusions, a wavefront of cell death moves from the subendocardial zone across the wall to involve progressively more of the transmural thickness of the ischemic zone. In contrast, the lateral margins in the subendocardial region of the infarct are established as early as 40 minutes after occlusion and are sharply defined by the anatomic boundaries of the ischemic bed. Early reperfusion salvages some of the ischemic tissue and thereby limits the transmural extent of infarct. *AP*, anterior papillary muscle; *PP*, posterior papillary muscle. Reproduced with permission of the authors and publishers of Ref. 26.

ischemia caused by sudden proximal occlusion of a major coronary artery that was not previously severely stenotic.[6] Although unproved, the time course of ischemic cell death could be slower in the human than in the dog heart, if the degree of ischemia was less severe or if ischemia was gradual or intermittent in onset. For example, ischemia could be less severe if the involved coronary artery was obstructed only partially, if prior coronary disease had induced the growth of functionally important collateral interconnections, or if infarction was caused by intermittent coronary spasm or platelet aggregation. Also, the hemodynamic determinants of cardiac metabolic rate (heart rate, blood pressure, and contractility) often are lower in human patients than in anesthetized dogs. Finally, the phenomenon of preconditioning (see later section) could delay cell death in acute ischemia.

The Lateral "Borderzone"

Several studies have shown that intermediate levels of collateral blood flow and biochemical derangement as well as intermediate functional impairment in myocardium occurs at the lateral margins of an ischemic region. Such data have been interpreted to indicate the existence of a lateral "borderzone," where salvage of ischemic myocardium might be possible. However, studies of the myocardial microvasculature have shown few, if any, interconnections between capillary loops perfused by adjacent epicardial arteries.[51] Thus, there is no anatomic basis for any true lateral gradient of collateral blood flow and measured gradients of collateral blood flow, metabolites, etc., are explained as averages of values from samples containing both ischemic and nonischemic myocardium. The lack of lateral limitation of infarct size by early reperfusion in dogs is direct evidence against the existence of a lateral zone of less severe ischemic injury.[26] Furthermore, studies of human infarcts have shown marked intrinsic variation in the transmural extent of necrosis, but a constant relationship of infarct boundaries to the anatomic boundaries of the occluded vascular bed.[52]

Determinants of Ultimate Infarct Size

In hearts from patients studied at autopsy, as well as in dogs, there is great variation in infarct size. In part, this variation is due to differences in the size of the ischemic vascular bed (myocardium at risk of infarction).[26,53] In patients, the ischemic bed size varies according to the arteries involved (anterior descending supplying the greatest proportion of the left ventricle) and site of occlusion (distal occlusion involving less myocardium than a more proximal occlusion).[52] There also is considerable variation in the amount of myocardium actually supplied by a given artery. For example, considerable variation in ischemic vascular bed size occurs among experimental animals even when the artery and site of occlusion are constant.

In addition to the variation in size of the involved vasculature bed, there is variation in the amount of necrosis developing within the ischemic region. Infarcts bear a fairly constant relationship to the lateral boundaries of the occluded vascular bed (the myocardium at risk).[52,53] However, there is considerable variation in the transmural extent of myocardial infarcts within the area at risk. The possible factors contributing to the transmural extent of an infarct include hemodynamic determinants of myocardial metabolic demand, such as heart rate, left ventricular systolic pressure, wall tension and contractility, and most important, the availability of collateral blood flow. For example, in the dog model, there is an inverse correlation between the transmural extent of infarction and the amount of collateral blood flow to the subepicardial region (Fig. 3.16).[26] Because of this relationship, measurements of collateral blood flow are essential in studies attempting to test the effects of therapy on infarct size. It seems likely that collateral blood flow is a similarly important determinant of ultimate infarct size in patients but accurate quantitation of subepicardial collateral flow cannot be done in humans with currently available techniques.

EFFECTS OF REPERFUSION ON MYOCARDIAL INFARCTION

The recent widespread evaluation of thrombolytic therapy during the early hours of myocardial infarction has kindled much interest in the effects of reperfusion on ischemic myocardium.[6] The effects of reperfusion are variable and depend on the duration and severity of preceding ischemia.

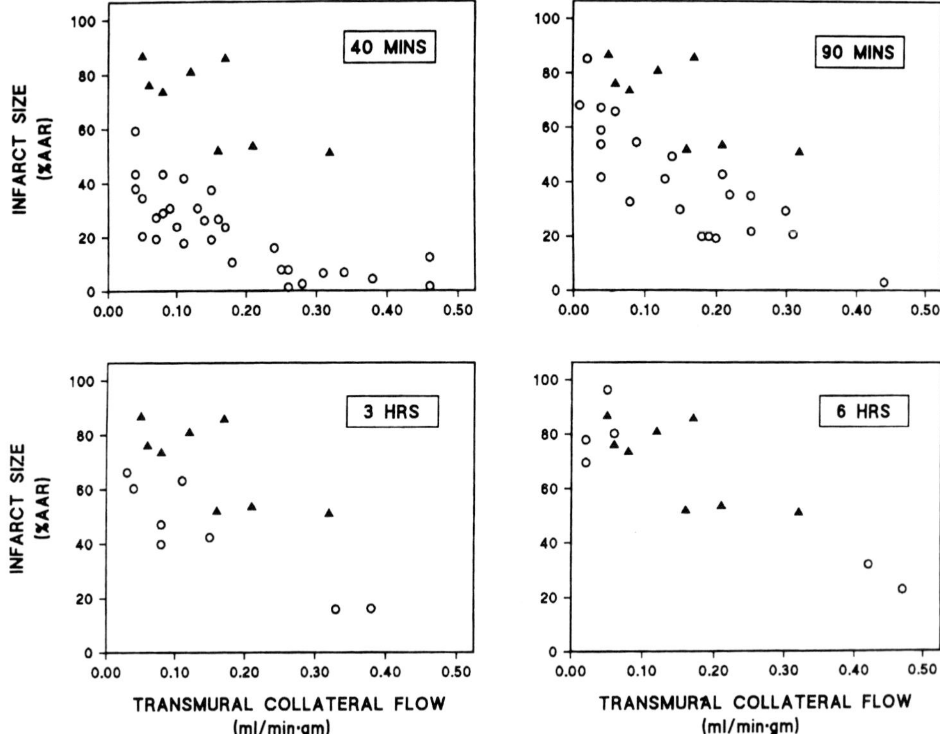

FIG. 3.16. Relation between infarct size and transmural mean collateral blood flow in dogs with various durations of circumflex coronary artery occlusion followed by 4 days of reperfusion. Flow was measured 10–20 minutes after coronary occlusion and infarct size was measured histologically after a 4-day survival period. In each panel, infarct size following reperfusion at the indicated time (o) is compared with nonreperfused infarct size (▲). Each regression line indicates a strong inverse relation between the transmural extent of the infarct and the amount of collateral blood flow to the subepicardial region. A significant downward shift of the regression was done at either 40, 90, or 180 minutes, but no effect was observed for reperfusion at 6 hours. As expected, the magnitude of the beneficial effect of reperfusion on infarct size was inversely related to the duration of ischemia prior to reperfusion. Reproduced with permission of the authors and publishers of Ref. 81.

Salvage of Reversibly Injured Myocytes

Most importantly, reperfusion of reversibly injured myocytes prevents subsequent necrosis. Within a period of 60–120 seconds of successful reperfusion of reversibly injured myocardium, aerobic respiration resumes and ATP becomes the dominant nucleotide in a smaller adenine nucleotide pool.[27] The restoration of aerobic metabolism and recharging of the adenine nucleotide pool is completed during the first 3 minutes of reperfusion.

Functional, metabolic, and ultrastructural recovery are not instantaneous. Ultrastructural recovery is virtually complete 20 minutes after a single 15-minute period of ischemia except for a rare permanently damaged mitochondrion.[27] On the other hand, many studies have shown that contractile function is depressed for several days after brief periods of ischemia.[54,55] Also, adenine nucleotides, which are reduced by 50% in areas subjected to only 15 minutes of ischemia, are not completely restored even 4 days later.[56] Thus, many ischemic changes require hours or days of reperfusion before recovery is complete. Nevertheless, myocardium salvaged by reperfusion eventually recovers all parameters evaluated.

Later reperfusion, at 40 minutes to 3 hours, does not prevent infarction entirely, but does limit the transmural extent of infarcts. In other words, reperfusion salvages reversibly injured myocardium in the subepicardial region (Fig. 3.15).

Persistent Functional Changes in Reversibly Injured Myocytes

Reperfused living reversibly damaged myocytes do not contract as efficiently as they did in the control state. This phenomenon is termed *stunning*[54,55,57] and persists for hours or days. Myocytes reperfused late in the reversible phase of ischemia still exhibit stunning 48–72 hours after being reperfused. Using spin-trapping techniques, Bolli[55,58] has shown that abundant products of oxygen-derived free radical reactions are present in coronary sinus blood beginning at the time tissue is reperfused. Moreover, part of the stunning phenomenon clearly is due to those oxygen-derived free radicals because stunning can be ameliorated greatly if free radical scavengers such as superoxide dismutase and catalase are given immediately before reperfusion.[55,57,58] Because necrotic myocardium does not contract, it is difficult to quantitate the impact of stunning on the function of reperfused hearts containing areas of necrosis. Nevertheless, stunning may contribute to power failure in humans with acute infarction if the infarct contains significant quantities of reversibly injured tissue.

Adaptation to Ischemic Stress (Ischemic Preconditioning)

Reversibly injured myocardium adapts to episodes of ischemia and reperfusion in such a way that myocytes destined to die during a prolonged test episode of ischemia survive if they are preconditioned with an episode of reversible ischemia and reperfusion. This adaptive response has been termed *ischemic preconditioning*[59]; however, the mechanism through which the myocardium is protected remains unknown. It is known to be associated with reduced energy demand during subsequent episodes of ischemia[60]. Recent studies suggest that Ado released during the preconditioning episodes of ischemia may be involved. This Ado is believed to bind to Ado (A1) receptors on the myocytes and sympathetic neurons. The receptor stimulation presumably alters the metabolic response of the myocardium to the subsequent episode of ischemia.[61]

It is of interest that a brief preconditioning episode of ischemia and reperfusion improves contractile function in the isolated perfused rodent heart when it is reperfused after a prolonged episode of ischemia.[62–64] Also, a similar preconditioning protocol reduces the incidence of arrhythmias.[65] Finally, *heat shock proteins* develop in hearts exposed to a preconditioning protocol *in vivo.*[66] These appear to be cardioprotective; however, these proteins form too slowly to account for the classic preconditioning response. The various adaptive responses of reversibly injured myocardium are currently the subject of intense investigation.

Accelerated Necrosis of Irreversibly Injured Myocytes (Contraction-Band Necrosis)

Most of the severely ischemic myocytes in the subendocardial region have been irreversibly injured by 40 minutes of ischemia. When these myocytes are successfully reperfused, dramatic ultrastructural and biochemical effects appear (Fig. 3.12).[31,42,45]

Defects in the plasmalemma become much more prominent in association with massive cell swelling that develops after only 1–2 minutes of reflow.[43] In addition, there is massive Ca^{2+} entry from the plasma Ca^{2+} reperfusing the tissue.[67] This causes massive myocyte contraction; the myofibrils shorten markedly. This change can be seen by either light or electron microscopy. Some of the excess Ca^{2+} is accumulated by the mitochondria, where it is precipitated as calcium phosphate (Fig. 3.12, inset)[68] and, in the process, inhibits oxidative phosphorylation.

Subsarcolemmal blebs result from the massive cell swelling. The disrupted trilaminar unit membrane reforms into little vesicles, leaving large stretches of denuded glycocalyx similar in structure to those seen in low-flow ischemia (Fig. 3.9).

Contraction-band formation begins at about the time of the massive calcium influx; it is detectable after only 2 minutes of reflow.[42] Moreover, this myofibrillar disruption is readily detectable by light and electron microscopy and is termed contraction-band necrosis.[69] Contraction-band necrosis should be contrasted to coagulation necrosis, which becomes detectable after much more extended episodes of ischemia. Because contraction-band necrosis is characteristic of infarcts caused by transient ischemia, this type of necrosis is seen frequently in hearts of patients with perioperative infarcts associated with cardiac surgery and in infarcts treated early with thrombolytic therapy. It is often found in the myocytes dying on the edge of infarcts caused by permanent occlusion of a coronary artery. Presumably, there is sufficient diffusible extracellular Ca^{2+} available at the periphery and enough intracellular ATP in cells dying in this zone to support mitochondrial accumulation of calcium phosphate (Fig. 3.14). This peripheral calcification is detectable by nuclear medicine techniques involving administration of technetium pyrophosphates.[70]

Sarcolemmal disruption also permits rapid washout of intracellular electrolytes, metabolites, cofactors, and enzymes. The rapid washout of creatine kinase provides an indirect indication that reperfusion has been achieved.

Hemorrhage and the No-Reflow Phenomenon

Microvascular damage and necrosis are components of most myocardial infarcts (Fig. 3.9*D*).[45] Restoration of systemic arterial pressure to an artery supplying an intact and patent microvasculature will restore blood flow. On the other hand, restoration of arterial pressure to an artery supplying a damaged capillary bed may have one of two additional effects: if the damaged microvasculature is patent, hemorrhage may occur into the infarct. Conversely, *no-reflow* may be possible if capillaries have been occluded by extravascular compression, cardiac rigor, endothelial swelling, or intravascular elements such as platelet aggregates.[46]

Hemorrhage is common in experimental infarcts associated with 60 minutes or more of ischemia (Fig. 3.17). These areas of hemorrhage are located in the center of the area of severe ischemia and are especially common in the subendocardial and midmyocardial zone. Evaluation of the significance of this hemorrhagic response has been complex. This most important clinical question is: Does hemorrhage increase infarct size? Because microvascular injury has been documented in the center of evolving infarcts but not at the advancing subepicardial edge of myocyte death,[71] it seems likely that the hemorrhage is related directly to vascular damage. The location of the hemorrhage, together with the

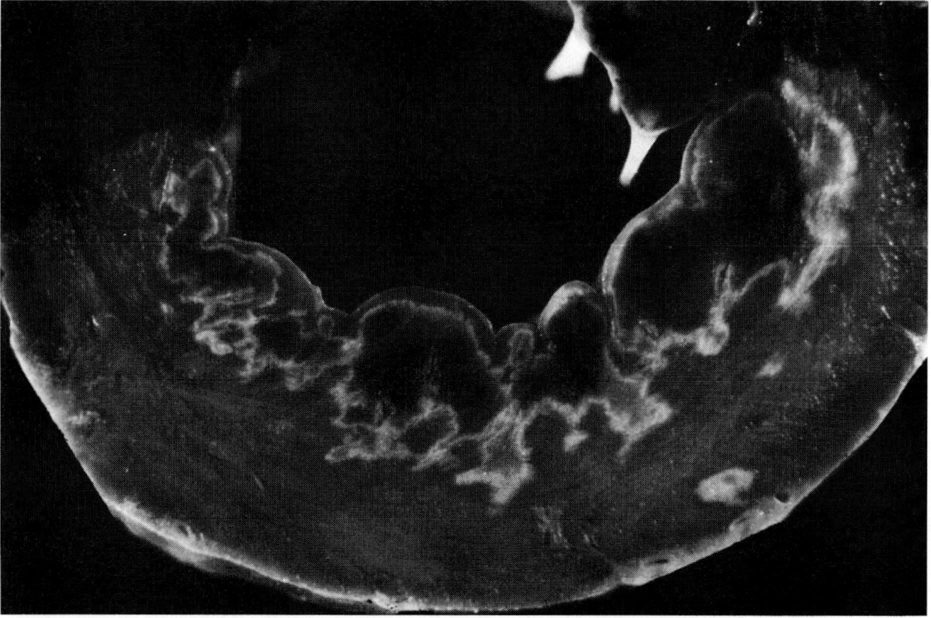

FIG. 3.17. Subendocardial myocardial infarct in a dog heart, delineated by dehydrogenase staining using triphenyl tetrazolium chloride (TTC). The illustration includes part of a cross-sectional slice of a dog left ventricle, viewed from the apex. Before sectioning, the ischemic and nonischemic vascular regions were identified by postmortem coronary perfusion with blue dye (nonischemic) and TTC (ischemic region). In viable subepicardial areas, TTC was reduced by tissue dehydrogenases from its colorless oxidized state to a brick-red color. The lighter subendocardial areas demarcate the infarct, caused by 40 minutes of circumflex coronary occlusion followed by 4 days of reperfusion. The dark areas within the confines of the infarct are due to hemorrhage. Note that whereas the subepicardial half of the ischemic regions was spared by reperfusion, lateral boundaries of viable myocardium within the previously ischemic vascular bed were narrow. Reproduced with permission of the authors and publishers of Ref. 82.

fact that myocardial perfusion occurs via arterioles that penetrate from the epicardial surface, make it highly unlikely that microvascular damage or hemorrhage, per se, accentuate ischemia in subepicardial areas where myocytes have not already been injured irreversibly. Thus, hemorrhage probably does not increase true infarct size. On the other hand, to the extent that hemorrhage and/or edema and the inflammatory response occur, infarct volume will be composed not only of edematous dead myocardium, but also of the added vascular elements. Thus, true infarct size (the dead myocardium) will be overestimated in anatomic studies involving measurement of this endpoint.[72] Also unknown is the effect of hemorrhage on the quality of scarring. It is possible that it alters scarring in such a way that the strength or volume of the ultimate infarct scar is affected.

Hemorrhage in Reperfused Human Infarcts

Hemorrhage is noted frequently in human hearts of patients dying after thrombolysis (Fig. 3.18). However, the degree of hemorrhage noted in patients surviving successful reperfusion is unknown. It seems likely that it is present in some of the successfully reperfused necrotic tissue, especially that tissue that has significant ischemic vascular injury. It seems likely that hemorrhage is not usually deleterious because morbidity and mortality both are reduced with thrombolytic treatment.

REPERFUSION INJURY

There has been much debate over whether reversibly injured myocytes, alive at the time of reperfusion, die as a consequence of some aspect of the reperfusion process. This phenomenon has been termed *lethal reperfusion injury*. Studies of stunning have shown that oxygen-derived free radicals are released by living reversibly injured myocytes during reperfusion with much of the release occurring during the first few minutes of reperfusion. These free radicals clearly are involved in stunning.[55,57,58] Thus, stunning represents a form of *sublethal reperfusion injury*. The question is: do oxygen-derived free radicals arising during reperfusion kill myocytes as well? This question has been addressed by infusing free radical scavengers before reperfusion and assessing the effect of such therapy on infarct size. Some groups have seen beneficial effects and others have not.[73] Our results have been negative.[73–76] Nevertheless, it is possible that lethal reperfusion injury does occur as a consequence of the development of new areas of ischemia secondary to vascular occlusion mediated by leukocytes emigrating into the area of ischemic injury. Endothelial damage by means of leukocyte-derived free radicals, thrombosis, or plugging of capillaries by leukocytes all could contribute.[35] This hypothesis has been difficult to test. We have reduced the number of leukocytes entering the area of injury by administering an antibody against a surface glycoprotein (CD18) involved in binding of leukocytes to endothelium. However, anti-CD18 treatment had no detectable beneficial effect on infarct size even though the number of leukocytes accumulating in the area of injury was cut substantially.[77]

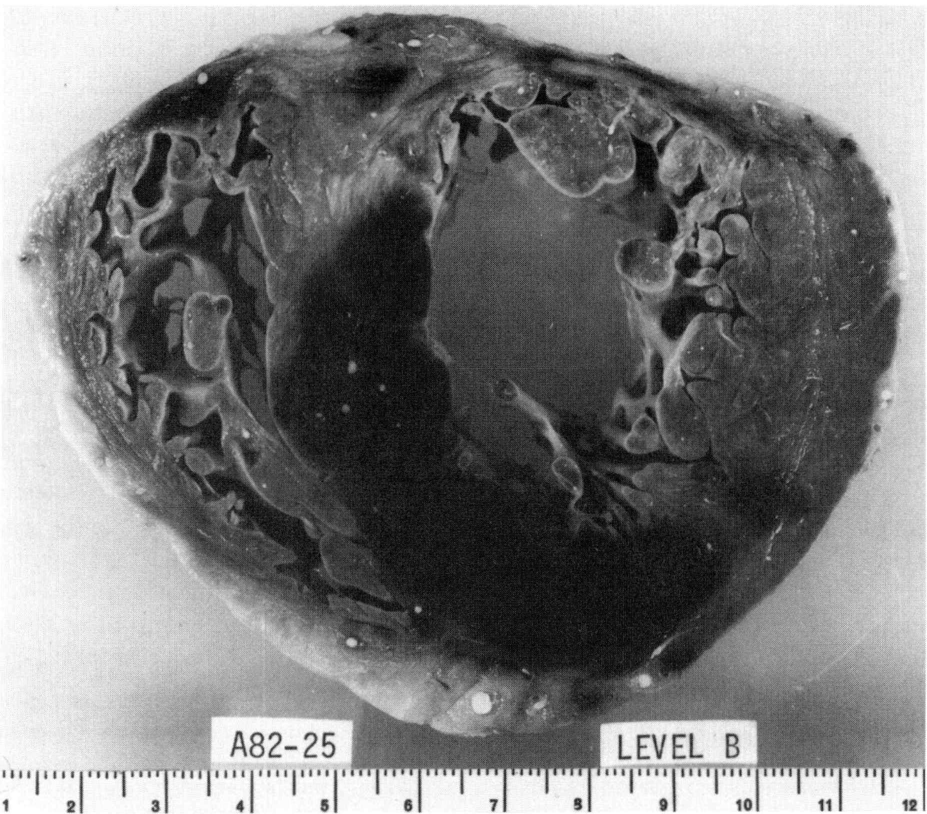

FIG. 3.18.   Hemorrhagic myocardial infarct. The illustration is of a cross-section through the ventricles of a heart from a patient who died after myocardial infarction and intracoronary administration of streptokinase. The section is viewed from the basal side (anterior wall at *bottom* of photo). There is extensive hemorrhage within a nearly transmural anteroseptal infarct (*dark area*). A scar from a prior posteroseptal (inferior) myocardial infarct also is present. Reproduced with permission of the authors and publishers of Ref. 83.

SUMMARY

Myocardial infarction is a dynamic process that begins with the transition from reversible to irreversible ischemic injury and culminates in the replacement of dead myocardium by a fibrous scar. Many biochemical and metabolic changes have been observed early after the onset of ischemia, but the precise cause of the transition to irreversibility has not been elucidated. However, disruption of the plasmalemma of the sarcolemma is an early event, the presence of which indicates that the ischemic myocytes are dead.

Not all ischemic myocytes become irreversibly injured simultaneously in experimental infarction in the canine heart; rather, myocytes die in a transmural wavefront of cell death proceeding from the subendocardial to the subepicardial myocardium with the subendocardial layer dying first and the subepicardial layer last. About 6 hours of ischemia are required to complete the wavefront. During the reversible phase of ischemic injury, reperfusion salvages all ischemic myocytes in all layers, but once lethal injury begins to develop, reperfusion salvages reversibly injured myocytes that are located chiefly in the subepicardial and midmyocardial layers and thereby limits the transmural extent of infarction. The gradual evolution of cell death in experimental acute ischemia provides a basis for limitation of infarct size by reperfusion with arterial blood in man.

Many functions of myocardium subjected to reversible episodes of ischemia return to the control condition a few seconds or minutes after the onset of reperfusion. Others, such as repletion of the adenine nucleotide pool, require hours to days to repair. Reversibly injured myocardium exhibits reduced contractile efficiency, termed stunning, which is a form of reperfusion injury. Stunning is reversible; it disappears after hours or days of reperfusion. Finally, reversibly injured myocardium develops adaptive changes that protect it against subsequent episodes of ischemia. One such change, termed ischemic preconditioning, persists for 1–2 hours and serves to delay the development of cell death if the tissue is subjected to a new prolonged episode of ischemia. Another, heat shock protein synthesis, does not appear until the tissue has been reperfused for 12–24 hours; it also protects the myocardium against subsequent ischemic injury. The molecular mechanisms underlying stunning, ischemic preconditioning, and heat shock protein synthesis remain to be established.

ACKNOWLEDGMENT

This work was supported by Grants HL23138, HL27416 and HL17670 from the National Heart, Lung, and Blood Institute of the National Institutes of Health.

REFERENCES

1. Jennings RB, Murry CE, Steenbergen C,Jr, Reimer KA. Development of cell injury in sustained acute ischemia. *Circulation* 1990;82(Suppl):II-2–II-12.
2. Jennings RB, Sommers H, Smyth GA, Flack HA, Linn H. Myocardial necrosis induced by temporary occlusion of a coronary artery in the dog. *Arch Pathol Lab Med* 1960;70:68–78.
3. DeWood MA, Spores J, Notske R, et al. Prevalence of total coronary occlusion during the early hours of transmural myocardial infarction. *N Engl J Med* 1980;303:897–902.
4. Davies MJ. A macro and micro view of coronary vascular insult in ischemic heart disease. *Circulation* 1990;82(suppl II):II-38–II-46.
5. Fuster V, Stein B, Ambrose JA, Badimon L, Badimon JJ, Chesbro JH. Atherosclerotic plaque rupture and thrombosis. Evolving concepts. *Circulation* 1990;82(Suppl II):II-47–II-59.
6. Yusuf S, Collins R, Peto R, et al. Intravenous and intracoronary fibrinolytic therapy in acute myocardial infarction: overview of results on mortality, reinfarction and side effects from 33 randomized controlled trials. *Eur Heart J* 1985;6:556–583.
7. Maseri A, L'Abbate A, Baroldi G, et al. Coronary vasospasm as a possible cause of myocardial infarction: a conclusion derived from the study of "preinfarction" angina. *N Engl J Med* 1978;229:1271–1277.
8. Bloor CM. Functional significance of the coronary collateral circulation. *Am J Pathol* 1974;76:562–587.
9. Elliot EC, Bloor CM, Jones EL, Mitchell WJ, Gregg DE. Effect of controlled coronary occlusion on collateral circulation in conscious dogs. *Am J Physiol* 1971;220:857–861.

10. Schaper W, Wusten B. Collateral Circulation. In: Schaper W, ed. *Pathophysiology of myocardial perfusion.* Amsterdam: Elsevier/North Holland Biomedical Press, 1979:415–470.

11. Jennings RB, Reimer KA. Biology of experimental, acute myocardial ischemia and infarction. In: Hearse DJ, de Leiris J, eds. *Enzymes in cardiology: diagnosis and research.* New York: John Wiley & Sons, 1979:21–57.

12. Jennings RB, Reimer KA. Factors involved in salvaging ischemic myocardium: effect of reperfusion of arterial blood. *Circulation* 1983;68(Suppl):I-25–I-36.

13. Gordon EE, Morgan HE. Principles of metabolic regulation. In: Fozzard HA, Haber JE, Jennings RB, Katz AM, Morgan HE, eds. *The heart and cardiovascular system.* New York: Raven Press, 1986:51–60.

14. Jennings RB, Hawkins HK, Lowe JE, Hill ML, Klotman S, Reimer KA. Relation between high energy phosphate and lethal injury in myocardial ischemia in the dog. *Am J Pathol* 1978;92:187–214.

15. Allison TB, Ramey CA, Holsinger JW, Jr. Transmural gradients of left ventricular tissue metabolites after circumflex artery ligation in dogs. *J Mol Cell Cardiol* 1977;9:837–852.

16. McDonough KH, Dunn RB, Griggs DM, Jr. Transmural changes in porcine and canine hearts after circumflex artery occlusion. *Am J Physiol* 1984;246:H601–H607.

17. Jennings RB, Reimer KA, Steenbergen C, Jr, Murry CE. Energy metabolism in myocardial ischemia. In: Dhalla NS, Innes IR, Beamish RE, eds. *Myocardial ischemia.* Boston: Martinus Nijhoff, 1987:185–198.

18. Jennings RB, Reimer KA, Hill ML, Mayer SE. Total ischemia, in dog hearts, *in vitro.* I. Comparison of high energy phosphate production, utilization and depletion and of adenine nucleotide catabolism in total ischemia *in vitro* vs severe ischemia *in vivo. Circ Res* 1981;49: 892–900.

19. Neely JR, Morgan HE. Relationship between carbohydrate and lipid metabolism and the energy balance of heart muscle. *Annu Rev Physiol* 1974;36:413–459.

20. Rovetto MJ, Lamberton WF, Neely JR. Mechanisms of glycolytic inhibition in ischemic rat hearts. *Circ Res* 1975;37:742–751.

21. Neely JR, Rovetto MJ, Whitmer JT. Rate-limiting steps of carbohydrate and fatty acid metabolism in ischemic hearts. *Acta Med Scand* 1976;587(Suppl):9–13.

22. Jennings RB, Reimer KA. Lethal myocardial ischemic injury. *Am J Pathol* 1981;102:241–255.

23. Reimer KA, Jennings RB. Myocardial ischemia, hypoxia, and infarction. In: Fozzard HA, Haber JE, Jennings RB, Katz AM, Morgan HE, eds. *The heart and cardiovascular system,* 2nd ed. New York: Raven Press, 1991:1875–1974.

24. Jennings RB, Reimer KA, Steenbergen C, Jr. Effect of inhibition of the mitochondrial ATPase on net myocardial ATP in total ischemia. *J Mol Cell Cardiol* 1991;23:1383–1395.

25. Rouslin W, Ericsson JLE, Solaro RJ. Effects of oligomycin and acidosis on rates of ATP depletion in ischemic heart muscle. *Am J Physiol* 1986;250:H503–H508.

26. Reimer KA, Jennings RB. The "Wavefront Phenomenon" of myocardial ischemic cell. II. Transmural progression of necrosis within the framework of ischemic bed size (myocardium at risk) and collateral flow. *Lab Invest* 1979;40:633–644.

27. Jennings RB, Schaper J, Hill ML, Steenbergen C, Jr, Reimer KA. Effect of reperfusion late in the phase of reversible ischemic injury. Changes in cell volume, electrolytes, metabolites, and ultrastructure. *Circ Res* 1985;56:262–278.

28. Jennings RB, Reimer KA. The cell biology of acute myocardial ischemia. *Annu Rev Med* 1991;42:225–246.

29. Jennings RB, Hawkins HK. Ultrastructural changes of acute myocardial ischemia. In: Wildenthal K, ed. *Degradative processes in heart and skeletal muscle.* Amsterdam/New York: Elsevier, 1980;295–344.

30. Jennings RB, Baum JH, Herdson PB. Fine structural changes in myocardial ischemic injury. *Arch Pathol Lab Med* 1965;79:135–143.

31. Jennings RB, Ganote CE. Structural changes in myocardium during acute ischemia. *Circ Res* 1974;35(Suppl):III-156–III-172.

32. Buja LM, Dees JH, Harling DF, Willerson JT. Analytical lectron microscopic study of mitochondrial inclusions in canine myocardial infarcts. *J Histochem Cytochem* 1976;24: 508–516.

33. Jennings RB, Shen AC, Hill ML, Ganote CE, Herdson PB. Mitochondrial matrix densities in myocardial ischemia and autolysis. *Exp Mol Pathol* 1978;29:55–65.
34. Steenbergen C, Jr, Jennings RB. Dissociation of tissue phospholipid alterations from plasma membrane injury during total in vitro ischemia in dog heart. *J Mol Cell Cardiol* 1983;15(Suppl 1):188.
35. Jennings RB, Reimer KA, Steenbergen C, Jr, Myocardial ischemia revisited. The osmolar load, membrane damage, and reperfusion. (Editorial). *J Mol Cell Cardiol* 1986;18:769–780.
36. Jennings RB, Ganote CE. Mitochondrial structure and function in acute myocardial ischemic injury. *Circ Res* 1976;38(Suppl):I-80–I-91.
37. Jennings RB, Reimer KA, Steenbergen C, Jr, Schaper J. Total ischemia. III. Effect of inhibition of anaerobic glycolysis. *J Mol Cell Cardiol* 1989;21(Suppl):I-37–I-54.
38. Steenbergen C, Jr, Hill ML, Jennings RB. Volume regulation and plasma membrane injury in aerobic, anaerobic, and ischemic myocardium *in vitro*. Effect of osmotic cell swelling on plasma membrane integrity. *Circ Res* 1985;57:864–875.
39. Steenbergen C, Jr, Hill ML, Jennings RB. Cytoskeletal damage during myocardial ischemia: changes in vinculin immunofluorescence staining during total in vitro ischemia in canine heart. *Circ Res* 1987;60:478–486.
40. Schliewa M. The cytoskeleton. An introductory survey. *Cell Biol Monogr* 1986;13:1–26.
41. Pardo JV, Siliciano JD, Craig SW. Vinculin is a component of an extensive network of myofibril-sarcolemma attachment regions in cardiac muscle fibers. *J Cell Biol* 1983;97:1081–1088.
42. Kloner RA, Ganote CE, Whalen D, Jennings RB. Effect of a transient period of ischemia on myocardial cells. II. Fine structure during the first few minutes of reflow. *Am J Pathol* 1974;74:399–414.
43. Whalen DA, Jr, Hamilton DG, Ganote CE, Jennings RB. Effect of a transient period of ischemia on myocardial cells. I. Effects on cell volume regulation. *Am J Pathol* 1974;74:381–398.
44. Steenbergen C, Jr, Jennings RB. Cytoskeletal damage and lethal myocardial ischemic injury. *J Mol Cell Cardiol* 1992;24(Suppl I):S.28.
45. Kloner RA, Ganote CE, Jennings RB. The "no-reflow" phenomenon after temporary coronary occlusion in the dog. *J Clin Invest* 1974;54:1496–1508.
46. Jennings RB, Kloner RA, Ganote CE, Hawkins HK, Reimer KA. Changes in capillary fine structure and function in acute myocardial ischemic injury. In: Tillmann H, Kubler W, Zebe H, eds. *Microcirculation of the heart. Theoretical and clinical problems.* Heidelberg: Springer-Verlag, 1982:87–97.
47. Kloner RA, Przylklenk K. Consequences of ischemia reperfusion on the coronary microvasculature. In: Yellon D, Jennings RB, eds. *Myocardial protection: the pathophysiology of reperfusion and reperfusion injury.* New York: Raven Press, 1992:85–103.
48. Sommers HM, Jennings RB. Experimental acute myocardial infarction. Histologic and histochemical studies of early myocardial infarcts induced by temporary or permanent occlusion of a coronary artery. *Lab Invest* 1964;13:1491–1503.
49. Lowe JE, Cummings RG, Adams DH, Hull-Ryde EA. Evidence that ischemic cell death begins in the subendocardium independent of variations in collateral flow or wall tension. *Circulation* 1983;68:190–202.
50. Fujiwara H, Ashraf M, Sato S, Millard RW. Transmural cellular damage and blood flow distribution in early ischemia in pig hearts. *Circ Res* 1982;51:683–693.
51. Factor SM, Kirk ES. Microcirculatory determinants of infarct dimensions. In: Tillmanns H, Kubler W, Zebe H, eds. *Microcirculation of the heart. Theoretical and clinical problems.* Heidelberg: Springer-Verlag, 1982:141–148.
52. Lee JT, Ideker RE, Reimer KA. Myocardial infarct size and location in relation to the coronary vascular bed at risk in man. *Circulation* 1981;64:526–534.
53. Lowe JE, Reimer KA, Jennings RB. Experimental infarct size as a function of the amount of myocardium at risk. *Am J Pathol* 1978;90:363–379.
54. Heyndrickx GR, Millard RW, McRitchie RJ, Maroko PR, Vatner SF. Regional myocardial functional and electrophysiological alterations after brief coronary artery occlusion in conscious dogs. *J Clin Invest* 1975;56:978–985.
55. Bolli R. Mechanism of myocardial "stunning." *Circulation* 1990;82:723–738.

56. Reimer KA, Hill ML, Jennings RB. Prolonged depletion of ATP and of the adenine nucleotide pool due to delayed resynthesis of adenine nucleotides following reversible myocardial ischemic injury in dogs. *J Mol Cell Cardiol* 1981;13:229–239.

57. Murry CE, Richard VJ, Jennings RB, Reimer KA. Myocardial protection is lost before contractile function recovers from ischemic preconditioning. *Am J Physiol (Heart Circ Physiol)* 1991;260:H796–H804.

58. Bolli R. Postischemic myocardial "stunning." Pathogenesis, pathophysiology, and clinical relevance. In: Yellon D, Jennings RB, eds. *Myocardial protection: the pathophysiology of reperfusion and reperfusion injury.* New York: Raven Press, 1992:105–149.

59. Murry CE, Jennings RB, Reimer KA. Preconditioning with ischemia: a delay of lethal cell injury in ischemic myocardium. *Circulation* 1986;74:1124–1136.

60. Murry CE, Richard VJ, Reimer KA, Jennings RB. Ischemic preconditioning slows energy metabolism and delays ultrastructural damage during sustained ischemia. *Circ Res* 1990;66:913–931.

61. Downey JM, Thornton JD, Van Winkle DM, Stanley AWH, Olsson RA. Protection against infarction afforded by preconditioning is mediated by A_1 adenosine receptors in rabbit heart. *Circulation* 1990;84:350–356.

62. Hendrikx M, Toshima Y, Mubagwa K, Flameng W. Improved functional recovery after ischemic preconditioning in the globally ischemic rabbit heart is not mediated by adenosine A_1 receptor activation. *Circulation* 1992;84:I-433 (Abstr).

63. Asimakis GK, Inners-McBride K, Medellin G, Conti VR. Ischemic preconditioing attenuates acidosis and postischemic dysfunction in isolated rat heart. *Am J Physiol* 1992;263:H887–H894.

64. Steenbergen C, Jr, Perlman ME, London RE, Murphy E. Mechanism of preconditioning. Ionic alterations. *Circ Res* 1993;72:112–125.

65. Shiki K, Hearse DJ. Preconditioning of ischemic myocardium: reperfusion-induced arrhythmias. *Am J Physiol* 1987;253:H1470–H1476.

66. Yellon DM, Latchman DS. Stress proteins and myocardial protection during ischemia and reperfusion. In: Yellon DM, Jennings RB, eds. *Myocardial protection: the pathophysiology of reperfusion and reperfusion injury.* New York: Raven Press, 1992:185–195.

67. Shen AC, Jennings RB. Kinetics of calcium accumulation in acute myocardial ischemic injury. *Am J Pathol* 1972;67:441–452.

68. Shen AC, Jennings RB. Myocardial calcium and magnesium in acute ischemic injury. *Am J Pathol* 1972;67:417–440.

69. Ganote CE. Contraction band necrosis and irreversible myocardial injury. (Editorial). *J Mol Cell Cardiol* 1983;15:67–73.

70. Reimer KA, Martonffy K, Schumacher BL, Henkin RE, Quinn JL, Jennings RB. Localization of 99mTc-labeled pyrophosphate and calcium in myocardial infarcts after temporary coronary occlusion in dogs. *Proc Soc Exp Biol Med* 1977;156:272–276.

71. Reimer KA, Lowe JE, Rasmussen M, Jennings RB. The wavefront phenomenon of ischemic cell death. I. Myocardial infarct size vs duration of coronary occlusion in dogs. *Circulation* 1977;56:786–794.

72. Reimer KA, Jennings RB. The changing anatomic reference base of evolving myocardial infarction. Underestimation of myocardial collateral blood flow and overestimation of experimental anatomic infarct size due to tissue edema, hemorrhage, and acute inflammation. *Circulation* 1979;60:866–876.

73. Reimer KA, Murry CE, Richard VJ. The role of neutrophils and free radicals in the ischemic-reperfused heart. Why the confusion and controversy? *J Mol Cell Cardiol* 1989;21:1225–1239.

74. Richard VJ, Murry CE, Jennings RB, Reimer KA. Therapy to reduce free radicals during early reperfusion does not limit the size of myocardial infarcts caused by 90 minutes of ischemia in dogs. *Circulation* 1988;78:473–480.

75. Richard VJ, Murry CE, Jennings RB, Reimer KA. Oxygen-derived free radicals and postischemic myocardial reperfusion: pharmacological implications. *Fundam Clin Pharmacol* 1990;4:85–103.

76. Tanaka M, Richard VJ, Murry CE, Jennings RB, Reimer KA. Superoxide dismutase plus catalase therapy delays neither cell death nor the loss of TTC reaction in experimental myocardial infarction in dogs. *J Mol Cell Cardiol* 1993;25:367–378.

77. Tanaka M, Brooks SE, Richard VJ, et al. Effect of anti-CD18 antibody on myocardial neutrophil accumulation and infarct size after ischemia and reperfusion in dogs. *Circulation* 1992;87:526–535.

78. Jennings RB, Murry CE, Steenbergen C, Jr, Reimer KA. The acute phase of regional ischemia. In: Cox RH, ed. *Acute myocardial infarction: emerging concepts of pathogenesis and treatment.* New York: Praeger Scientific, 1989:67–84.

79. Jennings RB, Reimer KA, Jones RN, Peyton RB. High energy phosphates, anaerobic glycolysis and irreversibility in ischemia. In: Spitzer JJ, ed. *Myocardial ischemia.* New York: Plenum, 1983;403–419.

80. Jennings RB, Reimer KA, Steenbergen C, Jr. Myocardial ischemia and reperfusion. Role of calcium. In: Parratt JR, ed. *Control and manipulation of calcium movement.* New York: Raven Press, 1985;273–302.

81. Reimer KA, Vander Heide RS, Richard VJ. Reperfusion in acute myocardial infarction: effect of timing and modulating factors in experimental models. *Am J Cardiol* 1993;72:13G–21G.

82. Reimer KA, Jennings RB. Effects of reperfusion on infarct size: experimental studies. *Eur Heart J* 1985;6(Suppl E):97–108.

83. Kao R, Hackel DB, Kong Y. Hemorrhagic myocardial infarction after streptokinase treatment for acute coronary thrombosis. *Arch Pathol Lab Med* 1984;108:121–124.

Chapter 4

Surgical Pathology of the Heart: Endomyocardial Biopsy, Valvular Heart Disease, and Cardiac Tumors

HENRY D. TAZELAAR

The variety of specimens removed from the heart by interventional cardiologists and at operative procedures continues to expand. Some of these specimen types are covered in other portions of this volume, such as atherectomy material and biopsies from patients undergoing cardiac transplantation or suspected of having vasculitis. This update on surgical pathology of the heart will focus on three areas: (1) experience with the Dallas criteria for myocarditis by pathologists for the myocarditis treatment trial funded by the National Institutes of Health, (2) current trends in the surgical pathology of native aortic and mitral valves, and (3) selected aspects of cardiac tumor pathology.

MYOCARDITIS

The criteria for and significance of myocarditis diagnosed by endomyocardial biopsy have been controversial. To address this problem and in anticipation of a proposed multicenter immunosuppressive therapy trial in patients with biopsy-proven myocarditis, a group of eight cardiac pathologists formulated what have come to be known as the "Dallas criteria" for idiopathic lymphocytic myocarditis.[1] Such a study was eventually funded by the National Institutes of Health with Dr. Jay Mason as the principal investigator and is known as the "Multicenter Myocarditis Treatment Trial." Patients older than 18 years were enrolled in the study if they had undergone an endomyocardial biopsy showing lymphocytic myocarditis within 2 years of the onset of unexplained left ventricular dysfunction (defined by a left ventricular ejection fraction of less than 45% in the absence of significant coronary artery disease, renal dysfunction, or hypertension). During the early months of the study, patients were enrolled on the basis of the local pathologist's diagnosis and, later, on the basis of confirmation by one of the participating pathologists. After enrollment, patients were randomized to no immunosuppression *versus* treatment with cyclosporine and prednisone. Clinical follow-up and additional biopsies were performed at 6 months and 1 year after randomization. The enrollment period for the study was from October 1986 to October 1990, and follow-up ended in October 1991.

Although not all of the clinicopathologic correlation has been completed, initial results recently have been reported in abstract form.[2]

According to the Dallas criteria, a diagnosis of myocarditis requires the presence of nonischemic myocyte damage accompanied by an adjacent, predominantly lymphocytic, inflammatory infiltrate.[1] For the trial, cases were subdivided into focal and diffuse myocarditis based on the number of pieces involved and the extent of the infiltrate in involved pieces. Biopsies showing either focal or diffuse myocarditis were considered "positive" for myocarditis. A diagnosis of focal myocarditis was rendered if there was a scant infiltrate present involving one to three pieces; myocyte damage was, by definition, present but difficult to find (Fig. 4.1). Diffuse myocarditis, in contrast, was usually a low-power diagnosis, with an abundant interstitial infiltrate in one or more pieces and readily recognizable myocyte damage (Fig. 4.2). "Borderline" myocarditis was diagnosed if there was a scant interstitial infiltrate without evidence of myocyte damage (Fig. 4.3). Cases classified as negative showed either no abnormality, nonspecific changes, or changes of cardiomyopathy, ischemia, or other specific diseases.[3] If giant cells or large numbers of eosinophils were present, the case was excluded from the study. Several publications focus on specific aspects of differential diagnosis of myocarditis, including the significance of giant cells and numerous eosinophils, and the interested reader is referred to these for additional information.[3–5] In a system analogous to that used for cardiac transplant biopsy interpretation, the Dallas criteria use a systematized nomenclature (Table 4.1) for initial and follow-up biopsies, although results on the natural history of the disease utilizing these criteria in the treatment trial are not yet available.

Among 2224 patients, 9.8% had "positive" initial biopsies according to the Dallas criteria. Of these 224 cases, 102 were reviewed by the Pathology Panel, and only 58 were confirmed as myocarditis. These results suggest that the in-

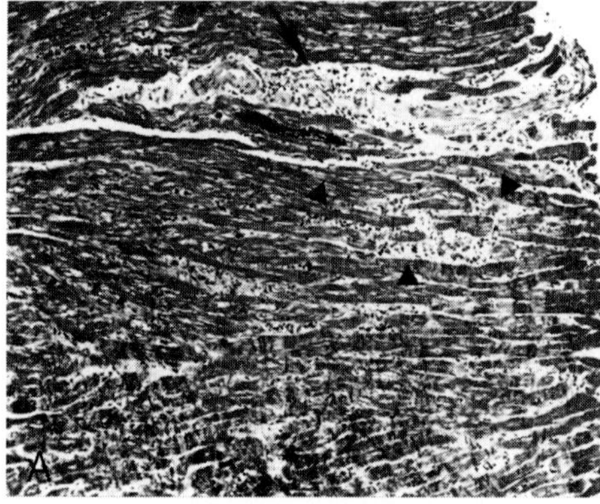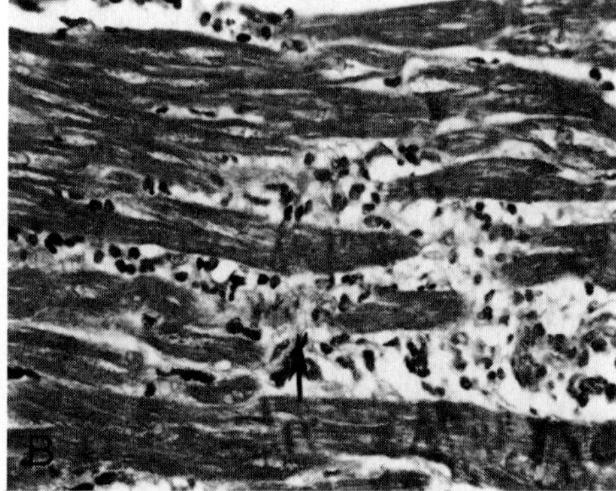

FIG. 4.1.   Focal myocarditis. *A.* The majority of the myocardium is normal. A mild lymphocytic infiltrate is present in the perivascular interstitial space (*arrow*) as well as focally within the myocardium (*arrowheads*). *B.* A small focus of myocardial damage is identified at higher power (*arrow*). This focus is sufficient for a diagnosis of focal myocarditis.

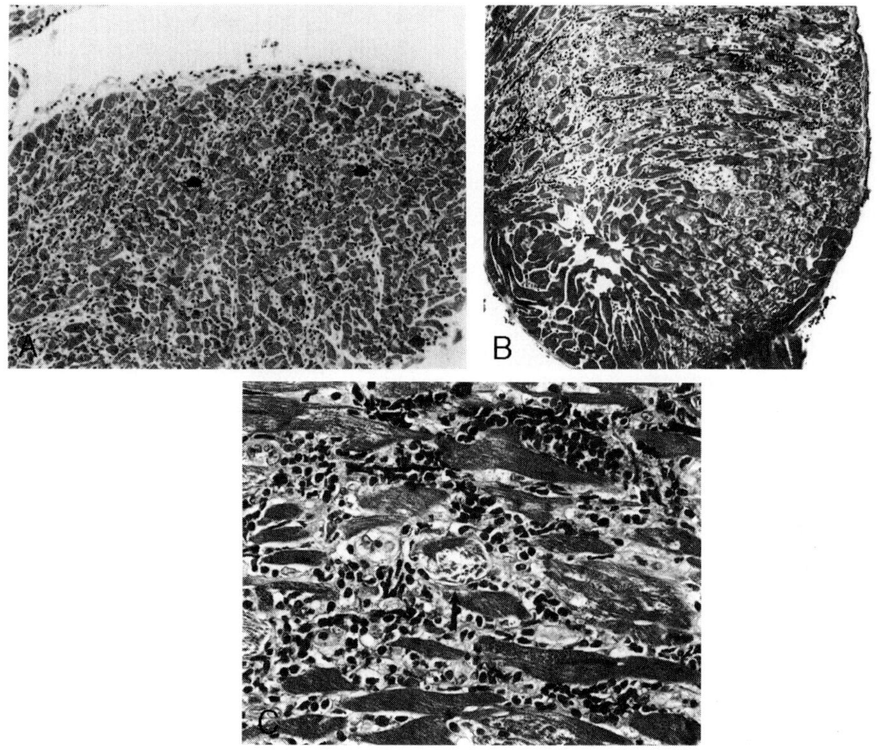

FIG. 4.2.   Diffuse myocarditis. *A.* The interstitium and endocardium contain a sparse but diffuse infiltrate of lymphocytes. Foci of myocyte damage are present (*arrows*). *B.* Another example of diffuse mild myocarditis, this one involving only a portion of the biopsy piece. *C.* Higher power shows myocyte damage with vacuolization (*arrow*).

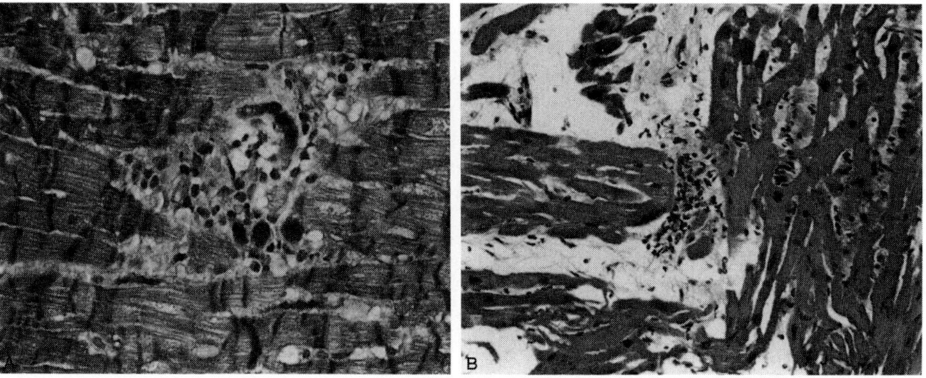

FIG. 4.3.   Borderline myocarditis. *A.* A perivascular focus of lymphocytes is present but is unassociated with myocyte damage. *B.* An interstitial collection of lymphocytes unassociated with myocyte damage.

TABLE 4.1. DALLAS CRITERIA FOR DIAGNOSIS OF MYOCARDITIS

First biopsy
Myocarditis, with or without fibrosis
Borderline myocarditis (rebiopsy may be indicated)
No myocarditis
Subsequent biopsies
Ongoing (persistent) myocarditis ± fibrosis
Resolving (healing) myocarditis ± fibrosis
Resolved (healed) myocarditis ± fibrosis

cidence of histologically confirmed active myocarditis in the appropriate clinical setting (excluding borderline myocarditis) is approximately 5–7%. Thus, although a wide range of rates for myocarditis diagnosed by endomyocardial biopsy has been reported (as high as 67%),[6–10] when strict criteria are used, myocarditis can be confirmed infrequently in patients with unexplained congestive heart failure.

Although not addressed in the currently available treatment trial data, another recent study has shown that if a diagnosis of borderline myocarditis is followed by a second biopsy, a diagnosis of definite myocarditis can be achieved in as many as 67% of cases.[11] Cutting and staining additional levels of the paraffin block can also be helpful in such circumstances.

The prime goal of the myocarditis treatment trial was to determine whether immunosuppressive therapy would benefit patients with lymphocytic myocarditis, as had been suggested anecdotally in the literature.[12] As stated earlier, the analysis is just being completed and complete verification of the data is necessary. However, the initial results indicate that patients randomized to no treatment *versus* treatment with cyclosporine and prednisone show no statistically different changes in left ventricular ejection fraction at either 28 or 52 weeks. This suggests that immunosuppressive therapy in most patients with biopsy-proven myocarditis does not appear beneficial. Results comparing follow-up of patients with focal *versus* diffuse myocarditis, however, are not yet available, and it is therefore still possible that further analysis may show a subset of patients who do benefit from immunosuppressive therapy.

In summary, the Dallas criteria do appear to be useful and reproducible in the morphologic diagnosis of myocarditis, particularly in diffuse cases. The reproducibility of a diagnosis of myocarditis falls off as the disease process becomes more focal, and in such instances, additional biopsy may be indicated. The results of the myocarditis treatment trial suggest that until there is clear evidence of a benefit of immunosuppressive therapy (perhaps in certain subsets of patients), most patients with myocarditis should not receive immunosuppressive drugs. Endomyocardial biopsy may be necessary to exclude other disease processes and therefore is still useful in the setting of unexplained heart failure.

CARDIAC VALVE DISEASE

Cardiac valve replacement is undertaken for dysfunction due to calcification, fibrosis, scar retraction, perforation, dilatation, congenital malformations, and other less common diseases. Changing disease patterns, an aging United States population, and changing operative procedures, however, have altered the frequency of the major causes of valve disease etiologies during the past quarter-century.[13–16] This update will focus on the recent changes observed and on their implications for pathologic diagnosis.[14,16]

AORTIC VALVE DISEASE

Based on gross examination, aortic valves can be etiologically classified as degenerative, postinflammatory, congenitally bicuspid, posttherapeutic, associated with aortic root dilatation, involved by active or healed endocarditis, or involved by other specific disorders.[17,18] Table 4.2 summarizes the major categories and salient diagnostic features that have been described in detail by other authors.[13,17,20–26] In the majority of cases, histology is unnecessary, only adding time and cost to the examination; gross examination alone is usually sufficient for diagnosis. Specific instances where histology is required are when infective endocarditis or an active inflammatory process is suspected clinically or by gross examination. The surgical pathology report is most complete when the anatomic diagnosis and functional status of the valve are combined. This practice is highly recommended. At the Mayo Clinic, the functional status of the valve is available at the time a diagnosis is rendered because the surgeon checks off the major clinical data and the functional status of the valve and its severity on a preprinted card submitted with the specimen.[16] Utilizing

TABLE 4.2. AORTIC VALVE DISEASE: GROSS DIAGNOSTIC FEATURES BY ETIOLOGIC CATEGORY

Degenerative ("senile")
  Arch-shaped calcification along aortic aspect (usually sparing free edge)
  Variable amounts of diffuse fibrosis
  No or minimal commissural fusion
Postinflammatory (most commonly postrheumatic)
  Commissural fusion (1–3 cusps may be involved)
  Variable amounts of fibrosis, often diffuse ("dripped candle wax" appearance common)
  Variable amounts of nodular calcification (may involve free edge)
Congenitally bicuspid
  Two cusps usually of unequal size
  Raphe frequently calcified (with stenosis)
  Mild to moderate annular dilation
Aortic root dilatation
  Thinned stretched transparent cusps
  Annular circumference usually more than 8.5 cm[a]
Infective endocarditis
  Underlying valve may be normal or have features of any of the above valves
  Cusp perforations or destruction
  Cusp aneurysms
  Adherent thrombi or vegetations
  Minimal calcification
Posttherapeutic ("iatrogenic")
  Most frequently has features of either degenerative or postinflammatory valve
  Can be difficult without history to distinguish from postinflammatory valve

[a]Age- and gender-related (see Ref. 19).

this information, the diagnosis line includes the etiology as well as the functional status of the valve. A typical diagnosis might read: "tricuspid aortic valve with severe degenerative (senile) calcification and fibrosis, clinically associated with severe aortic stenosis and mild aortic insufficiency."

An ongoing Mayo Clinic study of the temporal changes in relative frequency of the etiologic categories of aortic valve disease (at 5-year intervals spanning 26 years) recently showed that several new trends in the frequency of etiologies identified previously have continued and some new ones have emerged.[13,14] Among 236 valves surgically excised at the Mayo Clinic in 1990, the mean patient age was 66 years (range, 10–92 years). This compared to a mean of 49 years in 1965. Stenotic valves in 1990 comprised 65% of the total group; 25% were insufficient and 10% were both stenotic and insufficient (Fig. 4.4).

Degenerative (senile) aortic valve disease was the most common cause of aortic stenosis in 1990 (Table 4.3). Among 187 valves studied between 1965 and 1990, 93% were purely stenotic and 7% were both stenotic and incompetent (Fig. 4.5). None were purely regurgitant. It is not surprising that degenerative calcification has become the most common cause of aortic valve stenosis based on aging trends in the United States.

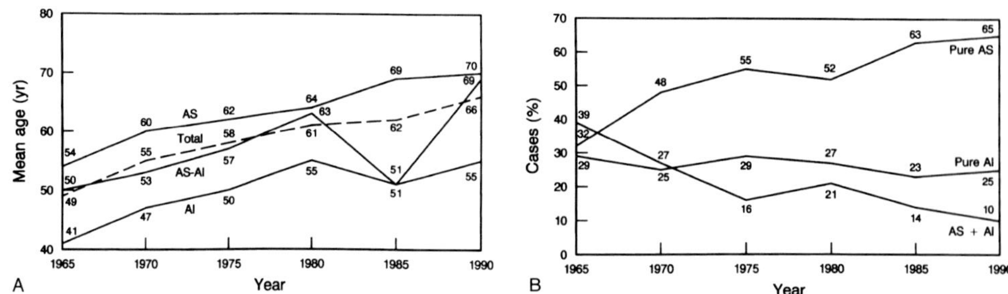

FIG. 4.4.   Temporal changes in aortic valve disease from 1965 to 1990 (1221) cases). *A.* Patient age. *B.* Functional status of the aortic valve. *AS,* aortic stenosis; *AI,* aortic insufficiency; *AS + AI,* combined aortic stenosis and aortic insufficiency. (From Ref. 14, with permission.)

TABLE 4.3.   AORTIC STENOSIS, 1990 (154 CASES)[a]

Etiology	No. of Cases (%)	Gender		Mean Age, yr (Range)
		M	F	
Degenerative	79 (51)	49	30	74 (49–92)
Postinflammatory	55 (36)	32	23	65 (20–84)
Bicuspid	14 (9)	7	7	70 (49–80)
Posttherapeutic	2 (1)	1	1	74 (69–79)
Mucopolysaccharidosis type VI	1 (1)	0	1	34
Indeterminate	3 (2)	2	1	68 (58–78)
Total	154 (100)	91	63	70 (20–92)

[a]Data from Ref. 14.

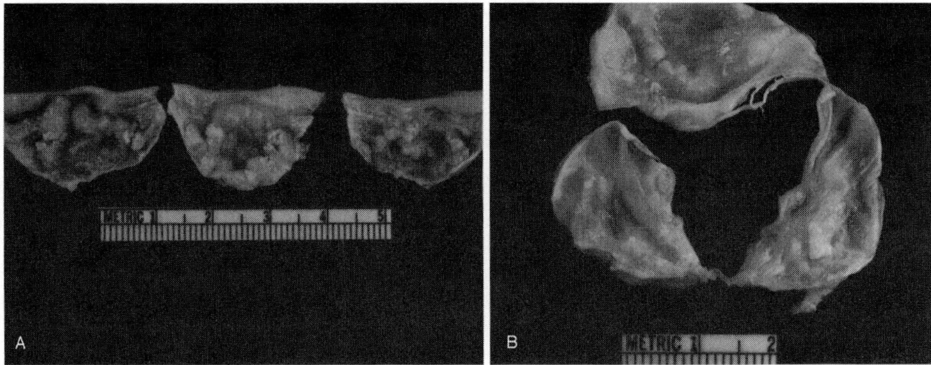

FIG. 4.5. Degenerative ("senile") aortic valve disease. *A.* Arch-shaped calcifications are present in the aortic aspect of the valve (valve "pocket") along the lines of "wear and tear" resulting in severe aortic stenosis. *B.* Similar pattern of calcification in valve with combined aortic insufficiency and stenosis.

Congenitally bicuspid aortic valves were the second most common cause of aortic valve dysfunction among all 1221 valves studied from 1965 to 1990 accounting for 32%, similar to the findings of other authors[17,26,27] and to the data from the 1990 Mayo series alone (28%). Bicuspid valves (Fig. 4.6) are most often stenotic (68%) but can become regurgitant (19%) or be both stenotic and regurgitant (13%) (Tables 4.3–4.5). They can also be associated with aortic dissection.[28] Calcification of the raphe, calcification in the valve pockets, cusp fibrosis, and secondary commissural fusion may all contribute to stenosis. Incompetent valves are generally not calcified but may develop cusp prolapse and annular dilatation. Bicuspid valves may also become regurgitant secondary to infective endocarditis. In fact, bicuspid valves were present in 42% of cases of infective endocarditis cases in the 1221 valve Mayo Clinic series.[14]

Postinflammatory disease continues to decline as a cause of aortic valve dysfunction. Whereas it accounted for 58% of cases in 1965, in 1990 it accounted for only 11%. This appears to represent a true decline of such patients in the surgical population rather than an artifact of referral bias, because the frequency of congenitally bicuspid valves in the series has remained relatively stable.

Aortic root dilatation has now become relatively more common than postinflammatory aortic valve disease (Table 4.5). Aortic root dilatation is now the leading cause of aortic insufficiency at the Mayo Clinic. Dilatation of the ascending aorta causes stretching of the commissures and a lack of cusp coaptation. Consequently, the valve cannot close completely, producing regurgitation. Patients under 40 years old tend to develop aortic root dilatation in association with Marfan syndrome (Fig. 4.7), other connective tissue disorders, or operated congenital heart disease (a newly emerging group of patients who develop aortic insufficiency). Over the age of 40, the aortic root dilation ap-

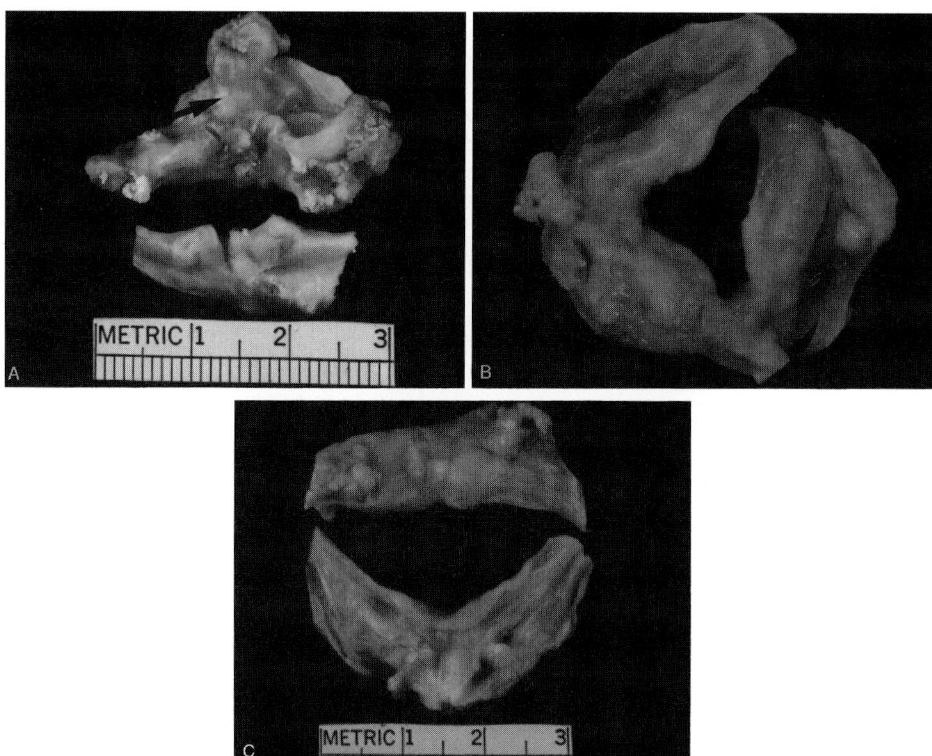

FIG. 4.6. Congenitally bicuspid aortic valves. *A.* Heavily calcified raphe (*arrow*) and diffuse valve calcification resulting in aortic stenosis. *B.* Calcification, fibrosis, and leaflet edge retraction resulting in aortic stenosis and combined aortic stenosis and insufficiency. *C.* Bicuspid aortic valve with minimal calcium deposition resulting in aortic insufficiency characteristically leading to the "rolled edge" appearance (*lower leaflet*).

TABLE 4.4. COMBINED AORTIC STENOSIS AND INSUFFICIENCY, 1990 (24 CASES)[a]

Etiology	No. of Cases (%)	Gender M	Gender F	Mean Age, yr (Range)
Degenerative	11 (46)	7	4	74 (64–84)
Postinflammatory	4 (17)	3	1	58 (42–64)
Bicuspid	4 (17)	4	0	70 (54–82)
Posttherapeutic	3 (13)	2	1	64 (39–78)
Indeterminate	2 (8)	1	1	77 (74–79)
Total	24 (100)	17	7	69 (39–84)

[a]Data from Ref. 14.

pears due to age-related medial aortic degeneration (cystic medial "necrosis"). Aortic tissue that typically shows variable amounts of medial degeneration may also be resected in some patients along with the valve.

Surgical resection of aortic valve tissue may be performed in patients with active or healed endocarditis (Fig. 4.8). Actively infected aortic valves are ex-

TABLE 4.5. AORTIC INSUFFICIENCY, 1990 (58 CASES)[a]

Etiology	No. of Cases (%)	Gender M	F	Mean Age, yr (Range)
Aortic root dilatation	29 (50)	23	6	57 (10–80)
≤40 yr	8 (14)	5	3	29 (10–39)
≥40 yr	21 (36)	18	3	68 (47–80)
Bicuspid	8 (14)	8	0	53 (32–73)
Postinflammatory	8 (14)	3	5	48 (13–69)
Posttherapeutic	8 (14)	2	6	54 (23–83)
Endocarditis	1 (1.5)	1	0	65
Uncommissural	1 (1.5)	0	1	29
Indeterminate	3 (5)	2	1	69 (57–76)
Total	58 (100)	39	19	55 (10–83)

[a]Data from Ref. 14.

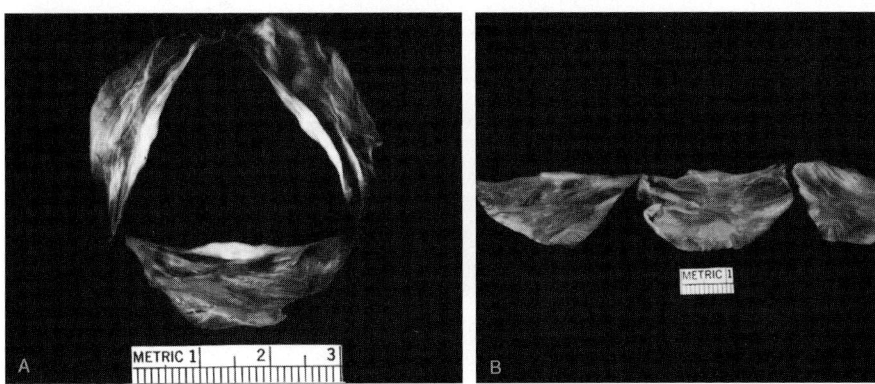

FIG. 4.7. Aortic insufficiency secondary to Marfan syndrome (*A* and *B*). Note thinned and stretched appearance of valve with rolled leaflet edges, particularly in *A,* indicating the presence of insufficiency.

cised if they are infected with *Staphylococcus aureus* or producing emboli. Most endocarditis values tend to be regurgitant (77%) or regurgitant and stenotic. The underlying valve condition before infection can be normal (42%), bicuspid (42%) (Fig. 4.8), postinflammatory (10%), or degenerative or unicommissural (3% each).[14]

Before 1990, surgical replacement of the dysfunctional aortic valve secondary to previous irradiation, operation, or drug therapy occurred in only 2 of 985 patients. In 1990, this accounted for 6% of all aortic valve replacements involving all three functional categories (Table 4.6). Gross examination of such valves may allow a determination of the underlying valve condition, but this is often impossible, especially after decalcification procedures (Fig. 4.9). An appropriate history is absolutely essential to the proper interpretation of these valves.

Other less common diseases may also necessitate aortic valve replacement (Fig. 4.9), but the study summarized here has shown that age-related degenerative calcification and degenerative dilation of the ascending aorta

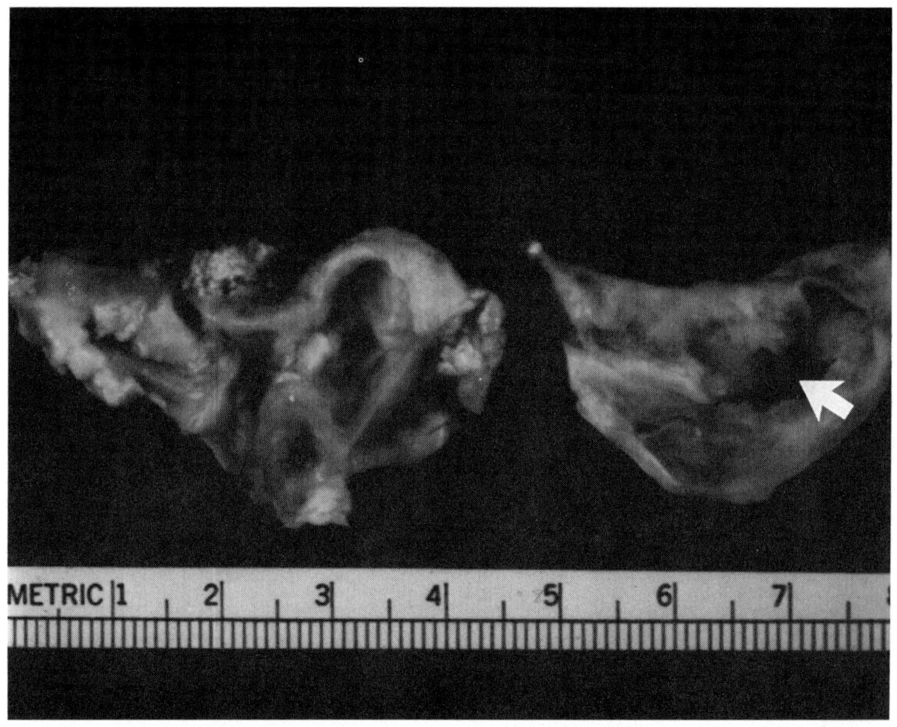

FIG. 4.8. Healed infective endocarditis associated with severe combined aortic stenosis and insufficiency. Note the markedly irregular calcium deposition and the presence of a perforation (*arrow*).

TABLE 4.6. POSTTHERAPEUTIC AORTIC VALVE DYSFUNCTION: ETIOLOGIES AND FUNCTIONAL STATUS[a]

Therapy	AS	AI	AS+AI
Surgical decalcification of stenotic value	+	++	+
Ventricular septal myectomy for hypertrophic cardiomyopathy		+	
Mediastinal irradiation		+	+
Ergot alkaloids		+	
Balloon or surgical valvotomy		+	+

[a]AS, aortic stenosis, AI, aortic insufficiency, AS + AI, combined aortic stenosis and aortic insufficiency.

have become by far the most frequent causes of aortic valve dysfunction. Although the frequency of valves replaced following decalcification procedures may go down (because of abandonment of the procedure because of a lack of long-term success),[29] the increasing number of patients surviving mediastinal irradiation, operated congenital heart disease, and other interventional procedures will likely increase. Again, communication with clinicians and surgeons is vital to correct pathologic interpretation of these specimens.

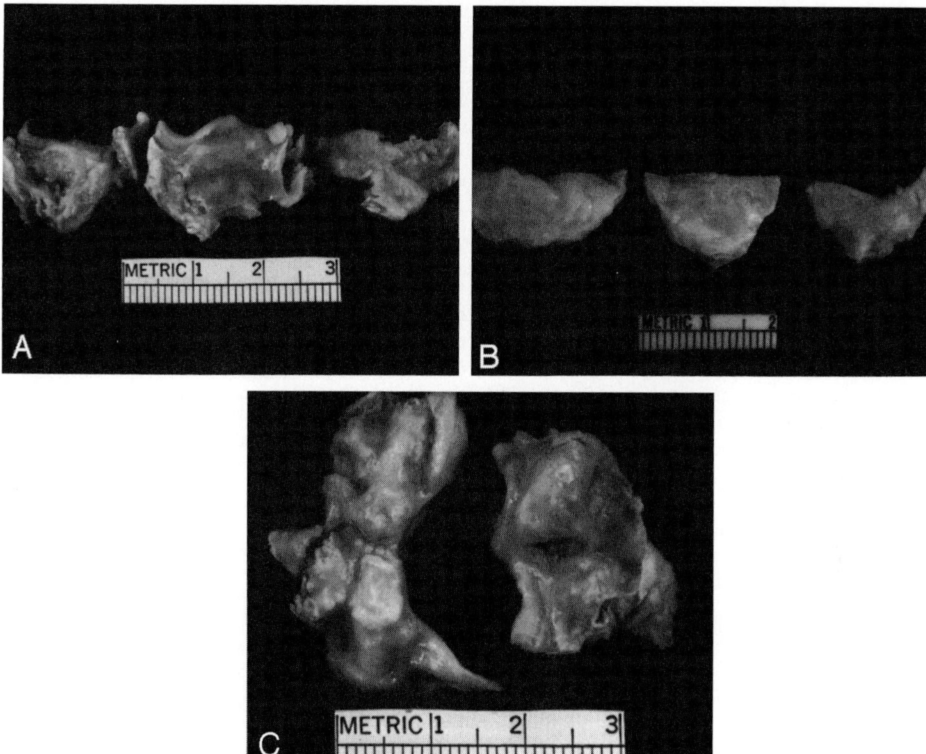

FIG. 4.9.   Aortic valve disease. *A.* Aortic stenosis after therapeutic decalcification for degenerative (senile) calcification. The underlying cause of the aortic valve disease, however, is unrecognizable. *B.* Combined aortic stenosis and insufficiency after removal of degenerative calcific deposits. *C.* Aortic insufficiency after surgical decalcification of a bicuspid valve originally associated with aortic stenosis.

Mitral Valve

As for the aortic valve, the evaluation of mitral valve pathology is also best done on the basis of gross examination.[17,18] The surgical pathologic features characteristic of the major diseases affecting the mitral valve have been well described[15,30–33] and are summarized in Table 4.7. Ongoing Mayo Clinic studies of the etiology of mitral valve disease have shown some recent changes in the frequency of diseases leading to mitral valve operation. Furthermore, because of changing operation techniques, the entire mitral valve may no longer be removed at the time of surgery, thus making determination of the underlying etiology by gross inspection alone more difficult than in the past. Both aspects of mitral valve pathology are addressed here.

A recent study examined all surgically excised mitral valves at the Mayo Clinic in 1990.[16] In comparison with the previous studies on mitral valve pathology, several trends were noted. Although there continues to be a decline

TABLE 4.7. MITRAL VALVE DISEASE: GROSS DIAGNOSTIC FEATURES BY ETIOLOGY CATEGORY

Postinflammatory (commonly rheumatic)
    Commissural and chordal fusion
    Diminished orifice area (slitlike, "fish-mouth" appearance)
    Diffuse leaflet fibrosis, with or without vascularization ("dipped candle wax"
       appearance common)
    Nodular calcifications anywhere on valve
    Fibrotic retraction of chordae and leaflets
Floppy
    Leaflet redundancy (posterior more than anterior), with hooding deformity
    Annular dilatation (mean circumference more than 10 cm)
    Fibrosis of chordal anchoring sites or leaflet margin
    Diffuse myxomatous thickening ("rubbery" texture)
    Thin, elongated, attenuated chordae most common (thick and even focally fused
       chordae occasionally seen)
    Focal annular calcium
Ischemic heart disease
    Usually normal or mildly thickened leaflets and chordae
    Occasionally papillary muscle attached (either ruptured acutely or with old infarction)
    Occasionally thickened chordae
Infective endocarditis
    Underlying valve may be normal or abnormal and:
       Leaflet perforation
       Focal leaflet destruction along free edge ("rat bite")
       Ruptured chordae
       Adherent thrombi or vegetations

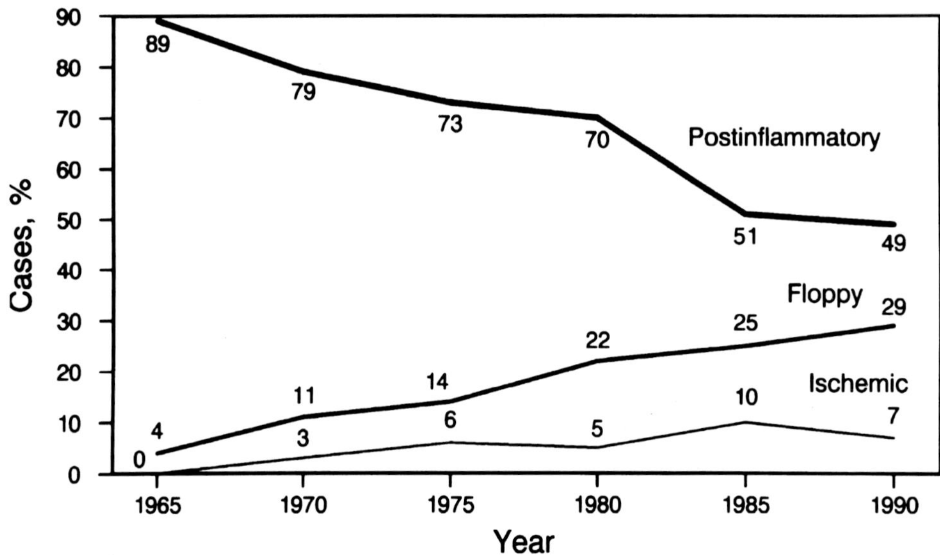

FIG. 4.10. Temporal changes in mitral valve disease from 1965 to 1990 for 807 cases. (From Ref. 16, with permission.)

in the incidence of postinflammatory mitral valve disease (Fig. 4.10), it is still the most common cause responsible for the excision of mitral valve tissue (49%). The second most common cause is floppy valve disease (29%), a trend other authors have noted as well.[30–33]

Among mitral valves with a component of stenosis, *i.e.,* valves with either pure stenosis or combined stenosis and insufficiency, there continues to be a striking preponderance of postinflammatory disease with only 2 of 40 cases in the 1990 series[16] due to other causes (ergotamine-induced disease and type VI mucopolysaccharidosis). Combining the results of several series of stenotic mitral valves,[15,16,31,33] only 0.02% were due to causes other than postinflammatory disease (Table 4.8).

Mitral valve regurgitation has a more varied etiology (Table 4.9), but several series, including the 1990 Mayo Clinic series,[16,30,31,33] have shown that floppy valve disease is the most common cause, followed by postinflammatory disease.

The most significant surprise observed in the 1990 Mayo series was in the type of mitral valve tissue submitted to surgical pathology in comparison with prior years. Between the years 1965 and 1985, 87% of the valves were removed entirely in one or two pieces.[15] In contrast, during 1990, only 32% were entirely excised (Fig. 4.11). This meant that only portions of the valve were received in the majority of cases (Table 4.10): the anterior leaflet alone, the anterior leaflet and a portion of posterior leaflet, posterior leaflet with or without chordae, or chordae alone (Fig. 4.12). The changing practice of removing only the anterior leaflet may better preserve left ventricular function and appears to be one factor leading to the virtual elimination of fatal left ventricular rupture after mitral valve replacement.[66,67] The success of mitral valve repair rather than replacement, when possible, is responsible for the increased number of isolated pieces of posterior leaflet and chordae received in pathology.

To facilitate interpretation of portions of a valve, clinical history is often required. Information on the presence of annular dilation, the functional

---

TABLE 4.8. ETIOLOGY OF EXCISED STENOTIC MITRAL VALVES WITH OR WITHOUT REGURGITATION

Postinflammatory disease (almost all cases)
Ergotamine-induced disease[34,35]
Congenital[15,16]
Massive annular calcification[36,37]
Infective endocarditis with obstructive vegetations[38]
Systemic lupus erythematosus[39]
Rheumatoid arthritis[40]
Gout[41]
Amyloidosis[42]
Whipple's disease[43]
Carcinoid syndrome[44]
Mucopolysaccharidosis[16,45–48]
Fabry's disease[49]
Pseudoxanthoma elasticum[50]

TABLE 4.9.   ETIOLOGY OF MITRAL REGURGITATION

Fifty-five total cases from 1990[a]

Floppy mitral valve	49%
Postinflammatory	16%
Ischemic heart disease	13%
Endocarditis	9%
Carcinoid heart disease	3%
Radiation-induced disease	2%
Hypertrophic cardiomyopathy	2%
Congenitally dysplastic	2%
Indeterminate	4%

Other rare causes

Idiopathic chordal rupture[15]
Dilated cardiomyopathy[51]
Restrictive cardiomyopathy[52]
Annular calcification[50,51]
Left atrial myxoma[53]
Systemic lupus erythematosus[54–56]
Rheumatoid athritis[57]
Anklyosing spondylitis[18,51]
Trauma[58]
Kawasaki disease[59]
Marfan or Ehler-Danlos syndromes, pseudoxanthoma
   elasticum, osteogenesis imperfecta[60–64]
Mucopolysaccharidosis[46,47]
Fabry's disease[65]

[a]Data from Ref. 16.

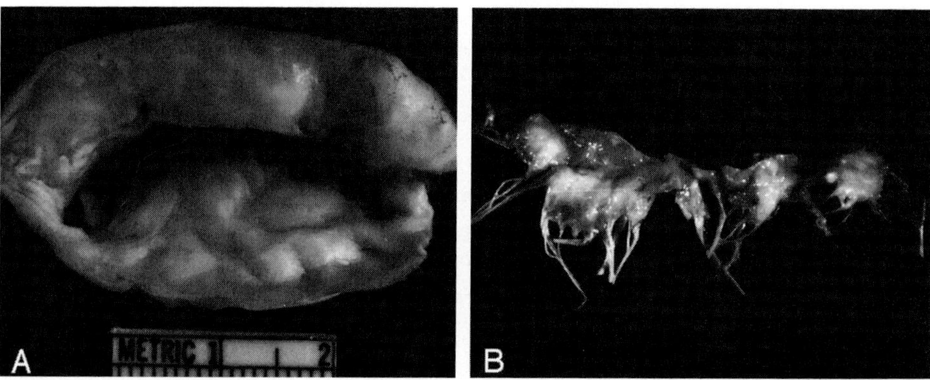

FIG. 4.11.   Completely excised valves from the two most common diseases resulting in mitral valve surgery. *A.* Diffusely fibrotic and thickened mitral valve from a patient with rheumatic fever and combined mitral stenosis and mitral regurgitation. *B.* Floppy mitral valve with elongated, thin chordae and hooding.

TABLE 4.10. MITRAL VALVE DISEASE, 1990A

	No. of Cases	Tissue Received vs. Etiology (%)				
		Postinfl	Floppy	Isch	IE	Other
Entire valve	30 (32)	(87)	(3)	(0)	(3)	(7)
AL ± PPL	42 (44)	(50)	(19)	(14)	(3)	(14)
PPL ± chordae	21 (22)	(0)	(77)	(5)	(13)	(5)
Chordae	2 (2)	(0)	(50)	(50)	(0)	(0)

[a]Data from Ref. 14. AL, anterior leaflet; PPL, portion of posterior leaflet; Postinfl, postinflammatory; Isch, ischemia related; IE, infective endocarditis.

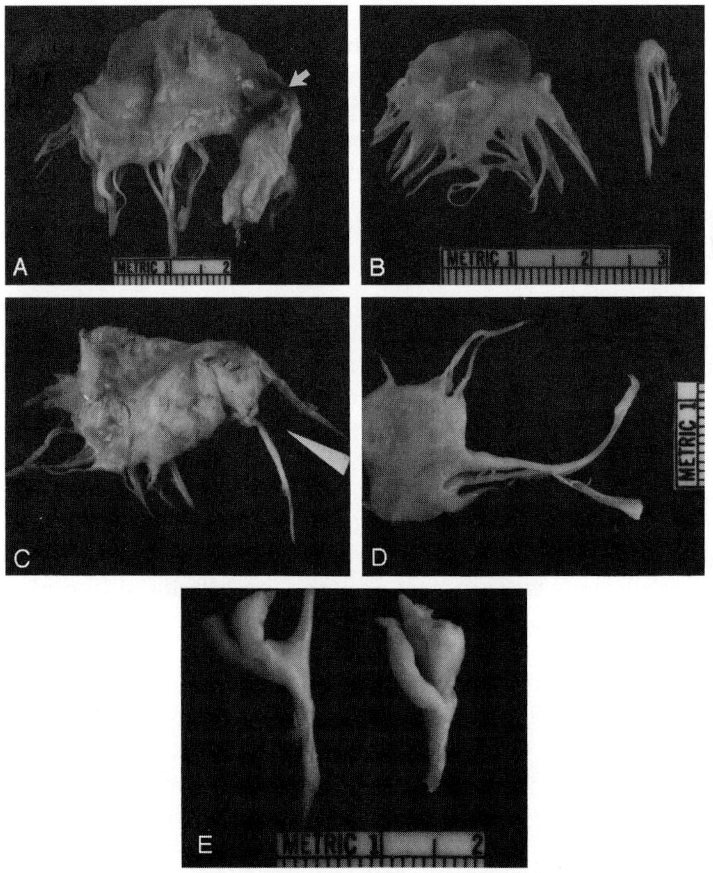

FIG. 4.12. The changing faces of surgically excised mitral valves. *A.* Anterior leaflet and portion of posterior leaflet removed from a 52-year-old patient with postrheumatic scarring. The degree of stenosis is difficult to appreciate when the whole valve is not available for examination, but the commissural fusion (*arrow*) and thickened and fused chordae are clues to the diagnosis. *B.* Anterior leaflet and chordae from a 79-year-old man with mitral regurgitation secondary to ischemic heart disease. The valve is diffusely thickened, as are the chordae, features that suggest the possibility of a postinflammatory etiology. Therefore, the history is essential in arriving at the correct diagnosis. *C.* Anterior leaflet of mitral valve with moderate diffuse thickening. The chordae are extremely long and thin, suggesting floppy mitral valve disease. The *arrow* shows where an attempted repair of chordal rupture was performed. *D.* Posterior leaflet of mitral valve with moderate diffuse thickening and elongated chordae characteristic of floppy mitral valve disease. *E.* Thickened chordae and fused chordae alone from a patient with floppy mitral valve disease and mitral regurgitation.

TABLE 4.11. MITRAL VALVE DISEASE, 1990A

| | | Tissue Received *vs.* Functional Status (%) | | |
Tissue	No. of Cases	MS	MS+MR	MR
Entire valve	30 (32)	(27)	(50)	(23)
AL ± PPL	42 (44)	(19)	(21)	(60)
PPL ± chordae	21 (22)	(0)	(0)	(100)
Chordae	2 (2)	(0)	(0)	(100)

[a]Data from Ref. 14. AL, anterior leaflet; PPL, portion of posterior leaflet; MS, mitral stenosis; MS+MR, combined mitral stenosis and regurgitation; MR, mitral regurgitation.

status of the valve (Table 4.11), the presence of leaflet prolapse or chordal rupture, the coexistence of other valvular or cardiac disease, and a history of endocarditis or rheumatic fever should be provided. As emphasized in the aortic valve discussion, this information can be obtained most readily by the use of specially printed forms that are made available to the cardiac operating room personnel.[16] These have proved to be invaluable at the Mayo Clinic and allow rapid, cost-effective, and sensible interpretation of cardiac valves.

CARDIAC TUMORS

Several recent articles and reviews have appeared discussing common cardiac tumors.[68–71] Two lesions of recent interest will be discussed here.

Mesothelial/Monocytic Incidental Cardiac Excrescences: Cardiac MICE

In 1990, Luthringer *et al.*[72] reported the presence of a lesion originally thought to resemble a histiocytoid (epithelioid) hemangioma[73] occurring within the cardiovascular system, particularly the heart. The authors suggested that the lesions were in part showing mesothelial differentiation. Two additional reports[74,75] have been published recently confirming the presence of mesothelial cells in these lesions. The most recent evidence[75] suggests that these lesions are probably best regarded as "pseudotumors" and may, in some instances, be artifactually produced. Herein these lesions will be referred to as cardiac MICE.

Twenty examples of cardiac MICE have been reported occurring in patients from 5 to 76 years of age (11 male, 9 female). All were incidental findings, and some were found to be "free-floating" by the surgeon. Lesions were found in cardiac chambers or on cardiac valves (11 cases) in right ventricular endomyocardial biopsy specimens (3), in the pericardial sac (3), in the specimen jars submitted to pathology (2), and in the ascending aorta (1). The lesions ranged in size from microscopic (in the case of those found in endomyocardial biopsy specimens) up to 3 cm. All lesions have been solitary. Grossly, they are dark-red to brown and frequently associated with obvious thrombus.

In the first reported examples of this lesion, they were referred to as histiocytoid hemangiomas.[72] Additional cases have originally been diagnosed as "chemoreceptor tissue" and "metastatic adenocarcinoma." Thus, it is clear that these lesions have caused at least some confusion to experienced surgical and cardiovascular pathologists. The nodules are usually discrete (Fig. 4.13) and distinct from the myocardium in cases in which myocardium is also present. The lesions are composed of two predominant cell types, an epithelioid or histiocytoid cell and a taller, columnar or cuboidal cell frequently present in strips (Fig. 4.14). The epithelioid/histiocytoid cells are round to oval and have a pink cytoplasm, well-defined nuclei with prominent nuclear grooves, and occasional nucleoli. They have a low nuclear-to-cytoplasmic ratio. These cells are positive for leukocyte common antigen, CD68 (KP-1), and lysozyme (Fig. 4.15). Electron microscopically, these cells have features typical of histiocytes with convoluted nuclei, prominent nucleoli, cytoplasm rich in rough endoplasmic reticulum, and surface pseudopodia. The second less common cells are usually present in small groups, strips, or tubular arrangements, have smaller amounts of eosinophilic cytoplasm, and have small round, noncleaved nuclei, with inconspicuous nucleoli. These cells are positive for keratin and negative for CEA (Carcinoembryonic antigen), leu-M1, Factor VIII-related antigen, and the hematolymphoid markers CD68 (KP-1), lysozyme, and leukocyte common antigen, (Fig. 4.15). Electron microscopically, these cells have haphazardly arranged intermediate filaments, and surface microvilli. Well-developed desmosomes and intercellular connections may also be present. These are features consistent with mesothelial cells. Both cell types are set in a fibrin-rich stroma containing small numbers of neutrophils, occasional lymphocytes, and eosinophils, sometimes arranged around spaces or adipocyte-like vacuoles. Occasional cases have shown foci of calcification and the presence of intermixed foreign material, including cotton fibers.

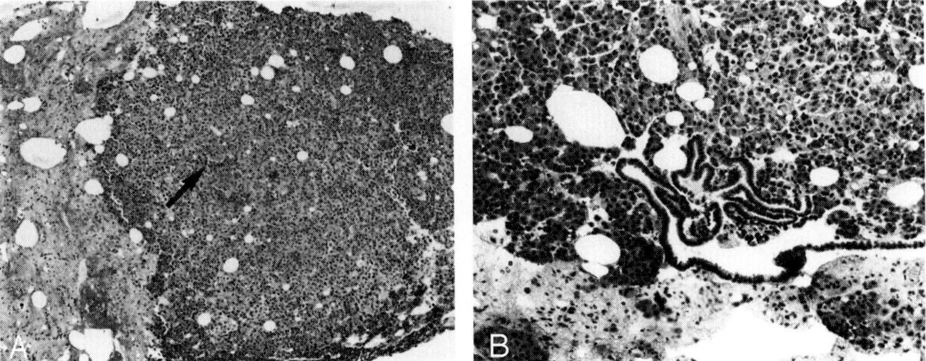

FIG. 4.13. Low power appearance of cardiac MICE. *A.* Rare strips of cuboidal cells are present (*arrow*). Note the vacuolated adipocytelike spaces. *B.* Prominent strip of cuboidal cells adjacent to epithelioid/histiocytoid cells.

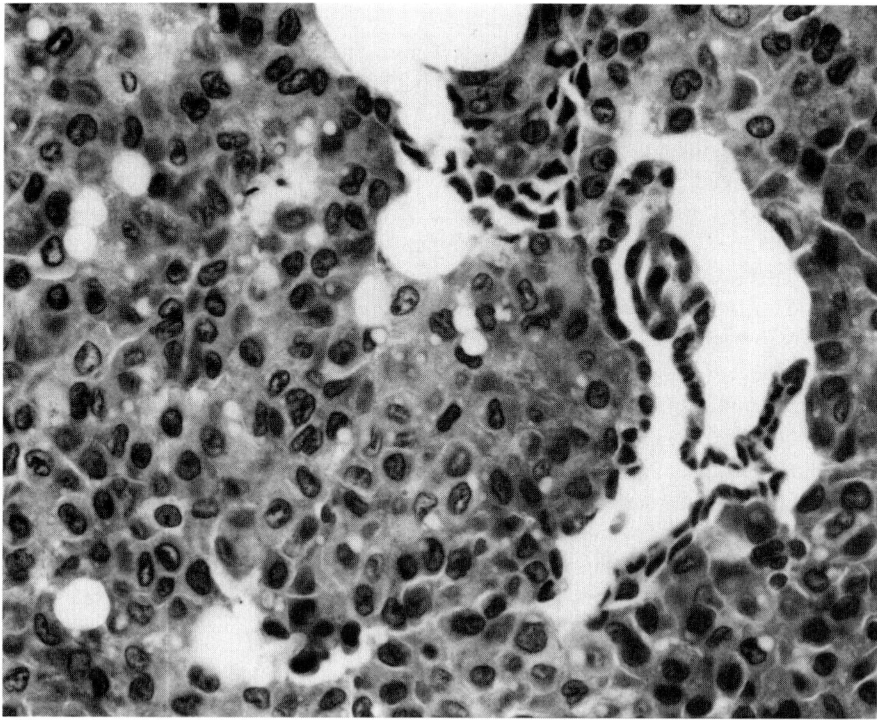

FIG. 4.14. A cardiac "mouse." The cuboidal cells have small round oval nuclei with inconspicuous nucleoli. These cells are somewhat smaller than the epithelioid/histiocytoid cells with convoluted nuclei.

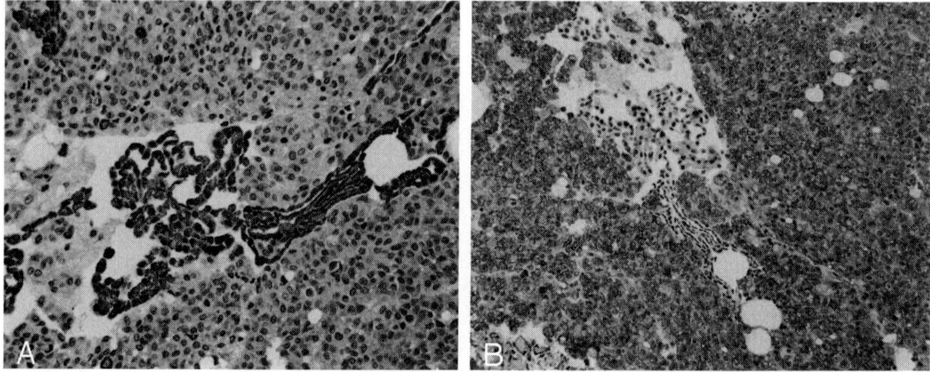

FIG. 4.15. Immunoperoxidase stains on cardiac MICE. *A.* The cuboidal cells are positive for keratin, and the epithelioid cells are negative. *B.* The cuboidal cells are negative for leukocyte common antigen, and the epithelioid/histiocytoid cells are positive.

The authors of the original two studies[72,74] suggested that cardiac MICE might represent a form of mesothelial hyperplasia, possibly representing a reactive process in response to previous cardiac catheterization, and 75% of the patients in one series had such a previous history. A perforation of the right ventricle, particularly during catheterization or even right ventricular endomyocardial biopsy, might cause subsequent migration and/or displacement of epicardial mesothelial cells into cardiac chambers. An additional hypothesis has been put forward by Cortice *et al.*[75] as a result of their examination material found in extracorporeal bypass pumps and material adherent to mediastinal and pericardial drains. Based on their study (in which cardiac MICE were found in the filters of 82% of extracorporeal bypass pumps investigated and 13% of mediastinal and pericardial drains following cardiac surgery), they suggested that these lesions were produced during cardiac surgery by the cardiotomy suction tip. Compaction of friable mesothelial strips, other tissue, debris, and fibers may then be agglomerated and transported around the operative site and, thus, be found "free-floating" in a large proportion of cases by either the surgeon or the pathologist. This is certainly an intriguing hypothesis and may well explain the majority of examples of this lesion. It does not, however, account for cases found on right ventricular endomyocardial biopsy; therefore, rare examples of this lesion are most likely the result of perforation of the right ventricle and subsequent displacement of mesothelial cells into the cardiac chamber which along with fibrin and previously circulating macrophages and rare inflammatory cells coalesce to form a pseudotumor. Either pathogenetic theory would explain how these MICE may occur within the heart. As emphasized by Cortice *et al.*,[75] the lack of histologic evidence of attachment to underlying tissues and a lack of supporting stroma highlight the fact that the fibrin meshwork previously described is not only a prominent feature of cardiac MICE but is likely an essential element in their formation and adherence to other tissues. The lack of a supporting stroma also makes it unlikely that these lesions actually have any capacity to "grow" other than by increasing the number of cells that adhere to the fibrin meshwork.

Follow-up on all of the cases of cardiac MICE has shown a benign behavior, as would be expected for an essentially artifactual lesion.

INFANTILE HISTIOCYTOID CARDIOMYOPATHY

The lesion terms "infantile histiocytoid cardiomyopathy" was originally reported as multiple rhabdomyomas by Wegmen and Egbert in 1935 in a 10-month-old girl who died with atrial tachycardia.[76] Since that time, approximately 45 cases have been reported under a variety of names including idiopathic infantile cardiomyopathy,[77,78] cardiac lipidosis,[79] infantile xanthomatous cardiomyopathy,[80] focal myocardial degeneration,[81] oncocytic cardiomyopathy,[82] and multifocal Purkinje-like tumor of the heart.[83] Despite the variety of names, the clinicopathologic setting associated with these nodules has been relatively consistent.[76–94] The lesions occur in children, from 1 to 28 months of age. The most common clinical presentations include congestive heart failure, incessant ventricular tachycardia, or sudden death. The first reports of these lesions were autopsy reports. More recently, however, these lesions have been surgically biopsied or, in some instances, excised; thus, they have now made their way into the purview of the cardiac surgical pathologist.[91–93]

The lesions are small (1–12 mm), ill-defined white-yellow nodules that occur on the endocardial, epicardial, or valve surfaces. They are occasionally elevated. Histologically, they are characterized by the presence of small clusters and sheets of abnormal cells that are 2–3 times the diameter of the adjacent normal myocytes (Fig. 4.16). The clusters are most often subendocardial in a distribution suggested to be reminiscent of conduction fibers. The edges of the nodules are usually discrete, but in some areas may interdigitate with normal myocardial cells (Fig. 4.17). The cells have clear to slightly eosinophilic vacuolated to granular cytoplasm, with one or two centrally placed nuclei and occasionally prominent eosinophilic nucleoli (Fig. 4.18). The cells are positive for muscle specific actin and desmin (Fig. 4.19) but are negative for smooth muscle actin, CD34, CD68 (KP-1), lysozyme, and viral proteins. Electron micro-

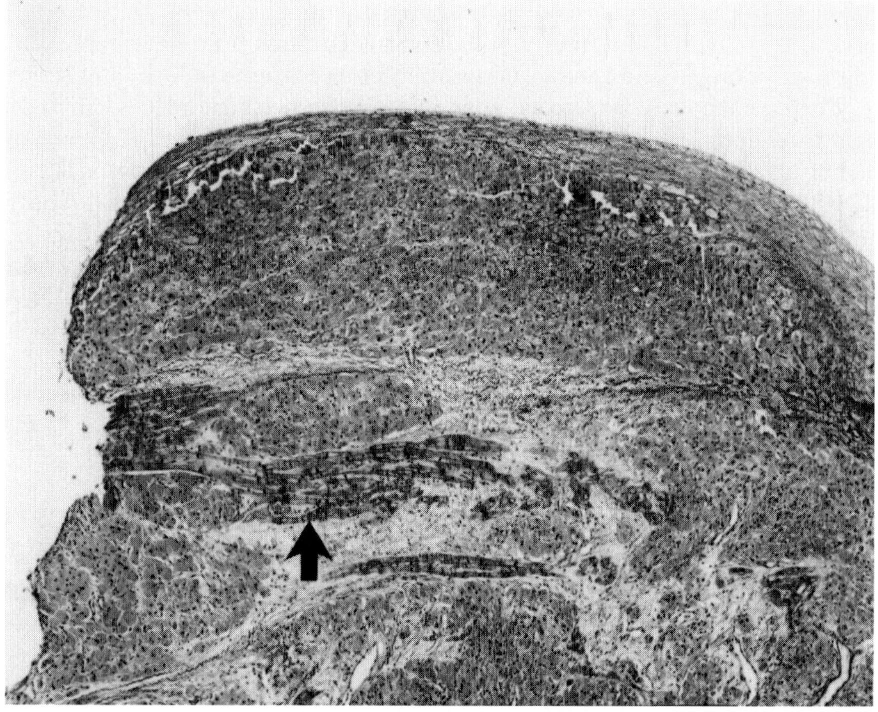

FIG. 4.16.   Infantile histiocytoid cardiomyopathy (myocardial hamartoma) showing characteristic subendocardial location of nodule and interdigitating myocytes (*arrow*).

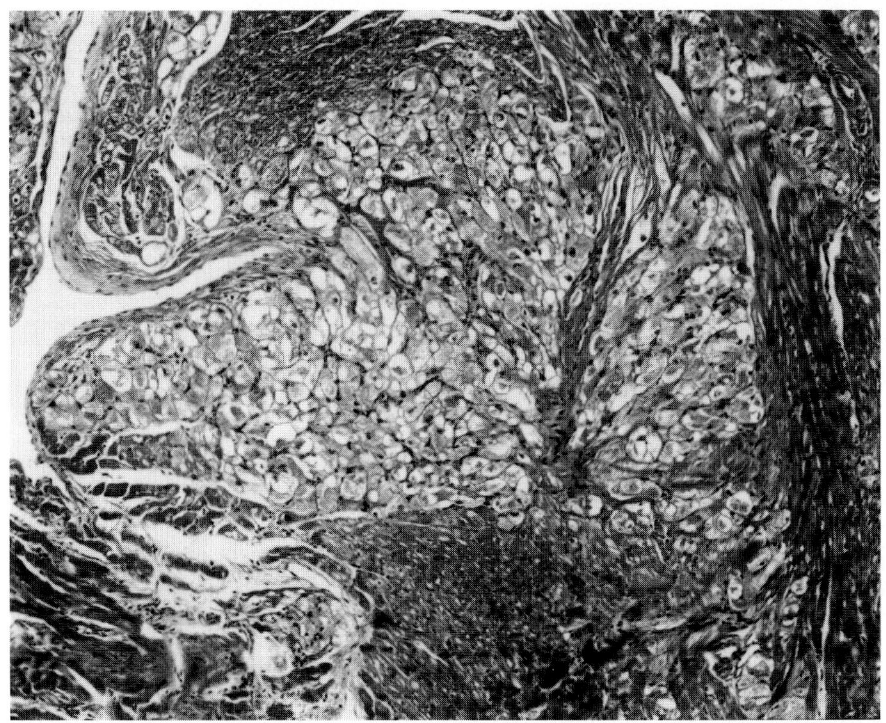

FIG. 4.17. Infantile histiocytoid cardiomyopathy. The abnormal cells are 2–3 times the size of the adjacent myocytes and contain cleared, focally vacuolated, and granular cytoplasm.

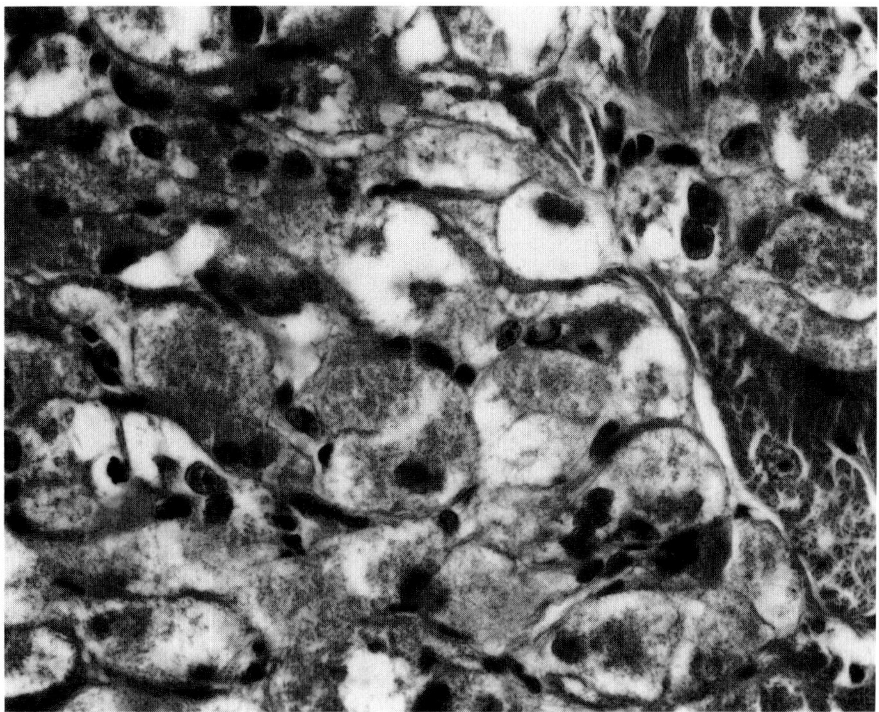

FIG. 4.18. Infantile histiocytoid cardiomyopathy. The abnormal cells contain round oval nuclei with occasionally prominent nucleoli. Again, note the character of the cytoplasm.

scopically, the cells have abundant mitochondria with abnormal cristae, lipid droplets, and intercellular junctions consistent with desmosomes. A few myofibrils may be present in these cells but appear to be small, disorganized, and peripherally located. Leptofibril-like structures also have been described in the cytoplasm.[91,93]

Although these lesions were originally fatal, further experience with these children has shown that they can be treated conservatively. Ziegler *et al.*[94] have successfully treated 14 children with incessant ventricular tachycardia with a combination of antiarrhythmic therapy (including amiodarone) and cryoablation of the lesions; 79% of their patients are free of the need for any antiarrhythmic medication.

The nature of the abnormal cells and whether they represent a hamartoma or developmental disorder is currently a matter of debate. Histologically and ultrastructurally the atypical cells resemble immature Purkinje cells, but the possibility that they represent primitive myocardial cell precursors nevertheless remains. Gelb *et al.*[93] recently suggested the lesions best be interpreted as a developmental anomaly, which seems to have some appeal given the fact that without surgical treatment many of these patients are able to apparently "outgrow their disease."

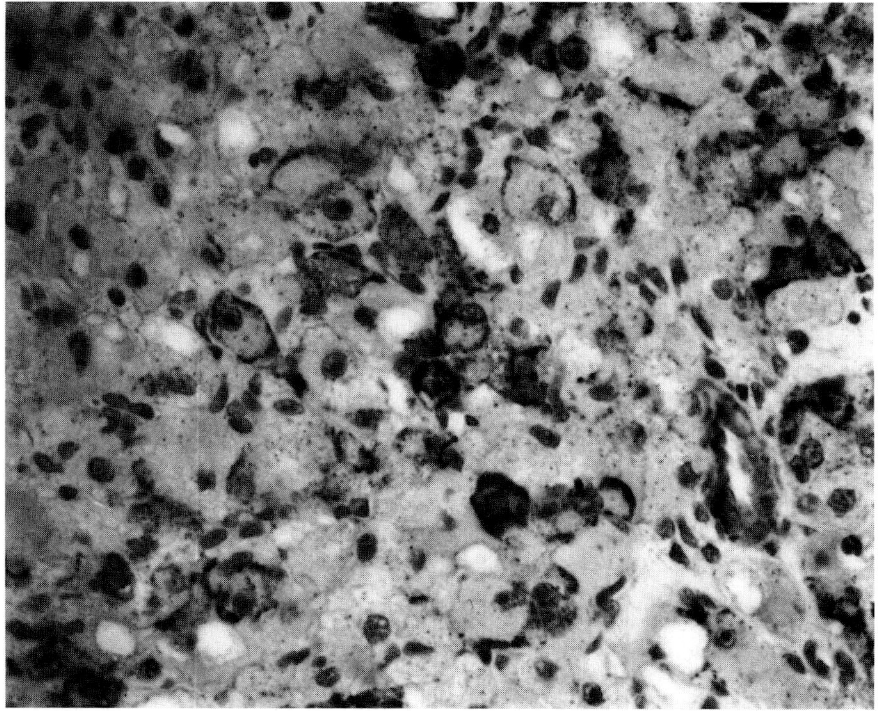

FIG. 4.19. Infantile histiocytoid cardiomyopathy. Desmin positivity is present in the cytoplasm in many of the involved cells, some with peripheral accentuation of staining.

ACKNOWLEDGMENTS

I thank Dr. H. T. Aretz and Dr. J. W. Mason for data from the myocarditis treatment trial, Dr. W. D. Edwards for helpful comments, Dr. P. J. Harrity and Dr. J. P. Veinot for photographic assistance, and Lisa Hurley for secretarial assistance.

REFERENCES

1. Aretz HT, Billingham ME, Edwards WD, et al. Myocarditis: a histopathologic definition and classification. *Am J Cardiovasc Pathol* 1987;1:3–14.
2. Aretz HT, Billingham ME, Edwards WD, et al. The utility of the Dallas criteria for the histopathological diagnosis of myocarditis in endomyocardial biopsy specimens *Circulation* 1993;88(Abstr):I-552.
3. Edwards WD. Pathology of endomyocardial biopsy. In: Waller BF, ed. *Pathology of the heart and great vessels.* New York: Churchill Livingstone, 1988:191–275.
4. Billingham ME. The role of endomyocardial biopsy in the diagnosis and treatment of heart disease. In: Silver MD, ed. *Cardiovascular pathology.* 2nd ed. New York: Churchill Livingstone, 1991:1465–1486.
5. Schoen FJ. *Interventional and surgical cardiovascular pathology: clinical correlations and basic principles.* Philadelphia: WB Saunders, 1989:183–186.
6. Zee-Cheng C-S, Tsai CC, Palmer DC, Codd JE, Pennington DG, Williams GA. High incidence

of myocarditis by endomyocardial biopsy in patients with idiopathic congestive cardiomyopathy. *J Am Coll Cardiol* 1984;3:63–70.

7. Nippoldt TB, Edwards WD, Holmes DR, Jr., Reeder GS, Hartzler GO, Smith HC. Right ventricular endomyocardial biopsy: clinicopathologic correlates in 100 consecutive patients. *Mayo Clin Proc* 1982;57:407–418.

8. Fenoglio JJ Jr., Ursell PC, Kellogg CF, Drusin RE, Weiss MB. Diagnosis and classification of myocarditis by endomyocardial biopsy. *N Engl J Med* 1983;308:12–18.

9. Parrillo JE, Aretz HT, Palacios I, Fallon JT, Block PC. The results of transvenous endomyocardial biopsy can frequently be used to diagnose myocardial diseases in patients with idiopathic heart failure: endomyocardial biopsies in 100 consecutive patients revealed a substantial incidence of myocarditis. *Circulation* 1984;69:93–101.

10. Billingham ME, Mason JW. Endomyocardial biopsy diagnosis of myocarditis and changes following immunosuppressive treatment. In: Bolte H-D, ed. *Viral heart disease.* Berlin: Springer-Verlag, 1984:200–210.

11. Dec GW, Fallon JT, Southern JF, Palacios I. "Borderline" myocarditis: an indication for repeat endomyocardial biopsy. *J Am Coll Cardiol* 1990;15:283–289.

12. Mason JW, Billingham ME, Ricci DR. Treatment of acute inflammatory myocarditis assisted by endomyocardial biopsy. *Am J Cardiol* 1980;45:1037–1044.

13. Passik CS, Ackermann DM, Pluth JR, Edwards WD. Temporal changes in the causes of aortic stenosis. A surgical pathologic study of 646 cases. *Mayo Clin Proc* 1987;62:119–123.

14. Dare AJ, Veinot JP, Edwards WD, Tazelaar HD, Schaff HV. New observations on the etiology of aortic valve disease: a surgical pathologic study of 236 cases from 1990. *Hum Pathol* 1993;24:1330–1338.

15. Olson LJ, Subramanian R, Ackermann DM, Orszulak TA, Edwards WD. Surgical pathology of the mitral valve: a study of 712 cases spanning 21 years. *Mayo Clin Proc* 1987, 62:22–34.

16. Dare AJ, Harrity PJ, Tazelaar HD, Edwards WD, Mullany CJ. Evaluation of surgically excised mitral valves: revised recommendations based on changing operative procedures in the 1990s. *Hum Pathol* 1993;24:1286–1293.

17. Davies MJ. *Pathology of cardiac valves* Boston: Butterworth Publishers, 1980.

18. Roberts WC, Morrow AG. Cardiac valves and the surgical pathologist. *Arch Pathol* 1966;82:309–313.

19. Kitzman DW, Scholz DG, Hagen PT, Ilstrup DM, Edwards WD. Age-related changes in normal human hearts during the first 10 decades of life. Part II (maturity): a quantitative anatomic study of 765 specimens from subjects 20 to 99 years old. *Mayo Clin Proc* 1988;63:137–146.

20. Subramanian R, Olson LJ, Edwards WD. Surgical pathology of pure aortic stenosis: a study of 374 cases. *Mayo Clin Proc* 1984;59:683–690.

21. Olson LJ, Subramanian R, Edwards WD. Surgical pathology of pure aortic insufficiency: a study of 225 cases. *Mayo Clin Proc* 1984;59:835–41.

22. Subramanian R, Olson LJ, Edwards WD. Surgical pathology of combined aortic stenosis and insufficiency: a study of 213 cases. *Mayo Clin Proc* 1985;60:247–254.

23. Pomerance A. Isolated aortic stenosis. In: Pomerance A, Davies MJ, eds. *The pathology of the heart.* London: Blackwell Scientific Publications, 1975:327–341.

24. Edwards JE. Pathology of aortic incompetence. In: Silver MD, ed. *Cardiovascular pathology.* 2nd ed. New York: Churchill Livingstone, 1991:1013–1027.

25. Edwards WD. Surgical pathology of the aortic valve. In: Waller BF, ed. *Pathology of the heart and great vessels.* New York: Churchill Livingstone, 1988:43–100.

26. Peterson MD, Roach RM, Edwards JE. Types of aortic stenosis in surgically removed valves. *Arch Pathol Lab Med* 1985;109:829–832.

27. Roberts WC. Congenitally bicuspid aortic valve: a study of 85 autopsy cases. *Am J Cardiol* 1970;26:72–83.

28. Larson EW, Edwards WD. Risk factors for aortic dissection: a necropsy study of 161 cases. *Am J Cardiol* 1984;53:849–855.

29. Craver JM. Aortic valve debridement by ultrasonic surgical aspirator: a word of caution. *Ann Thorac Surg* 1990;49:746–753.

30. Waller BF, Morrow AG, Maron BJ, et al. Etiology of clinically isolated, severe, chronic, pure mitral regurgitation: analysis of 97 patients over 30 years of age having mitral valve replacement. *Am Heart J* 1982;104:276–288.
31. Hanson TP, Edwards BS, Edwards JE. Pathology of surgically excised mitral valves: one hundred consecutive cases. *Arch Pathol Lab Med* 1985;109:823–828.
32. Van der Bel-Kahn J, Becker AE. The surgical pathology of rheumatic and floppy mitral valves: distinctive morphologic features upon gross examination. *Am J Surg Pathol* 1986;10:282–292.
33. Agozzino L, Falco A, de Vivo F, et al. Surgical pathology of the mitral valve: gross and histological study of 1288 surgically excised valves. *Int J Cardiol* 1992;17:79–89.
34. Hauck AJ, Edwards WD, Danielson GK, Mullany CJ, Bresnahan DR. Mitral and aortic valve disease associated with ergotamine therapy for migraine. *Arch Pathol Lab Med* 1990;114:62–64.
35. Redfield MM, Nicholson WJ, Edwards WD, Tajik AJ. Valve disease associated with ergot alkaloid use: echocardiographic and pathologic correlations. *Ann Intern Med* 1992;117:50–52.
36. Hammer WJ, Roberts WC, deLeon AC Jr. "Mitral stenosis" secondary to combined "massive" mitral annular calcific deposits and small, hypertrophied left ventricles: hemodynamic documentation in four patients. *Am J Med* 1978;64:371–376.
37. Osterberger LE, Goldstein S, Khaja F, Lakier JB. Functional mitral stenosis in patients with massive mitral annular calcification. *Circulation* 1981;64:472–476.
38. Ghosh PK, Miller HI, Vidne BA. Mitral obstruction in bacterial endocarditis. *Br Heart J* 1985;53:341–344.
39. Buckley BH, Roberts WC. The heart in systemic lupus erythematosus and the changes induced in it by corticosteroid therapy: a study of 36 necropsy patients. *Am J Med* 1975;58:243–264.
40. Bortolotti U, Valente M, Agozzino L, Mazzucco A, Thiene G. Rheumatoid mitral stenosis requiring valve replacement. *Am Heart J* 1984;107:1049–1051.
41. Scalapino JN, Edwards WD, Steckelberg JM, Wooten RS, Callahan JA, Ginsburg WW. Mitral stenosis associated with valvular tophi. *Mayo Clin Proc* 1984;59:509–512.
42. Shenoy UA, Peric-Golia L. Primary cardiovascular amyloidosis manifesting as mitral stenosis. *Hum Pathol* 1982;13:768–770.
43. McAllister HA Jr, Fenoglio JJ, Jr. Cardiac involvement in Whipple's disease. *Circulation* 1975;52:152–156.
44. Silver MD. *Cardiovascular pathology.* 2nd ed. Vol. 2. New York: Churchill Livingstone, 1991:954.
45. Blieden LC, Moller JH. Cardiac involvement in inherited disorders of metabolism. *Prog Cardiovasc Dis* 1974;16:615–631.
46. Schieken RM, Kerber RE, Ionasescu VV, Zellweger H. Cardiac manifestations of the mucopolysaccharidoses. *Circulation* 1975;52:700–705.
47. Renteria VG, Ferrans VJ, Roberts WC. The heart in the Hurler syndrome: gross, histologic and ultrastructural observations in five necropsy cases. *Am J Cardiol* 1976;38:487–501.
48. Ireland MA, Rowlands DB. Mucopolysaccharidosis type IV as a cause of mitral stenosis in an adult. *Br Heart J* 1981;46:113–115.
49. Leder AA, Bosworth WC. Angiokeratoma corporis diffusum universale (Fabry's disease) with mitral stenosis. *Am J Med* 1965;38:814–819.
50. Waller BF. Morphological aspects of valvular heart disease: part II. *Curr Prob Cardiol* 1984;9:1–74.
51. Roberts WC, Perloff JK. Mitral valvular disease: a clinicopathologic survey of the conditions causing the mitral valve to function abnormally. *Ann Intern Med* 1972;77:939–975.
52. Harley JB, McIntosh CL, Kirklin JJW, et al. Atrioventricular valve replacement in the idiopathic hypereosinophilic syndrome. *Am J Med* 1982;73:77–81.
53. Braunwald E. *Heart disease: a textbook of cardiovascular medicine.* 4th ed. Philadelphia: WB Saunders, 1992:1452.
54. Myerowitz PD, Michaelis LL, McIntosh CL. Mitral valve replacement for mitral valve regurgitation due to Libman-Sacks endocarditis: report of a case. *J Thorac Cardiovasc Surg* 1974;67:869–874.

55. Bulkley BH, Roberts WC. Systemic lupus erythematosus as a cause of severe mitral regurgitation: new problem in an old disease. *Am J Cardiol* 1975;35:305–308.
56. Benotti JR, Sataline LR, Sloss LJ, Cohn LH. Aortic and mitral insufficiency complicating fulminant systemic lupus erythematosus. *Chest* 1984;86:140–143.
57. Roberts WC, Kehoe JA, Carpenter DF, Golden A. Cardiac valvular lesions in rheumatoid arthritis. *Arch Intern Med* 1968;122:141–146.
58. Symbas PN. *Trauma to the heart and great vessels.* New York: Grune & Stratton, 1978:85–95.
59. Gidding SS, Shulman ST, Ilbawi M, Crussi F, Duffy CE. Mucocutaneous lymph node syndrome (Kawasaki disease): delayed aortic and mitral insufficiency secondary to active valvulitis. *J Am Coll Cardiol* 1986;7:894–897.
60. Roberts WC, Honig HS. The spectrum of cardiovascular disease in the Marfan syndrome; a clinico-morphologic study of 18 necropsy patients and comparison to 151 previously reported necropsy patients. *Am Heart J* 1982;104:115–135.
61. Leier CV, Call TD, Fulkerson PK, Wooley CF. The spectrum of cardiac defects in the Ehlers-Danlos syndrome, types I and III. *Ann Intern Med* 1980;92:171–178.
62. Jaffe AS, Geltman EM, Rodey GE, Uitto J. Mitral valve prolapse; a consistent manifestation of type VI Ehlers-Danlos syndrome: the pathogenetic role of the abnormal production of type III collagen. *Circulation* 1981;64:121–125.
63. Pickering NJ, Brody JI, Barrett MJ. Von Willebrand syndromes and mitral-valve prolapse: linked mesenchymal dysplasias. *N Engl J Med* 1981;305:131–134.
64. Lebwohl MG, Distefano D, Prioleau PG, Uram M, Yannuzzi LA, Fleischmajer R. Pseudoxanthoma elasticum and mitral-valve prolapse. *N Engl J Med* 1982;307:228–231.
65. Becker AE, Schoorl R, Balk AG, van der Heide RM. Cardiac manifestations of Fabry's disease: report of a case with mitral insufficiency and electrocardiographic evidence of myocardial infarction. *Am J Cardiol* 1975;36:829–835.
66. Azarides M, Lennox SC. Rupture of the posterior wall of the left ventricle after mitral valve replacement: etiological and technical considerations. *Ann Thorac Surg* 1988;46:491–494.
67. Karlson KJ, Ashraf MM, Berger RL. Rupture of left ventricle following mitral valve replacement. *Ann Thorac Surg* 1988;46:590–597.
68. Tazelaar HD, Locke TJ, McGregor CGA. Pathology of surgically excised primary cardiac tumors. *Mayo Clin Proc* 1992;67:957–965.
69. Herrmann MA, Shankerman RA, Edwards WD, Shub C, Schaff HV. Primary cardiac angiosarcoma: a clinicopathologic study of six cases. *J Thorac Cardiovasc Surg* 1992;103:655–664.
70. Burke AP, Virmani R. Cardiac myxoma. A clinicopathologic study. *Am J Clin Pathol* 1993;100:671–680.
71. Burke AP, Cowan D, Virmani R. Primary sarcomas of the heart. *Cancer* 1992;69:387–395.
72. Luthringer DJ, Virmani R, Weiss SW, Rosai J. A distinctive cardiovascular lesion resembling histiocytoid (epithelioid) hemangioma. *Am J Surg Pathol* 1990;14:993–1000.
73. Rosai J, Gold S, Landy R. The histiocytoid hemangioma: a unifying concept embracing several previously described entities of skin, soft tissue, large vessels, bone and heart. *Hum Pathol* 1979;10:707–730.
74. Veinot JP, Tazelaar HD, Edwards WD, Colby TV. Mesothelial/monocytic incidental cardiac excrescences: cardiac MICE. *Mod Pathol* 1994;7:9–16.
75. Courtice RW, Stinson WA, Walley VM. Tissue fragments recovered at cardiac surgery masquerading as tumoral proliferations: evidence suggesting iatrogenic or artefactual origin and common occurrence. *Am J Surg Pathol* 1994;18:167–174.
76. Wegman ME, Egbert DS. Congenital rhabdomyoma of the heart associated with arrhythmia. *J Pediatr* 1935;6:818–824.
77. Kauffman SL, Chandra N, Peress NS, et al. Idiopathic infantile cardiomyopathy with involvement of the conduction system. *Am J Cardiol* 1972;30:648–652.
78. Reid JD, Hajdu SI, Attah E. Infantile cardiomyopathy: a previously unrecognized type with histiocytoid reaction. *J Pediatr* 1968;73:335–339.
79. Ross CF, Belton BM. A case of isolated cardiac lipidosis. *Br Heart J* 1968;30:726–728.
80. MacMahon HE. Infantile xanthomatous cardiomyopathy. *Pediatrics* 1971;48:312–315.

81. Haese WH, Maron BJ, Mirowski M, et al. Peculiar focal myocardial degeneration and fatal ventricular arrythmias in a child. *N Engl J Med* 1972;287:180–181.
82. Silver MM, Burns JE, Sethi RK, et al. Oncocytic cardiomyopathy in an infant with oncocytosis in exocrine and endocrine glands. *Hum Pathol* 1980;11:598–604.
83. Rossi L, Piffer R, Turolla E, et al. Multifocal Purkinje-like tumor of the heart. Occurrence with other anatomic abnormalities in the atrioventricular junction of an infant with junctional tachycardia, Lown-Ganong-Levine syndrome, and sudden death. *Chest* 1985;87:340–345.
84. Bove KE, Schwartz DC. Focal lipid cardiomyopathy in an infant with paraxysmal atrial tachycardia. *Arch Pathol* 1973;95:26–36.
85. Ferrans VJ, McAllister HA, Haese WH. Infantile cardiomyopathy with histiocytoid change in cardiac muscle cells. Report of six patients. *Circulation* 1976;53:708–719.
86. Saffitz JE, Ferrans VJ, Rodriguez ER, et al. Histiocytoid cardiomyopathy: a cause of sudden death in apparently healthy infants. *Am J Cardiol* 1983;52:215–217.
87. McGregor CG, Gibson A, Caves P. Infantile cardiomyopathy with histiocytoid change in cardiac muscle cells: successful surgical intervention with prolonged survival. *Am J Cardiol* 1984;53:982–983.
88. Bruton D, Herdson PB, Becroft BM. Histiocytoid cardiomyopathy of infancy: an unexplained myofibre degeneration. *Pathology* 1977;9:115–122.
89. Zimmerman A, Diem P, Cottier H. Congenital "histiocytoid" cardiomyopathy: evidence suggesting a developmental disorder of the Purkinje cell system of the heart. *Virchows Arch A Pathol Anat Histopathol* 1982;396:187–195.
90. Van Creveld S, Van Der Linde HM. Cardiomegalia glycogenica circumscripta. *Arch Dis Child* 1939;14:14–21.
91. Kearney DL, Titus JL, Hawkins EP, et al. Pathologic features of myocardial harmartomas causing childhood tachyarrhythmias. *Circulation* 1987;75:705–710.
92. Ghargozloo F, Porter C-J, Tazelaar HD, Danielson GK. Multiple myocardial hamartomas causing ventricular tachycardia in young children: combined surgical modification and medical treatment. *Mayo Clin Proc* 1994;69:262–267.
93. Gelb AB, van Meter SH, Billingham ME, Berry GJ, Rouse RV. Infantile histiocytoid cardiomyopathy—myocardial or conduction system harmartoma: what is the cell type involved? *Hum Pathol* 1993;24:1226–1231.
94. Ziegler VL, Gillette PC, Crawford FA, Wiles HB, Fyfe DA. New approaches to treatment of incessant ventricular tachycardia in the very young. *J Am Coll Cardiol* 1990;16:681–685.

Chapter 5

Pathology of Human Cardiac Transplantation

MARGARET E. BILLINGHAM

The Registry of the International Society for Heart and Lung Transplantation in 1994 reports that 26,704 heart transplants have been performed since 1967 (Table 5.1)[1] Encouraging survival statistics have resulted in cardiac transplantation in neonates, infants, and children (Table 5.1), as well as cardiac recipients in the 6th and 7th decades. Patients with end-stage heart disease who are most likely to benefit from cardiac transplantation are those with less than a 6-month prognosis for survival, but who otherwise have reversible or minimal organ damage elsewhere, particularly in the liver and kidneys. The overall one-year survival for cardiac transplantation is now 80% and rates of higher than 85% are achieved in many major centers.[1] Over the years, different immunosuppressive regimens have been used and these in turn have affected not only the pathology of the transplanted heart, but the temporal relationship of rejection patterns as well. Although most centers now use cyclosporine, the unwanted side effects of hypertension, neurotoxicity, and nephrotoxicity have led to a reduction of the dose and the substitution of other immunosuppressive agents. At this time, most centers are using a combination of immunosuppressive agents including azathioprine, corticosteroids, and cyclosporine with or without OKT3 or OKT4 (monoclonal antibody to T cells; Ortho Pharmaceuticals, Inc.) or antithymocyte globulin (ATG) induction. In addition to these drugs, other new immunosuppressive drugs are emerging, such as FK506, rapamycin, mycophenolate mofetil, leflunomide, and others. Some of these drugs are undergoing clinical trials and may soon be available for use. There are also heart transplant survivors from the precyclosporine era (before 1981) who are still being treated with azathioprine and steroids only. Heart transplantation has allowed many patients with previous end-stage heart disease to return to satisfying and productive lives. There are many survivors over 10 years and the longest survivor died just recently, 21 years after transplant surgery.

CAUSES OF DEATH

Despite the wealth of experience over the last 25 years, the major causes of death in cardiac allografts remain acute cardiac rejection or infection in

TABLE 5.1 INTERNATIONAL SOCIETY FOR HEART AND LUNG TRANSPLANTATION (MODIFIED FROM REGISTRY DATABASE), ELEVENTH REPORT, 1994

Total heart transplants	26,704
Number of centers	251
Pediatric heart transplantation (0–18 yr)	1,918
Number of centers	200

TABLE 5.2 CAUSES OF DEATH IN CARDIAC RECIPIENTS (STANFORD CARDIAC TRANSPLANTATION)[a]

	First Postoperative Year		>1 yr Postoperation	
	CYA	AZA	CYA	AZA
Rejection	19	7	10	4
Infection	41	28	43	18
Graft vascular disease	3	0	30	7
Graft Failure	12	0	0	0
Lymphoproliferative disorder	4	0	5	4
Nonlymphoid				
Malignancy	3	0	11	3
Embolus (Pulmonary)	3	0	0	1
Pulmonary				
Hypertension	2	2	0	0
Cerebral Vascular Accident	3	0	2	0
Other	10	0	20	8
Total deaths	100	37	121	45

[a]CYA, cyclosporine A; AZA, Azathioprine.

the early postoperative years, or graft vascular disease in the later years (Table 5.2). Acute cardiac rejection may not manifest itself clinically until it is quite severe and therefore difficult to reverse. For this reason, the diagnosis of acute cardiac rejection has been monitored morphologically using the endomyocardial biopsy. Although noninvasive methods are being developed and many others have been tried, it is generally accepted that to monitor cardiac rejection, the most reliable method at present for diagnosing acute rejection is still the morphological one based on the endomyocardial biopsy findings.

ENDOMYOCARDIAL BIOPSY

The endomyocardial biopsy technique has been described in many previous articles.[2,3] From the pathologist's point of view, however, it is important that sufficient tissue is obtained to make a diagnosis of acute rejection or to rule out acute infection or lymphoproliferative disease. The International Society for Heart and Lung Transplantation, in their standardized cardiac biopsy grading, requires a minimum of 4 evaluable pieces of myocardial tissue. The sizes of the tissue obtained vary with the size of the bioptomes from a 5 French used for pediatric patients, up to a 9 French for adults. It has been published previously that with 4 pieces of tissue, using the large 9 French size, there is a 2% false-negative result, whereas with only 3 pieces, there is a 5% false-negative result.[4] It is suggested that 4 pieces be obtained, together with an extra piece, which is to be frozen for immunohistochemistry, immunofluorescence, or any other studies. The 4 pieces should be fixed immediately in 10% buffered formalin at room temperature (to prevent extra contraction artefact) and then paraffin-embedded in the conventional way. Paraffin sections obtained should be 4 μm thick; in those thicker than 6 μm, the apparent cellularity may be increased. The sections should be stained with hematoxylin and eosin and Masson's trichrome or another connective tissue stain. The tissue blocks should be "step-sectioned" to cut well into the block, so that maximum tissue is available for diagnosis. It is better to cut a few unstained sections for future staining, if required later (*e.g.,* Gomori silver stains), than to try to save the block. In centers where large numbers of biopsies are performed, it is recommended that the biopsies not be accessioned with consecutive numbers; the tissue slides look very similar and staggered numbering avoids mistakes. Endomyocardial biopsy is often performed on the diseased hearts of recipients before transplantation to rule out potentially recurrent conditions such as amyloidosis and sarcoidosis, as well as others listed in Table 5.3.

PATHOLOGY OF HEART TRANSPLANTATION

The pathology described is similar for orthotopic, heterotopic ("piggy-back" hearts), and pediatric heart transplants as well as for the donor hearts in combined heart-lung transplantation. The pathology of cardiac transplantation can best be summarized in a temporal fashion, as outlined in Table 5.4, although it should be understood that there is a good deal of overlap among groups.

TABLE 5.3   RECIPIENTS' DISEASES KNOWN TO RECUR IN THE DONOR HEART

Amyloidosis
Melanoma
Chagas disease
Sarcoidosis
Giant cell myocarditis

TABLE 5.4   PATHOLOGY OF HEART TRANSPLANTATION

Immediate (1–24 hr)
    a. Hyperacute rejection
    b. Right ventricular failure
Early (1–3 wks posttransplantation)
    a. Ischemic injury (with or without reperfusion)
    b. Pressor effect damage
Intermediate (1 mo–1 yr posttransplantation)
    a. Acute cellular rejection
    b. Humoral rejection
    c. Infectious myocarditis
    d. Epstein-Barr virus-related lymphoproliferative lesions
Late (1–22 yr)
    a. Graft hypertrophy and fibrosis
    b. Denervation
    c. Graft vascular disease (coronary and great vessels)

TEMPORAL PATHOLOGIC CHANGES

IMMEDIATE (1–24 HOURS POSTTRANSPLANTATION)

Hyperacute Rejection

This is an uncommon form of rejection that occurs immediately after transplantation.[5] It occurs in the setting of major blood group incompatibility between the donor and recipient (ABO mismatch) or as a result of other major histocompatibility differences. One group reported four cases of hyperacute rejection, secondary to circulating antiendothelial antibodies.[6] The myocardium becomes a deep red color as a result of diffuse ("global" as opposed to the patchy pattern in myocardial infarcts) hemorrhage into the interstitium (Fig. 5.1). Usually these changes occur shortly after the patient is weaned from the bypass pump and circulation is reestablished. The heart rapidly dilates, ventricular arrhythmias may develop, and cardiac failure ensues. Without emergent retransplantation or mechanical support, the patient will not survive because the graft will fail. If the patient survives for a few hours, early neutrophilic infiltrates may also be seen and fibrin thrombi may be found in small vessels, particularly capillaries, where "sludging" of red cells and platelets may occur.

Immediate Right Ventricular Failure

This is usually the result of a mechanical failure of a normal right ventricle from the recently placed donor heart that is unable to contract against a high

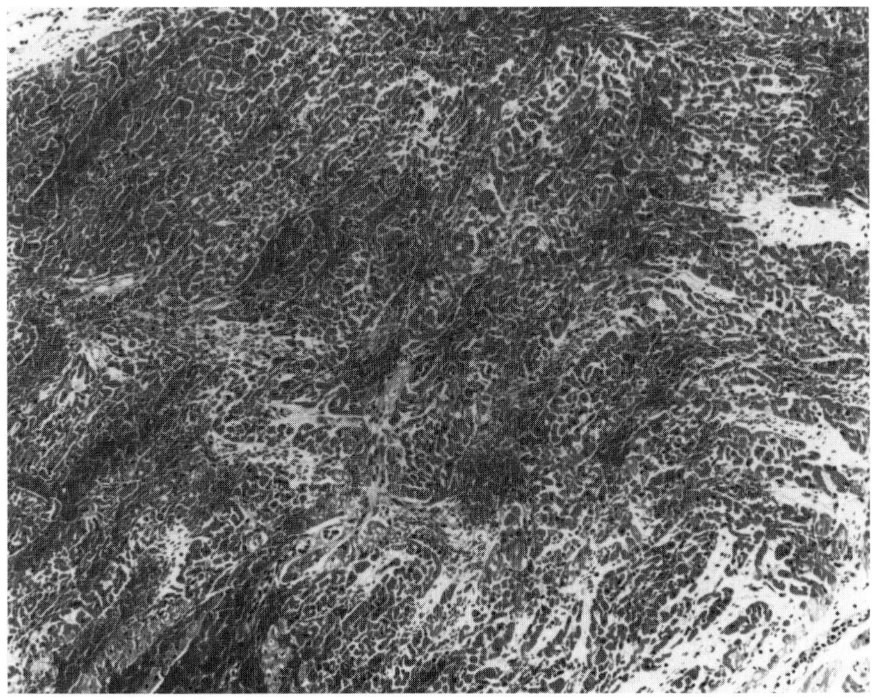

FIG. 5.1 Hyperacute rejection: Section of myocardium showing diffuse hemorrhage and edema. Hematoxylin and eosin; magnification × 100.

pulmonary vascular resistance in the recipient pulmonary bed. The nonhypertrophied normal right ventricle will become discolored, dilate, and fail. Histopathology at this stage is not helpful, although ischemic contraction bands may be seen. Recipients with known pulmonary hypertension will do better with a combined heart-lung transplant or if they obtain a donor heart from a recipient with known pulmonary hypertension (whose heart already has a hypertrophied right ventricle), for example, the heart of the recipient of a combined heart-lung transplant (the so-called "domino" heart transplantation).

Immediate right ventricular failure can also result from direct trauma to the heart in the case of an accident victim, or be due to an overly prolonged ischemic time between donor harvesting and *in situ* reperfusion. In rare instances, surgical trauma or inadvertent suture placement through a coronary artery will result in infarction and graft failure.

EARLY PATHOLOGY (1–3 WEEKS POSTTRANSPLANTATION)

Ischemic Injury (with or without Reperfusion)

Endomyocardial biopsies obtained within the first 3 weeks after transplantation may show pathologic evidence of ischemic injury and at a later phase this is replaced by granulation tissue; this should not be confused with acute rejection. In ischemic injury, the degree of myocyte damage is out of proportion to the number of inflammatory cells in the interstitium, which is in contrast to the predominantly lymphocytic infiltrates and the very focal, sometimes subtle, myocyte injury of acute rejection. Ischemic injury may be due to prolonged ischemic time due to transportation of the donor heart, ischemic injury followed by reperfusion with damage to capillaries, or due to failure to remove all air bubbles within the coronary circulation at transplantation. Although infarcts do occur, the ischemic necrosis is usually subendocardial and focal. The affected myocytes show shrinkage in size, hypereosinophilia with pyknotic nuclei, granular cytoplasm, and frequently, contraction bands. A trichrome stain will outline the ischemic focus with a grey/blue coloration of the affected myocytes. At a later stage, the necrotic myocardium is replaced by granulation tissue (Fig. 5.2).

"Pressor" Effect

Pressor effect is seen when there have been large doses of vasopressive drugs given to support the donor heart either before harvesting for transplantation or immediately posttransplantation. This may result in direct myocyte toxicity or "microinfarcts" due to constriction of the small "end vessels" of the coronary circulation. These are usually very small, focal insults with minimal acute inflammatory infiltrate (neutrophils), which also should not be confused with acute rejection.

INTERMEDIATE PATHOLOGY (1 MONTH–1 YEAR POSTTRANSPLANTATION)

Acute Cellular Rejection

Over the years several different grading systems for acute cardiac rejection have been described in the literature. To avoid the dilemma of understanding

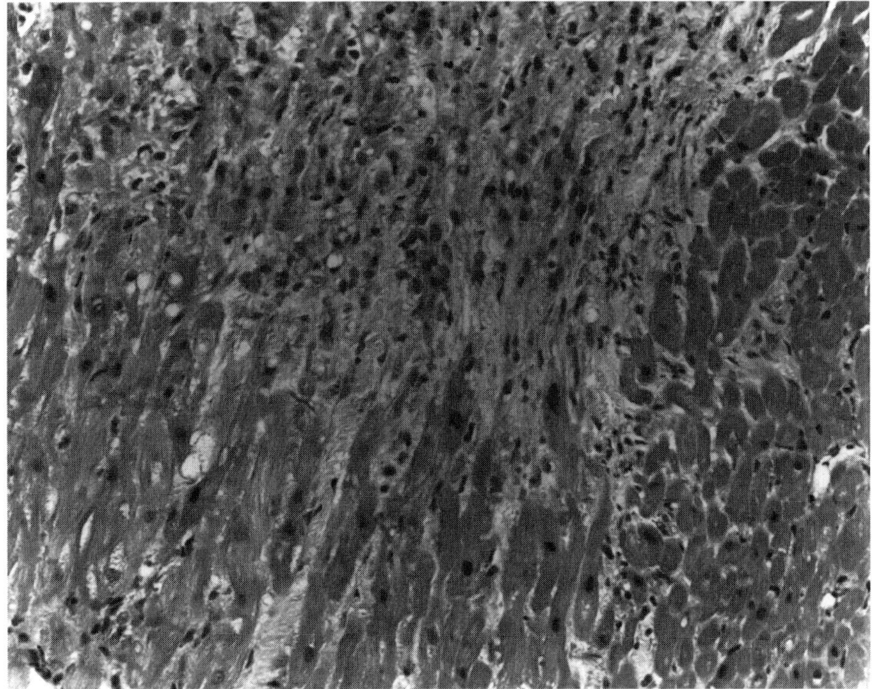

FIG. 5.2   Cardiac biopsy from cardiac recipient 1 week posttransplantation showing focal healing ischemic injury (paler area). Hematoxylin and eosin; magnification ×200.

and comparing results of cardiac transplantation from different institutions,[7] the International Society for Heart and Lung Transplantation (ISHLT) sponsored the Working Formulation for acute cardiac rejection (Table 5.5).[8] This grading system had already allowed multiinstitutional studies to take place and is generally conceded to have resulted in some uniformity among institutions and pathologists. As predicted, however, the Standardized Grading System after widespread use for 2 years will itself require modification.

The main morphological features of acute rejection, as described in Table 5.4, are a perivascular or interstitial inflammatory infiltrate of lymphocytes, with or without myocyte necrosis.

Grade 0 (ISHLT). Represents normal myocardium without an inflammatory infiltrate or myocyte damage.

Grade 1 (ISHLT). Represents either one or more focal perivascular infiltrates of activated lymphocytes without myocyte damage (Grade 1A) (Fig. 5.3) or similar focal infiltrates radiating into the surrounding interstitium in a "star burst" or "chicken wire" effect; also without myocyte damage (Grade 1B) (Fig. 5.4).

Grade 2 (ISHLT). One single focus in the entire collection of biopsy pieces of activated lymphocytes with myocyte damage. This may occur by itself or be accompanied by other forms of Grade 1, but no higher grades (Fig. 5.5).

Grade 3 (ISHLT). This represents multifocal lymphocytic infiltrates, obvious on low-power magnification, with myocyte damage or replacement (Fig.

TABLE 5.5 STANDARDIZED CARDIAC BIOPSY GRADING (MODIFIED) (INTERNATIONAL SOCIETY FOR HEART AND LUNG TRANSPLANTATION)[7]

Old Nomenclature	New Nomenclature	Grade
No rejection	No rejection	0
"Mild" rejection	A = Focal perivascular or focal interstitial infiltrate without myocyte damage	I
	B = Sparse focal interstitial infiltrate without myocyte damage	
"Focal" moderate rejection	One focus only with activated lymphocytes and myocyte damage	II
"Low" moderate rejection	A = Multifocal lymphocytic infiltrates with myocyte damage	III
"Borderline/Severe"	B = Diffuse (sometimes polymorphous) inflammatory process	
"Severe acute" rejection	Diffuse, polymorphous infiltrate with myocyte necrosis ± edema ± hemorrhage ± vasculitis	IV
"Resolving" rejection	Healing tissue with fibroblasts and pigmented macrophages	Denoted by a lesser grade
"Resolved" rejection	Mature scar tissue	Grade 0

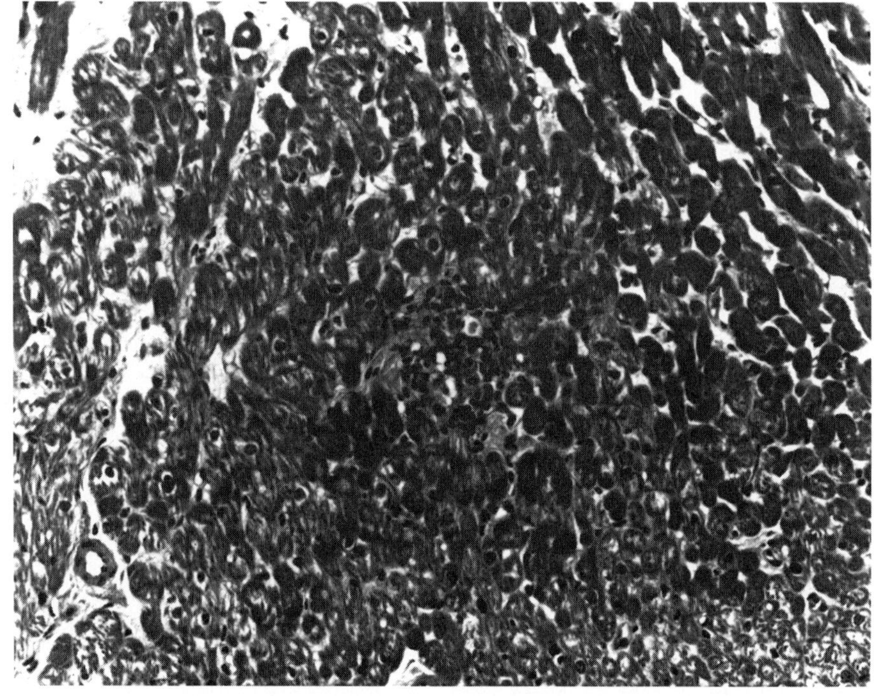

FIG. 5.3 Grade 1A (ISHLT Standardized Grading System). Cardiac biopsy showing a perivascular infiltrate of lymphocytes without myocyte damage (center) illustrating mild rejection. Hematoxylin and eosin; magnification ×200.

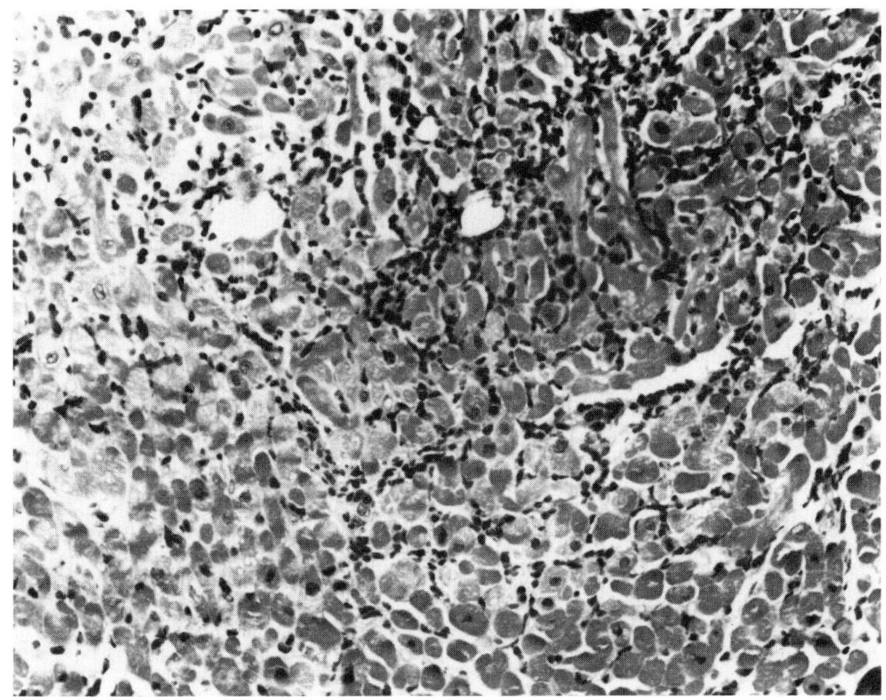

FIG. 5.4   Grade 1B (ISHLT Standardized Grading System). Cardiac biopsy showing a sparse interstitial infiltrate without myocyte damage. Hematoxylin and eosin; magnification ×200.

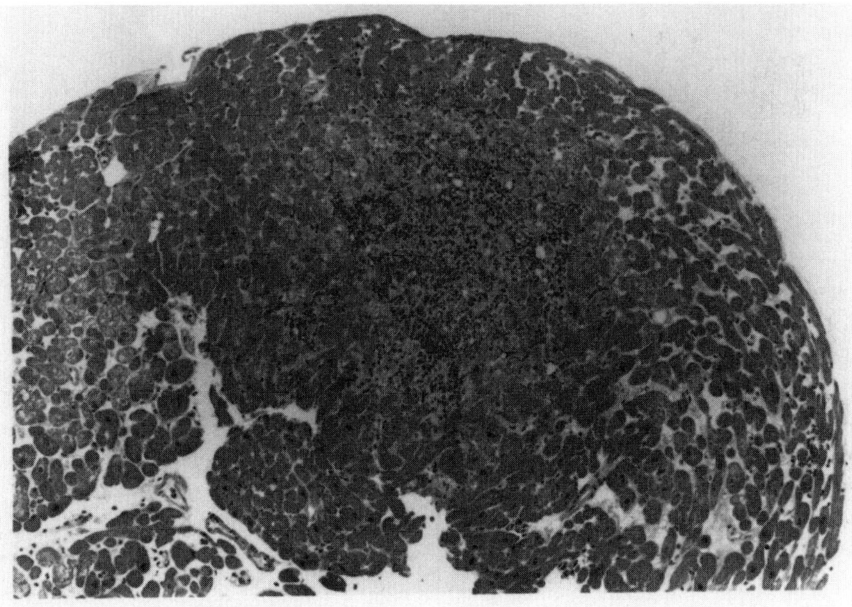

FIG. 5.5   Grade 2 (ISHLT Standardized Grading System). Cardiac biopsy with one aggregate of lymphocytes with myocyte damage. Hematoxylin and eosin; magnification ×200.

5.6). These infiltrates are usually in more than one fragment of myocardium and are often accompanied by a sparse, but definite endocardial infiltrate (Grade 3A). A more extensive and diffuse infiltrate, often polymorphous infiltrate with eosinophils, neutrophils, and sometimes red blood cells will suggest a "borderline severe" rejection (Grade 3B) (Fig. 5.7).

Grade 4 (ISHLT). This represents *severe* acute rejection with vasculitis, hemorrhage, and edema added to the changes seen in a Grade 3B. The endocardium is often infiltrated with inflammatory cells and hemorrhage.

Resolving Rejection. This is designated by a lesser grade than in the previous biopsy showing rejection. In addition to small inactivated lymphocytes, there are often fibroblasts and pigmented macrophages present.

Resolved Rejection. Again this is Grade 0 (ISHLT) after a documented rejection episode and shows only mature scar, but no inflammatory infiltrate.

To characterize the phenotype of the infiltrating lymphocytes for target selective immunosuppression in acute rejection, many centers are quantitating T-cell subsets in serial biopsies. Although there are trends in the T-cell population, some centers find that immunophenotyping is not particularly useful in the management or prediction of acute rejection, although it is useful for basic research. The reason for this is most likely because of sampling error inherent

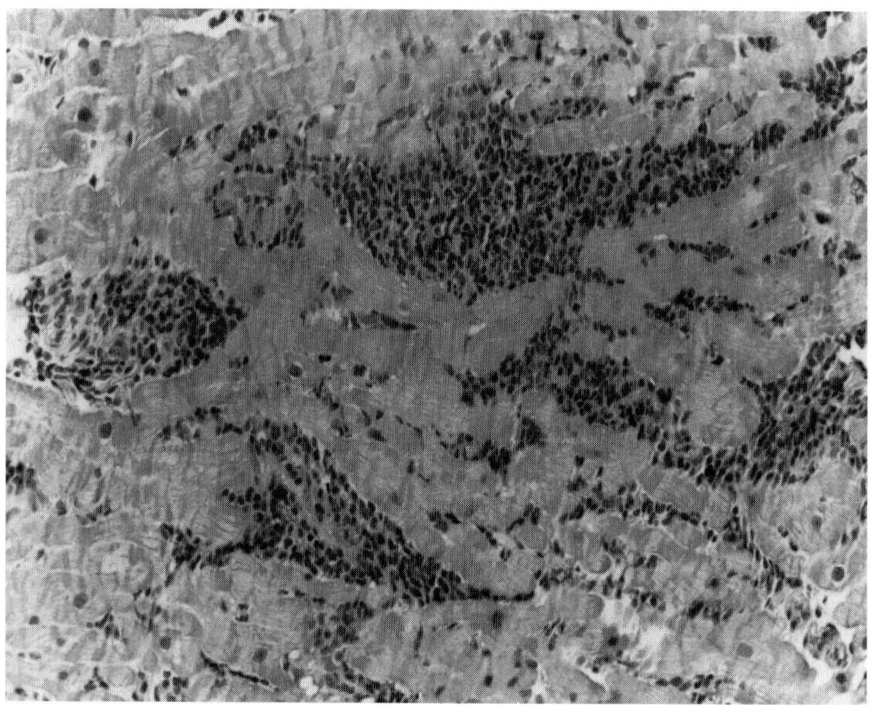

FIG. 5.6 Grade 3A (ISHLT Standardized Grading System). Cardiac biopsy with multifocal lymphocytic aggregates causing myocyte replacement and damage. Hematoxylin and eosin; magnification ×200.

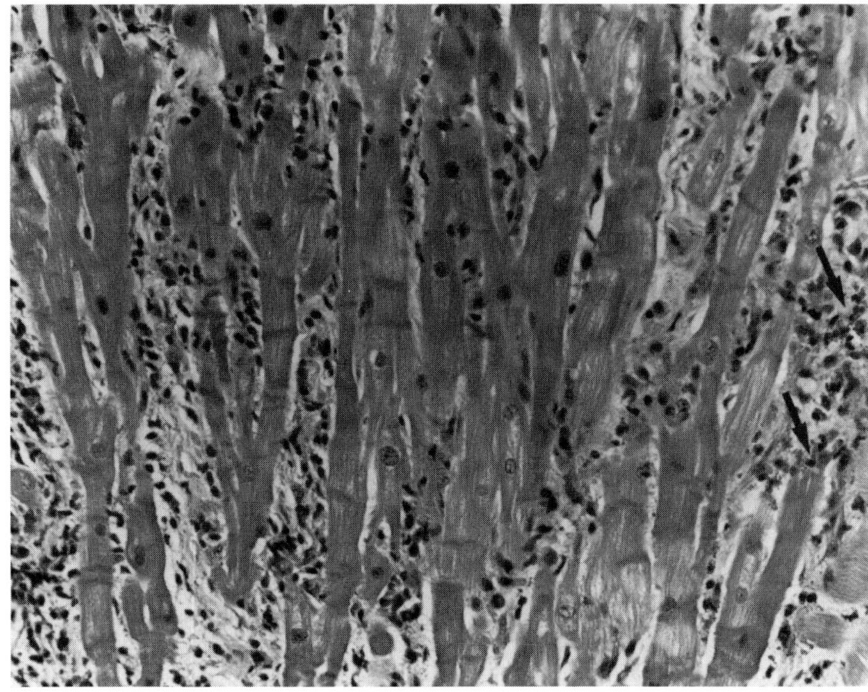

FIG. 5.7   Grade 3B (ISHLT Standardized Grading System). Cardiac biopsy with diffuse inflammatory infiltrate including eosinophils and causing myocyte damage (*arrows*). Hematoxylin and eosin; magnification ×200.

TABLE 5.6   ADDITIONAL REQUIRED INFORMATION IN STANDARDIZED
CARDIAC BIOPSY GRADING (ISHLT)[a]

Biopsy less than 4 pieces
Humoral rejection (positive immunofluorescence, vasculitis, or severe edema in absence of
  cellular infiltrate)
"Quilty" effect. A = no myocyte encroachment; B = with myocyte encroachment
Ischemia. A = up to 3 wk posttransplant; B = late ischemia
Infection present, biopsy therefore uninterpretable
Lymphoproliferative disorder
Other (specify)

[a]Modified from and reproduced with permission from Ref. 8.

in the biopsies and the use of monoclonal antibodies to T cells (OKT3/OKT4) as ongoing immunotherapy.

The Standardized Grading System also requires the tabulation of the presence of other changes (see Table 5.6).

MORPHOLOGICAL MIMICS OF ACUTE CELLULAR REJECTION.—Cellular infiltrates with myocyte damage may also be observed in a variety of lesions that affect the myocardium and must therefore be excluded before a definite diagnosis of acute rejection is made. The following are the more common pitfalls in the diagnosis of acute rejection: (1) healing of ischemic damage, (2) old biopsy sites, (3) the "Quilty" effect, and (4) infectious myocarditis.

1. Ischemic injury. This has been described in the preceding pages, and should not be confused with the changes of acute rejection.

2. Biopsy sites. Unfortunately, bioptomes are often guided back to the previous biopsy sites. These can be recent, within one or two weeks showing a crater-like area with fibrin and granulation tissue or older biopsy sites typically showing mature fibrous tissue scar with adjacent myocyte disarray (Fig. 5.8). Occasionally, aggregates of lymphocytes are trapped within the scar and these should not be confused with acute rejection.

3. "Quilty" effect. This is an aggregate of mononuclear lymphocytes, typically confined to the endocardium ("Quilty" A) containing small vascular channels (Fig. 5.9). These aggregates are polyclonal and consist mainly of T cells with some B cells, scattered marcophages, and plasma cells.[9] The "Quilty" effect may penetrate the underlying myocardium causing some myocardial damage ("Quilty" B) (Fig. 5.10). Some tangential cuts can be confused with acute rejection on biopsy samples, but the intensity of the focal infiltrate is more than that seen in acute rejection.

4. Infectious myocarditis. The distinction between rejection and infection is critical. The most common opportunistic infections see in cardiac allograft re-

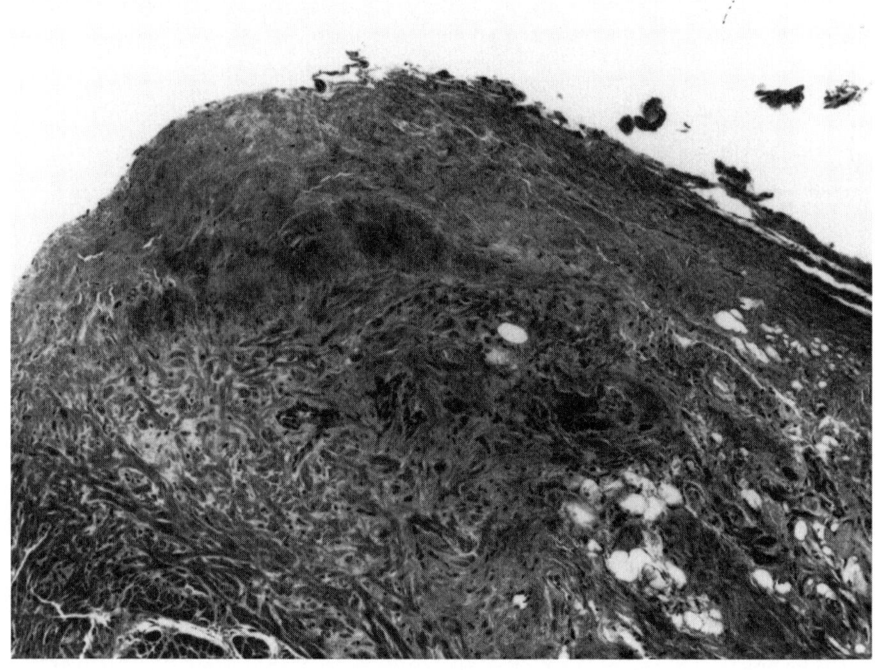

FIG. 5.8 Cardiac biopsy showing a previous (old) biopsy site with thick endocardial scar and subadjacent myocardial disarray with fatty infiltration. Masson's trichrome; magnification ×100.

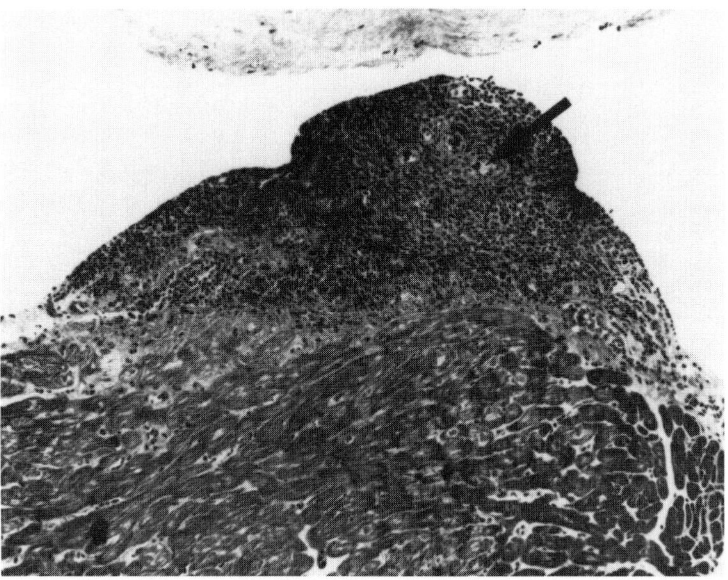

FIG. 5.9 "Quilty" A (ISHLT Standardized Grading System). Cardiac biopsy showing the characteristic focal endocardial infiltrate of mononuclear cells confined to the endocardium. Note the characteristic vascular spaces (*arrow*). Hematoxylin and eosin; magnification ×100.

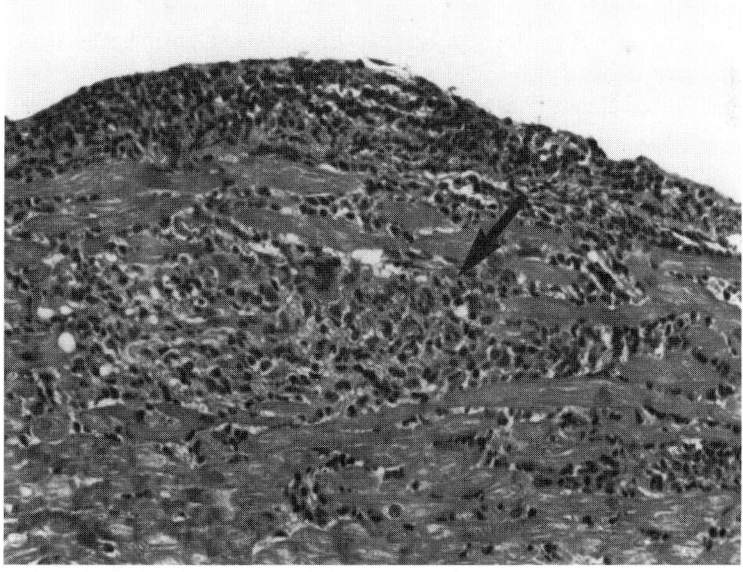

FIG. 5.10 "Quilty" B (ISHLT Standardized Grading System) lesion showing the mononuclear cell infiltrate extending into the subjacent myocardium (*arrow*). Hematoxylin and eosin; original magnification ×100.

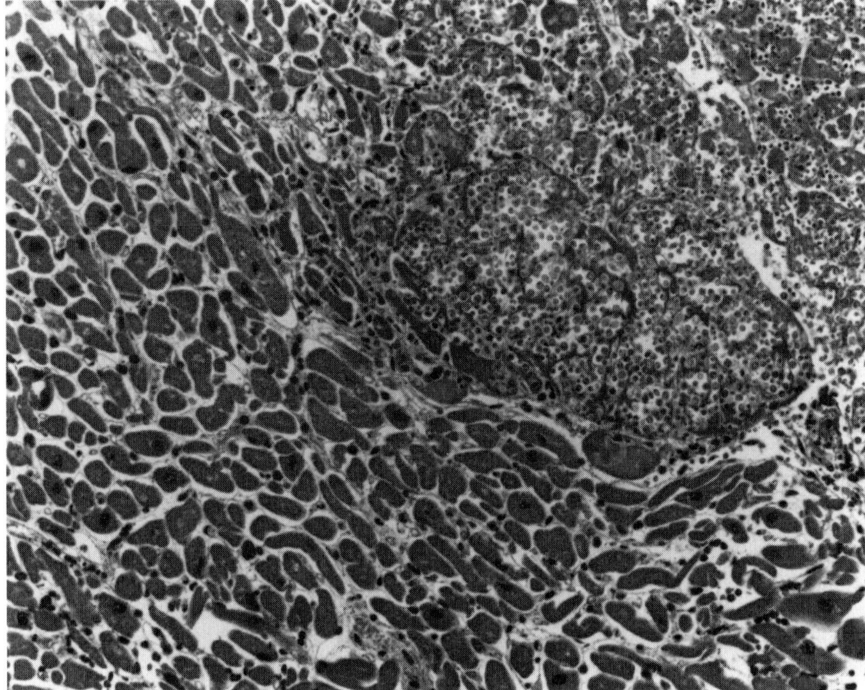

FIG. 5.11　Section of myocardium showing an infiltrate of candida spores (*top right*). Hematoxylin and eosin; magnification ×200.

cipients are viral, parasitic, and fungal (Fig. 5.11). Cytomegalovirus (Fig. 5.12) and *Toxoplasma gondii* induced myocarditis, often present with focal or dense mixed inflammatory infiltrates in the myocardium. In equivocal cases, serology, immunohistochemistry, or *in situ* hybridization may be indicated.[10] Fungal infections in the heart are less common since the advent of cyclosporine, rather than with the higher doses of corticosteroids given previously. The hematogenous dissemination of fungus may lead to vascular plaques causing discrete foci of infarction. It is recommended that cardiac recipients who are seronegative for cytomegalovirus and who receive a seropositive donor heart should have prophylactic antiviral treatment. After a cytomegalovirus infection, it has been observed that an acute rejection episode frequently follows. Infections in immunosuppressed cardiac recipients may affect other organs of the body.

Humoral Rejection or Acute Vascular Rejection

Recently, investigators have observed clinical examples of patients with hemodynamic and echocardiographic evidence of graft dysfunction, but without the cardinal histologic findings of cellular rejection. This is thought to represent "humoral" or antibody-mediated vascular rejection and this has been described in greater detail in the recent literature.[11,12] Endomyocardial biopsies taken at this time may show sparse acute inflammatory cells with

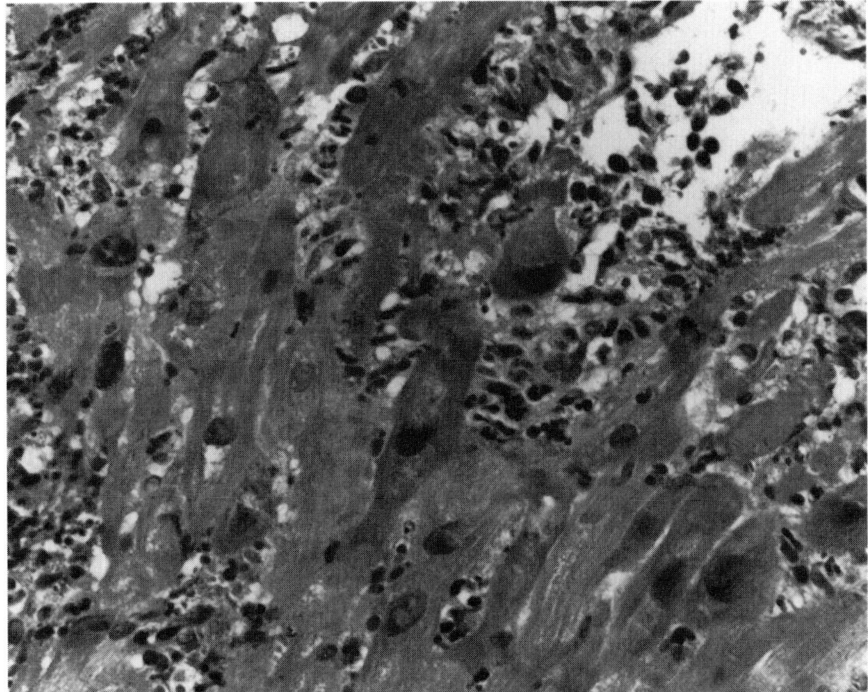

FIG. 5.12 Endomyocardial biopsy showing a mixed inflammatory (unlike that of rejection) infiltrate surrounding cytomegalovirus inclusions. Hematoxylin and eosin; magnification ×400.

an increase in interstitial edema (Fig. 5.13). Biopsies may also demonstrate evidence of endothelial swelling or injury of capillaries, venules, and arterioles that may be subtle.[11,12] At a later stage, the biopsies may also show evidence of a lymphocytic vasculitis. In addition to the histopathology described above, damage to small vessels in humoral rejection is often manifested by immunofluorescent evidence of deposition of immunoglobulins (IgG or IgM), complement (C3 and/or C1q), and fibrinogen in a linear staining pattern around small vessels (Fig. 5.14).[11,12] Some centers treat humoral rejection aggressively with a multiagent approach including cyclophosphamide, corticosteroids, intravenous heparin and plasmapheresis. Immunoglobulin deposition may, however, be seen in ischemia and other conditions, and it is not specific for humoral rejection.[13] In many centers this type of acute rejection is rare.

Epstein-Barr Virus-Related Lymphoproliferative Disease

In immunosuppressed organ donor recipients, Epstein-Barr virus related lymphoproliferative malignancies may occur particularly in younger patients and children. These lesions usually occur in other organs including the brain and gastrointestinal system or even in injection sites of antithymocyte globulin in the thighs.[14,15] Occasionally, lymphoproliferative infiltrates may be seen

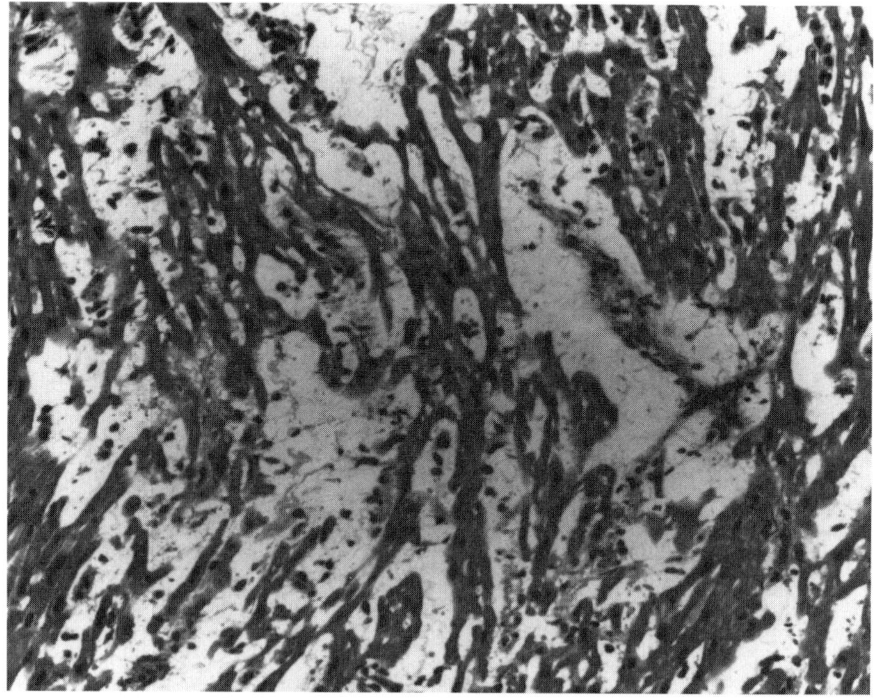

FIG. 5.13 Endomyocardial biopsy showing edema with sparse interstitial edema described in "humoral" rejection. Hematoxylin and eosin; magnification ×200.

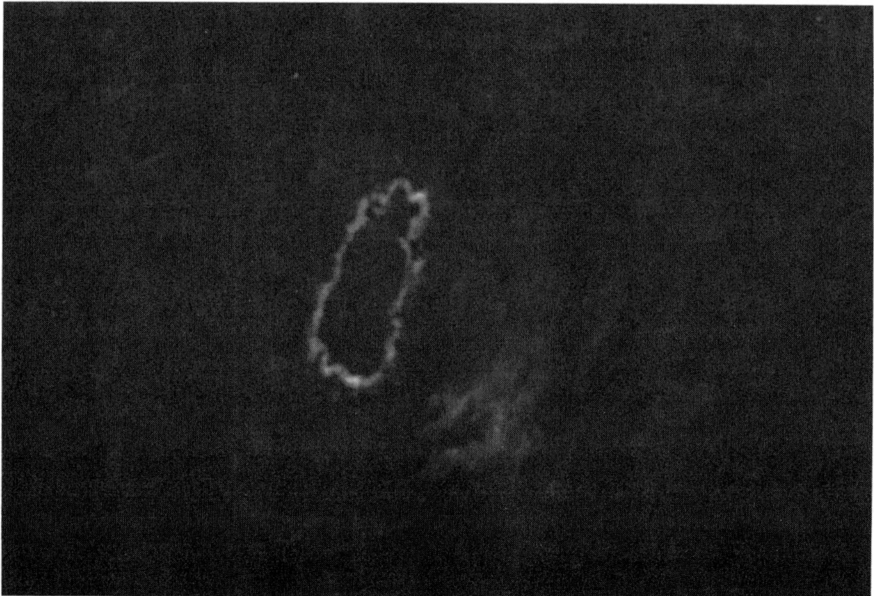

FIG. 5.14 Immunofluorescence (C′3) highlighting a small vessel in an endomyocardial biopsy. Hematoxylin and eosin; magnification ×200.

in endomyocardial biopsies or infiltrating into the myocardium at autopsy (Fig. 5.15). Lymphocytic infiltrates are more florid than in acute rejection, but may be confused with the "Quilty" effect. *In situ* hybridization for Epstein-Barr virus is now available to diagnose these lesions that can sometimes be reduced or "cured" by reduction in immunosuppression, particularly cyclosporine and antiviral agents.[16]

LATE PATHOLOGY OF HUMAN CARDIAC TRANSPLANTS (1–22) YEARS POSTRANSPLANTATION

Hypertrophy and Fibrosis

It has been observed that all cardiac allografts increase in size within weeks of transplantation, including those in children. One year after transplantation, most allografts show myocyte hypertrophy and an increase in interstitial fibrosis; several morphometric studies have been performed to support this.[17] This may partially result from donor ischemic time leading to myocardial and capillary damage causing fibrosis and compensatory hypertrophy. Restrictive and constrictive functional changes may also occur in long-term survivors of heart transplantation due to interstitial and pericardial fibrosis. Some reports suggest an increase in fine perimyocytic fibrosis due to cyclosporine.[18,19] With the reduced cyclosporine levels currently in use, the fine fibrosis is no longer seen so frequently.

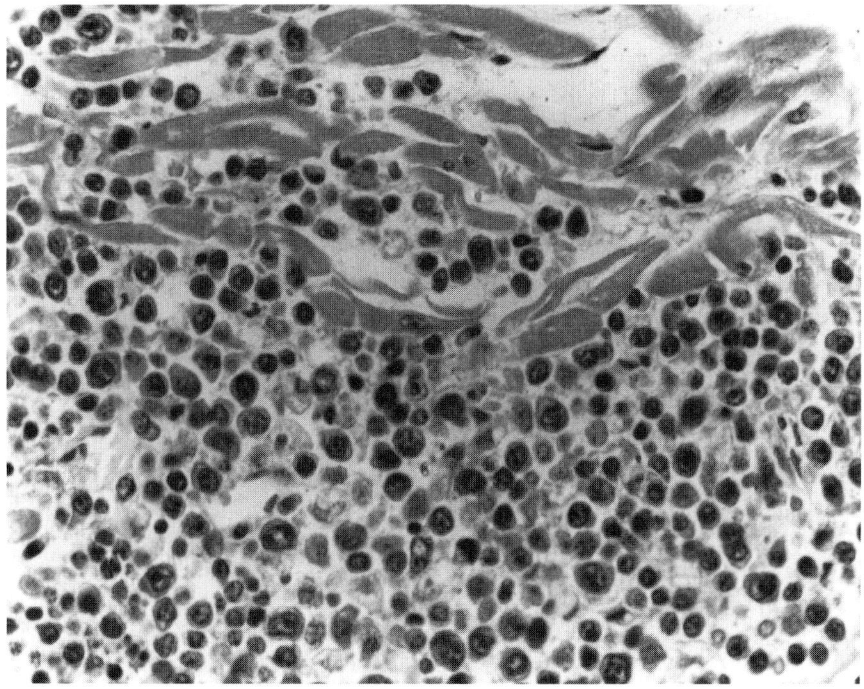

FIG. 5.15　Section of myocardium with infiltration by Epstein-Barr virus-induced lymphoma in a cardiac transplant recipient. Hematoxylin and eosin; magnification ×400.

Denervation

After cardiac transplantation, the allograft remains denervated and is not under the usual control of the sympathetic autonomic nervous system. Heart rate in response to dynamic exercise tends to be slower and not to achieve peak levels during maximum exercise when compared with age-matched normal controls. As judged by pharmacologic challenge and electrophysiologic studies on cardiac recipients, the transplanted heart remains denervated in long-term survivors. More recently, there have been reports of some physiologic evidence of reinnervation, although this has not yet been confirmed from the morphologic standpoint. Some nerves can be seen in the transplanted heart, although they are greatly reduced in number from normal.[20] These nerves most likely represent the postganglionic fibers of the intact parasympathetic ganglia left in the atrioventricular groove at transplantation.

Graft Vascular Disease

Although immunosuppressive therapy has greatly decreased and controlled allograft rejection, graft vascular disease is presently the major cause of death or retransplantation after the first postoperative year (Table 5.2). Gao *et al.*[21] reported 34.5% incidence in the Stanford experience in the first year, and 91% 5 years posttransplantation, as judged by coronary arteriography. Graft vascular disease may be evident as early as 3 months posttransplantation and may cause death in the recipient as late as 22 years postcardiac transplantation [22,23]. Graft vascular disease affects infants, children, and adults as well as the recipients of combined heart-lung transplants. The pathology of graft vascular disease is that of concentric intimal proliferation with minimal damage to the elastic lamina or minimal or no changes of the media of the coronary vessel walls (Fig. 5.16). The lesion may affect the entire length of the vessel and uniquely also affects the branches and small penetrating branches of the coronary system into the myocardium (Fig. 5.17). Because small vessels are involved, the resulting myocardial infarcts may be patchy and small. Correlation with acute rejection, although suspected, has not been definitely proved. As would be expected, graft vascular disease also affects the great vessels and adventitial vessels that remain attached to the allograft at transplantation.[24,25] Occasional plaques with cholesterol clefts and very focal calcification are sometimes seen in graft vascular disease[26] and it is not always clear whether these are legacies of the donor heart or whether they occur as "naturally occurring atherosclerosis" posttransplantation. The intimal proliferation appears to consist mainly of modified smooth muscle cells, lipid-filled macrophages, and sometimes T lymphocytes. Lymphocytes are not always present within the intimal proliferation. The lining of the endothelium is usually intact, but "endotheliolitis" has been described in cases with ongoing acute rejection (Fig. 5.18). The interactions of the intimal cells have been reviewed previously.[27] In general, it is thought that repetitive immunologic injury (by immunoglobulin or com-

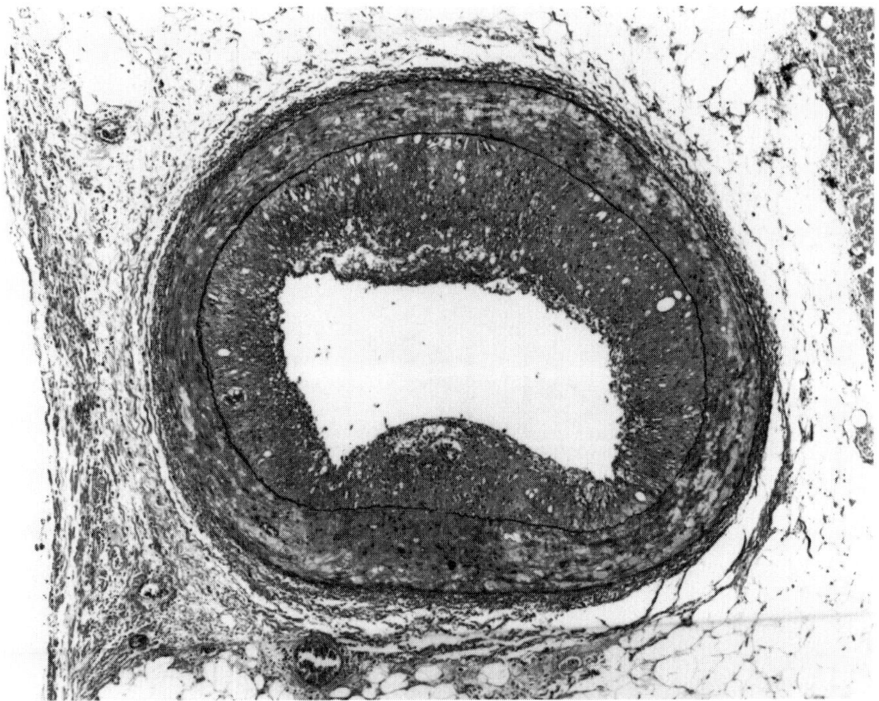

FIG. 5.16   Cross-section of epicardial coronary artery from a cardiac transplant recipient with intimal thickening characteristic of graft coronary disease. The internal elastic lamina is intact. Elastic van Giessen; magnification ×20.

plement) to the endothelial cells results in activated inflammatory and vascular wall cells releasing cytokines and growth factors that may stimulate smooth muscle cell proliferation.[28] Increased class II major histocompatability complex antigen expression in endothelial cells has also been postulated to play a role. These molecular studies have resulted in the development of new immunosuppressive drugs[29] that may reduce the development of graft coronary disease. Pathologic findings in the coronary vessels are similar in children and infants.[30] Currently the only satisfactory treatment for graft coronary disease is retransplantation of the affected organ. In a few cases, angioplasty has been successful for a limited time.

Despite the many pathologic changes that can occur, cardiac transplantation offers an excellent chance of long-term survival and functional rehabilitation for the carefully selected patient with end-stage heart disease.

ACKNOWLEDGMENT

This project was funded in part by National Heart, Lung, and Blood Institute Grant HL13108-24.

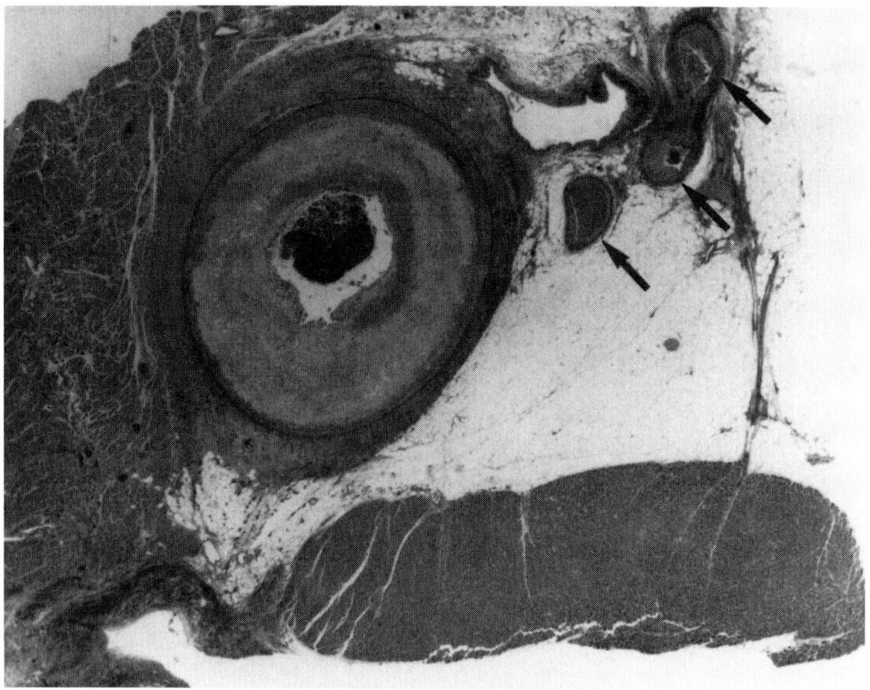

FIG. 5.17 Cross-section of epicardial coronary vessel from a transplant recipient showing marked intimal proliferation extending to small branches (*arrows*). Elastic van Gieson: magnification ×10.

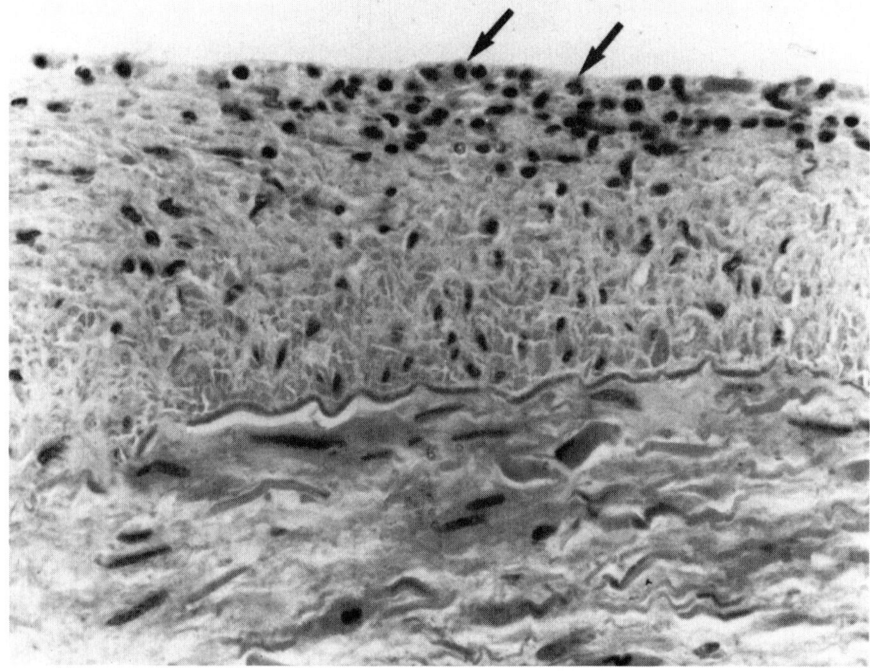

FIG. 5.18 Section of portion of coronary artery expanding intima showing an endothelialitis of lymphocytes (*arrow*). Hematoxylin and eosin; magnification ×400.

REFERENCES

1. Hosenpud JD. The Registry of the International Society for Heart and Lung Transplantation: Eleventh Official Report. Venice, March 1994.

2. Mason JW: Techniques for right and left endomyocardial biopsy. *Am J Cardiol* 1978; 41:887–892.

3. Tilkian AG, Daily EK. Endomyocardial biopsy. In: Tilkian AG, Daily EK, eds. *Cardiovascular procedures* St. Louis: CV Mosby 1986:180–203.

4. Spiegelhalter DJ, Stovin PGI. An analysis of repeated biopsies following cardiac transplantation. *Stat Med* 1983; 2:33.

5. Weil RR, Clarke D.R., Iwaki Y, Porteu KA. Hyperacute rejection of a transplanted human heart. *Transplantation* 1981; 32:71–72.

6. Basile L, Zerba T, Rabin B, Clarke J., Abrams A and Cerilli J. Identification of the antibody to vascular endothelial cells in patients undergoing cardiac transplantation. *Transplantation* 1985; 40:672–674.

7. Billingham, ME. Dilemma of variety of histopathologic grading systems for acute cardiac allograft rejection by endomyocardial biopsy. *J Heart Transplant* 1990; 9:272–276.

8. Billingham ME, Carey N.R.B., Hammond M.E., Kemnitz J., Marboe C, McAllister H.A. et al. A working formulation for the standardization of nomenclature in the diagnosis of heart and lung rejection: heart rejection study group. *J Heart Transplant* 1990; 9:587–592.

9. Joshi A, Masek MA, Billingham ME. Quilty revisited. *Mod Pathol.* 1993; 6:24A.

10. Weiss LM, Movahed LA, Berry GJ, Billingham ME. *In situ* hybridization studies for viral nucleic acids in heart and lung allograft biopsies. *Am J Clin Pathol.* 1990; 93:675–679.

11. Hammond EH, Yowell RL, Nunoda S, et al. Vascular (humoral) rejection in heart transplantation: pathologic observations and clinical implications. *J Heart Transplant* 1989; 8:430–443.

12. Hammond EH, Hansen JH, Spencer LS, et al. Vascular rejection in cardiac transplantation: histologic, immunopathologic and ultrastructural features. *Cardiovasc Pathol* 1993;2:1–14.

13. Bonnaud EN, Lewis NP, Masek MA, Billingham ME. Reliability and usefulness of immunofluorescence (IF) in cardiac transplantation. *J Heart Lung Transplant* 13 (Abstract 6):S33. 1994.

14. Cleary ML, Sklar J. Lymphoproliferative disorders in cardiac transplant recipients are multiclonal lymphomas. *Lancet* 1982; 2:489.

15. Cleary ML, Warnke R, Sklar J. Monoclonality of lymphoproliferative lesions in cardiac transplant recipients: clonal analysis based on immunoglobulin-gene rearrangements. *N Engl J Med* 1984;310:477.

16. Starzl TE, Porter KA, Iwatsuki S, et al. Reversibility of lymphomas and lymphoproliferative lesions developing under cyclosporine steroid therapy. *Lancet* 1984;1:583–587.

17. Rowan RA, Billingham ME. Pathologic changes in the long-term transplanted heart: a morphometric study of myocardial hypertrophy, vascularity and fibrosis. *Hum Pathol* 1990;21:767–772.

18. Karch SB, Billingham ME. Cyclosporine induced myocardial fibrosis: A uniquely controlled case report. *J Heart Transplant* 1985;4:210–212.

19. Tazelaar HD, Gay RE, Rowan RA, Billingham ME, Gay S. Collagen profile in the transplanted heart. *Hum Pathol* 1990;21:424–428.

20. Rowan RA, Billingham ME. Myocardial innervation in long-term cardiac transplant survivors: a quantitative ultrastructural survey. *J Heart Transplant* 1988;7:448–452.

21. Gao SZ, Alderman EL, Schroeder JS, et al. Accelerated coronary vascular disease in the heart transplant patient; coronary arteriographic findings. *J Am Coll Cardiol* 1988;12:334–340.

22. Billingham ME. Cardiac transplant atherosclerosis. *Transplant Proc.* 1987;19:19–25.

23. Billingham ME. Histopathology of graft coronary disease. Presented at the 1991 Transplant Coronary Artery Disease Symposium, St. Louis, Missouri. *J Heart Lung Transplant* 1992;11:S38–S44.

24. Russell ME, Fujita M, Masek MA, Rowan RA, Billingham ME. Cardiac graft vascular disease: nonselective involvement of large and small vessels. *Transplantation* 1993;56:762–764.

25. Fujita M, Russell M, Masek MA, Rowan RA, Nagashima K. Billingham ME. Graft vascular disease in the great vessels and vasa vasorum. *Hum Pathol* 1993;24:1067–1072.
26. Pucci A, Forbes RDC, Berry GJ, Billingham ME. Accelerated post-transplant coronary arteriosclerosis in combined heart-lung transplantation. *Transplant Proc* 1991;23:1228–1229.
27. Ross R. The pathogenesis of atherosclerosis: a perspective for the 1990s. *Nature* 1993;362:801–809.
28. Schoen FJ, Libby P. Cardiac transplant graft anteriosclerosis. *Trends Cardiovasc Med* 1991;1:216–223.
29. Gregory CR, Pratt RE, Huie P, et al. Effects of treatment with cyclosporine, FK 506, rapamycin, mycophenolic acid, or deoxyspergualin on vascular muscle proliferation *in vitro* in *in vivo*. *Transplant Proc* 1993;25:770–771.
30. Berry GJ, Rizeq MN, Weiss LM, Billingham ME. Graft coronary disease in pediatric heart and combined heart-lung transplant recipients: a study of fifteen cases. *J Heart Lung Transplant.* 1993;12:S309–S319.

Note Added in Proof
On December 9, 1994, many of the original pathologists who formulated the International Society for Heart and Lung Transplantation (ISHLT) Standardized Nomenclature for Heart Rejection met at Stanford to modify and simplify this system, based on experience gained since its introduction in 1990. A publication describing the changes is planned.

Chapter 6

Diagnostic Vascular Pathology: Still the Old Fashion Way

J. T. LIE

Although the underlying course and nature of the vascular lesions may differ according to geographic regions, diseases of the blood vessels accounts for more than 50% of the mortality and morbidity of people the world over, particularly among the aging populations. Effectual clinical management of any vascular disease must be based ultimately on sound knowledge of the pathology and correct diagnosis. A successful outcome in diagnostic vascular pathology is more assured when the answers to all the right questions are at hand.

Vascular disease affects not only the blood vessels but also the tissues and organs nourished by these blood vessels and, therefore, often results in serious or life-threatening consequences. The treatment of different types of vascular disease varies widely, from aspirin to the drastic immunosuppressive and cytotoxic agents, which are rarely without harmful side effects. The right choice cannot be made without a correct histopathologic diagnosis. The clinical and angiographic features of vasculopathies frequently overlap and the laboratory tests are seldom specific or diagnostic. It behooves the pathologist to master the art of diagnostic vascular pathology the old fashion way by practicing the same two essential elementary principles that Sir Arthur Conan Doyle (1859–1930) prescribed to immortalize the fictional super-sleuth, Sherlock Holmes: careful observation and analytical deduction.

WHAT TYPE OF BLOOD VESSELS ARE INVOLVED?

The family of blood vessels comprises structurally and functionally different elastic and muscular large, medium-sized, and small arteries, and the corresponding veins; arterioles and venules; and the capillaries; and each has its own unique normal histology and aging and reactive changes.[1,2] Some diseases occur only in blood vessels of certain size ranges and some involve only the arteries, whereas others affect both arteries and veins; this is true for both atherosclerotic and nonatherosclerotic degenerative vascular disease[3] and, especially, the various types of systemic, pulmonary, and cerebral vasculitides.[4–8]

In angiodysplasia, or the so-called arteriovenous malformation, either arteries or veins, or both, may be involved and, at times, the blood vessel appears morphologically to be a hybrid that resembles neither an artery nor a vein (Fig. 6.1).

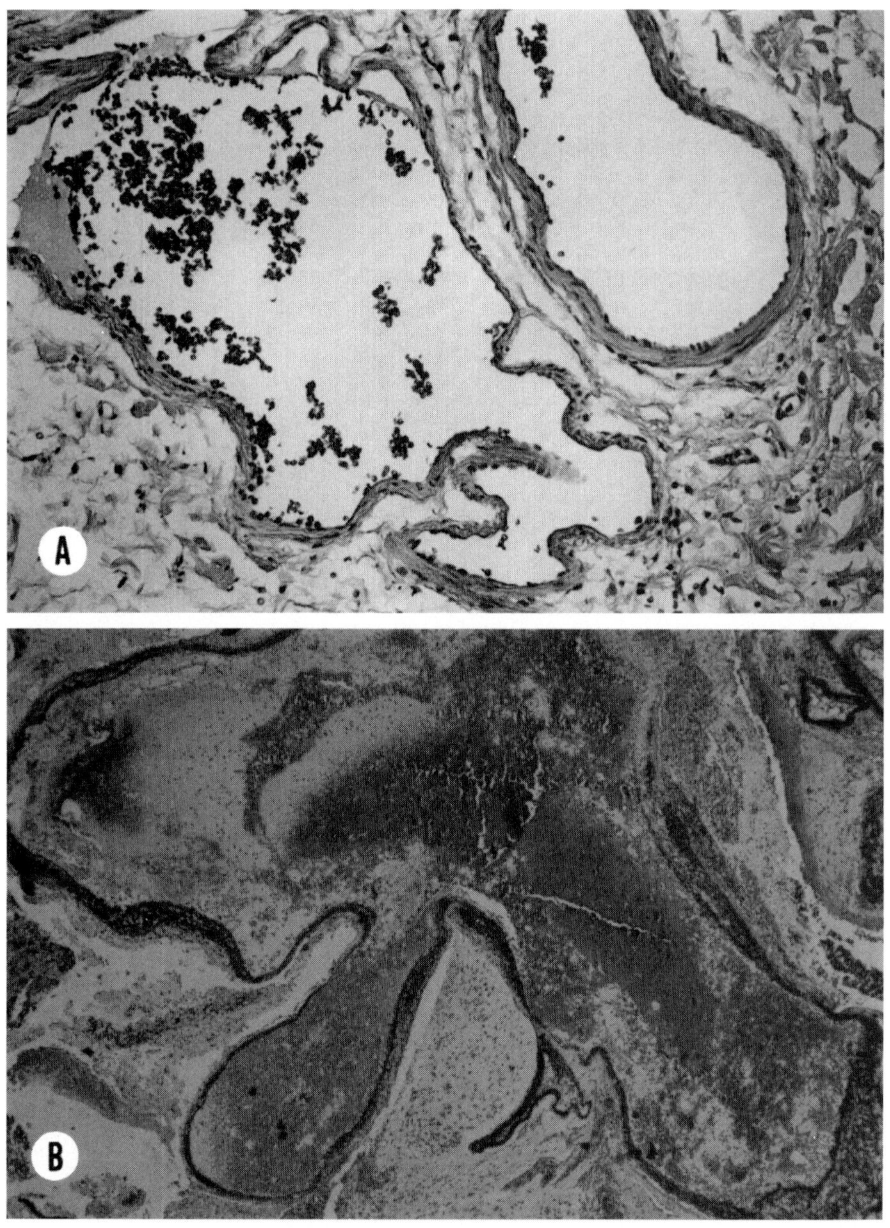

FIG. 6.1.   Photomicrographs of convoluted and dilated thin-walled nonartery/nonvein blood vessels in angiodysplasia of the gut (*A*) and brain (*B*). The lesions are commonly and still referred to by many as "arteriovenous malformation." Magnification: *A*, ×160; *B*, ×40.

In another situation, hemangioma is the vascular anomaly rather than arteriovenous malformation (Fig. 6.2). In Klippel-Trenaunay syndrome the pathologic lesions consist of both angiodysplasia and hemangiomas.[9]

WHAT HISTOLOGIC PREPARATIONS ARE NEEDED?

In diagnostic vascular pathology, the ability to recognize blood vessels in tissue sections and to distinguish arteries from veins is of paramount importance. It is imperative that all histologic preparations for the diagnosis of any vascular disease must routinely include elastin-stained sections to aid the identification of blood vessels and to facilitate the visual distinction between arteries and veins. The need is just as great for an experienced pathologist as for a novice.[6] In a cellularly crowded field of intense inflammation and tissue destruction, the small-caliber blood vessels are often obscured and altered beyond recognition in the hematoxylin-eosin sections. They can be revealed only by the stainable elastic fiber network pattern of the vessel walls, which often persists even after the cellular part of the blood vessel wall is damaged beyond recognition (Fig. 6.3).

It is the unique elastic fiber network pattern of the vascular wall matrix structure that distinguishes a vein from an artery, not the size, the wall thickness, or the presence or absence of an internal elastic lamina.[4–7] Elastin-stained sections are also essential for the diagnosis of medial degeneration (so-called cystic medionecrosis) in Marfan syndrome, Ehlers-Danlos syndrome, or idiopathic medionecrosis of Endheim, which may escape detection in the hematoxylin-eosin–stained sections. Likewise, the telltale marked medial atrophy and adventitial fibrosis of inflammatory aortic aneurysm[10,11] become readily apparent only in an elastin-stained section; without it, the lesion could be and has been misdiagnosed as aortitis (Fig. 6.4).

For the histological examination of vast majority of different types of vascular disease, cross-sections of the blood vessels are usually preferred and adequate for diagnosis. The examination of multiple or serial sections is necessary and highly desirable for the diagnosis of vasculitis, which is often focal and segmental in distribution and, thus, can be easily missed in a single histologic section.[6] In small biopsies, the identification or finding of a solitary focus of vasculitis may be more fortuitous than the pathologist's diagnostic acumen (Fig. 6.5 and 6.6).

Fibromuscular dysplasia (FMD) is a nonatherosclerotic and noninflammatory vascular disease.[12] The most common variety of FMD, medial dysplasia, is characterized by longitudinal corrugation of the vessel wall created by the hill-and-valley type, alternating segments of medial proliferation and deficiency. If FMD is suspected, the blood vessel in question should be sectioned longitudinally when the tissue sample is submitted for histological examination. Cross-sectional preparation, with rare exceptions, is unsuitable and may be misleading for a definitive diagnosis of FMD (Fig. 6.7).

WHAT IS KNOWN ABOUT THE VASCULAR DISEASE?

One is always more likely to find the right answer when one knows what evidence to look for, where to look, and how to look, in making a correct diagnosis of any vascular disease. This can be done only if one knows the disease in

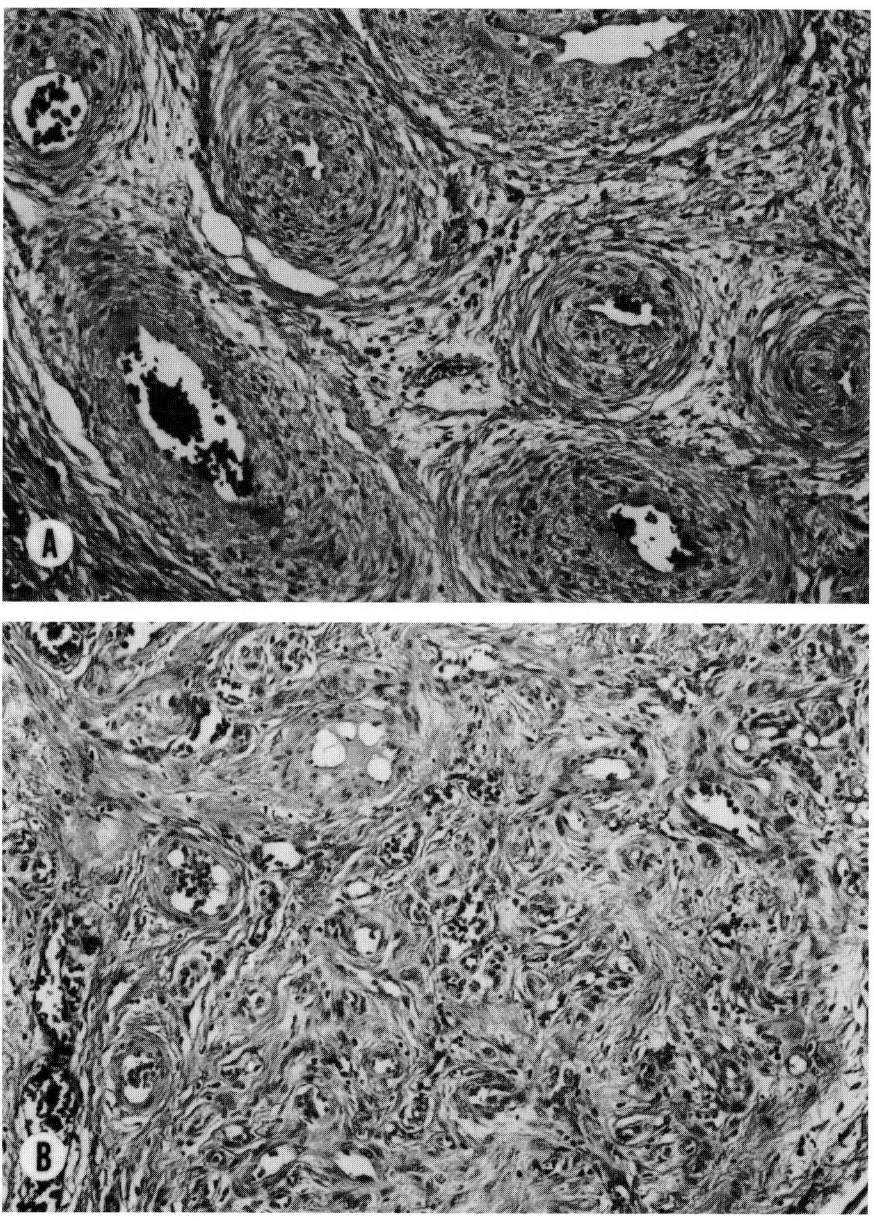

FIG. 6.2. Large (*A*) and small (*B*) arteriolar hemangioma variants of soft tissue angiodysplasia that may be diagnosed as "arteriovenous malformation" clinically and angiographically. Magnification: *A* and *B*, ×160.

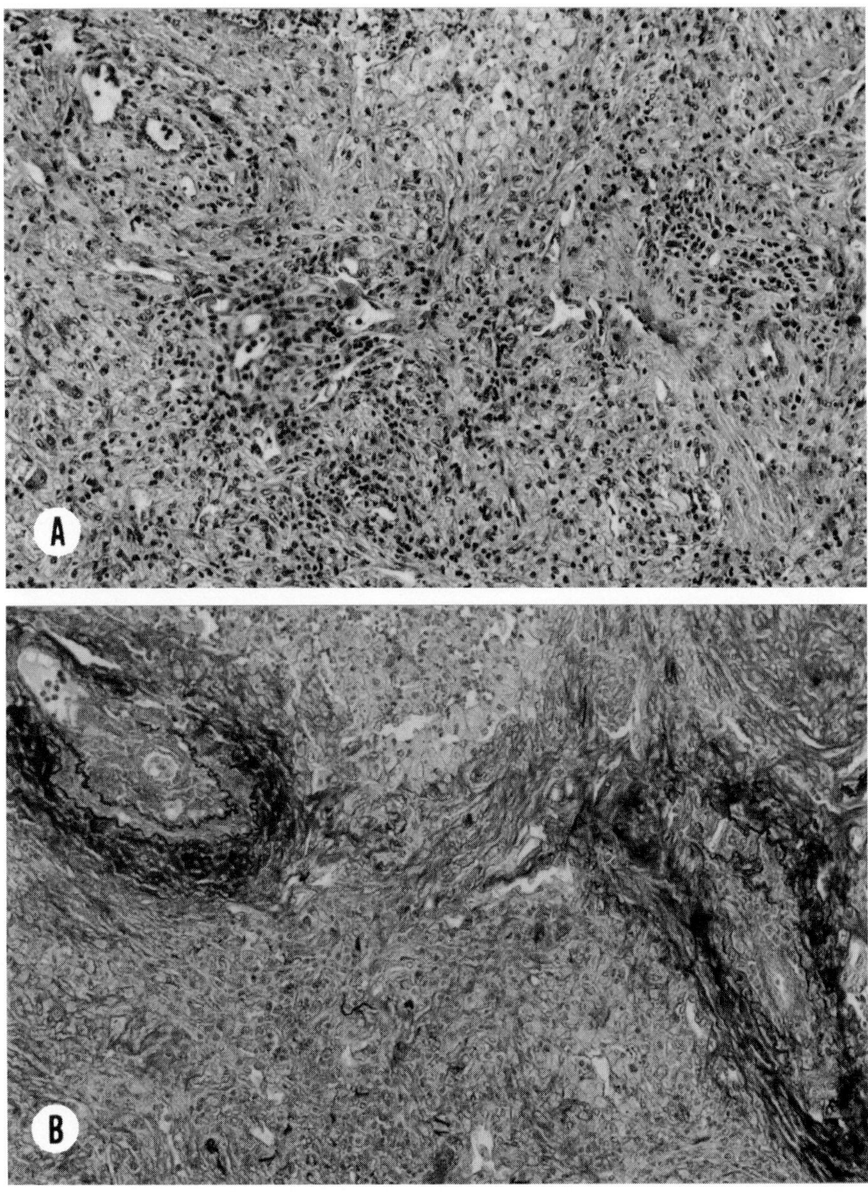

FIG. 6.3. Pulmonary vascular lesions may become obscured in a busy hypercellular background of intense inflammation and tissue destruction in a hematoxylin-eosin section (*A*). The vascular lesions become readily apparent in the companion elastin-stained section (*B*) as involving both small artery and small vein. Magnification: *A* and *B*, ×160.

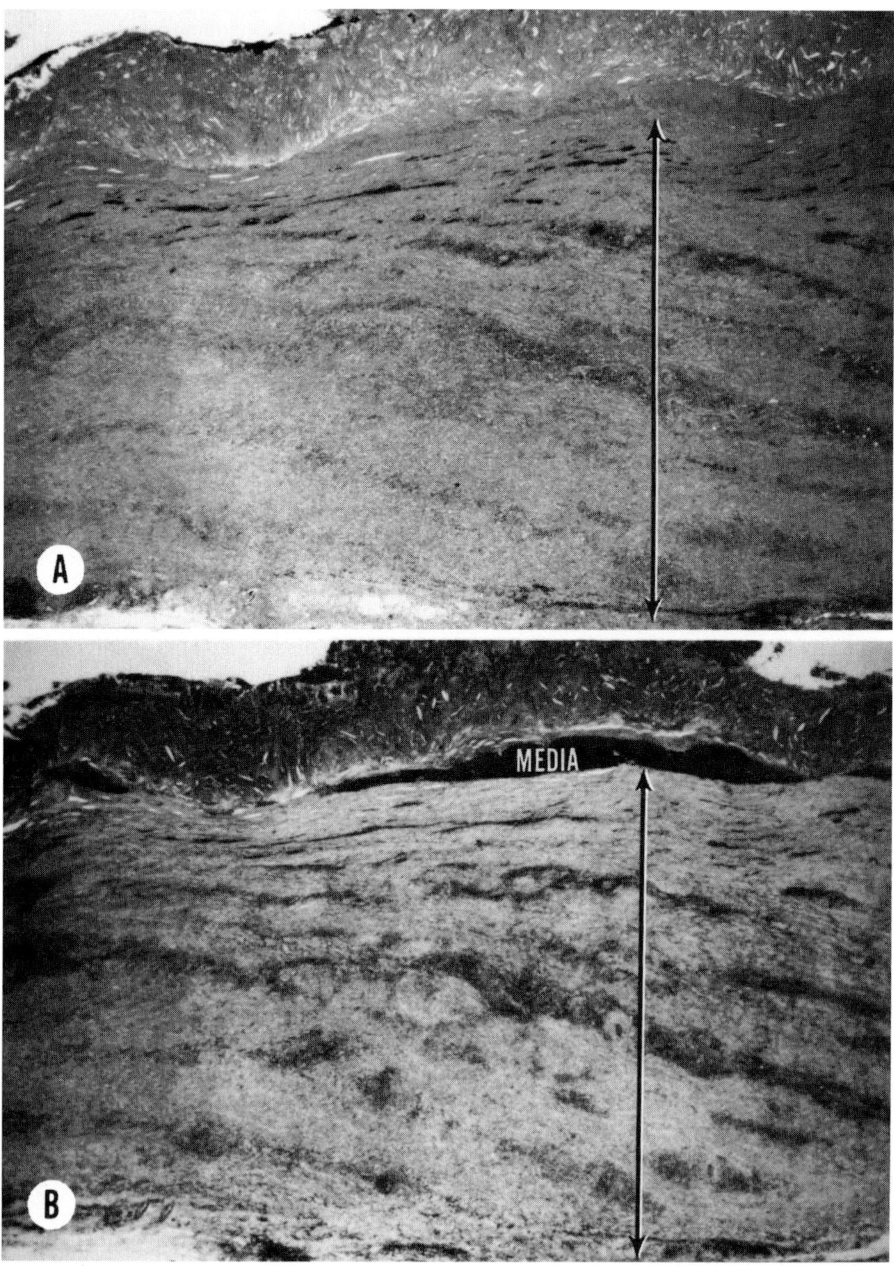

FIG. 6.4.   An aortic lesion was originally diagnosed as aortitis in a hematoxylin-eosin section
(*A*) based on the erroneous visual perception of diffuse cell infiltrate in the media (*arrow*). The
companion elastin stained section (*B*) correctly identify the atrophic media. What was thought to
be media with cell infiltrate (*arrows*) in the hematoxylin-eosin section is in fact marked adventitial fibrosis with lymphoplasmacytic infiltrate, diagnostic of inflammatory aneurysm of the aorta.
Magnification: *A* and *B*, ×16.

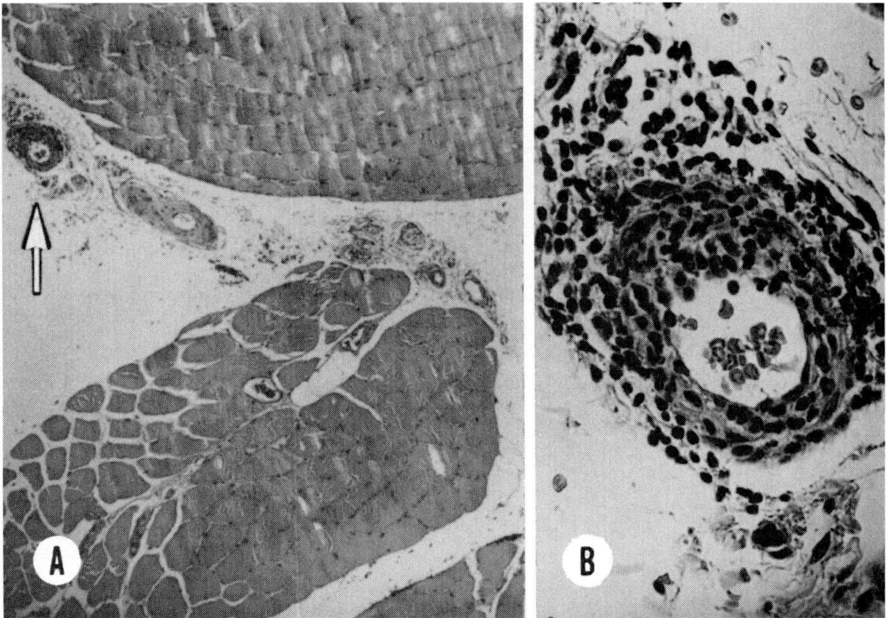

FIG. 6.5.   Serendipity in biopsy diagnosis of vasculitis. The solitary small blood vessel (*arrow*) that shows vasculitis is located right at the edge of a histologic section (*A*): the lesion could easily have not been included in the submitted tissue sample, seen at higher magnification in *B*. Magnification: *A*, ×40; *B*, ×400.

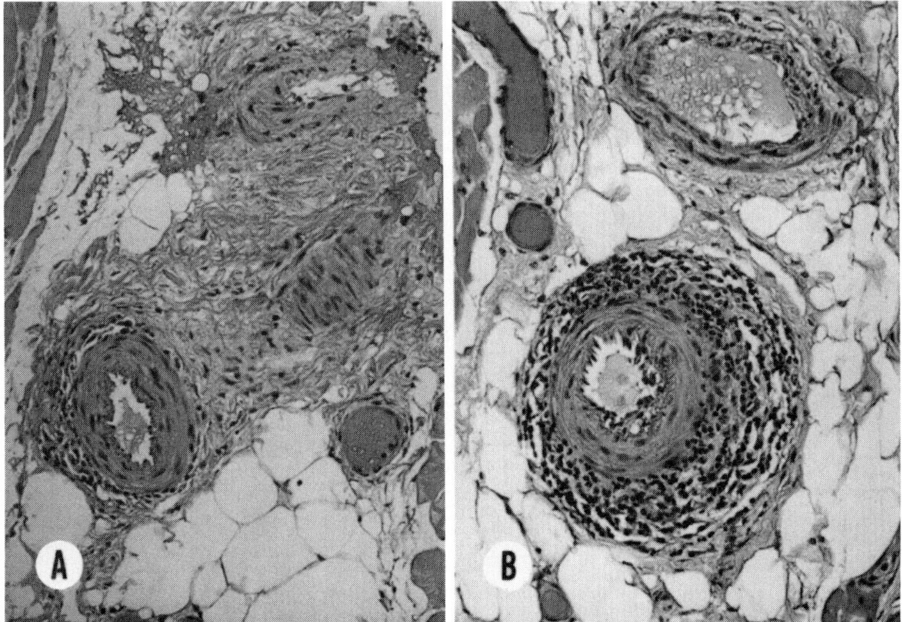

FIG. 6.6.   Small-vessel vasculitis as seen in serial sections of a muscle biopsy. What initially appears as a nondiagnostic or equivocal lesion (*A*) becomes an unequivocal positive vasculitis finding (*B*). The sections are 50 μm apart. Magnification: *A*, and *B*, ×160.

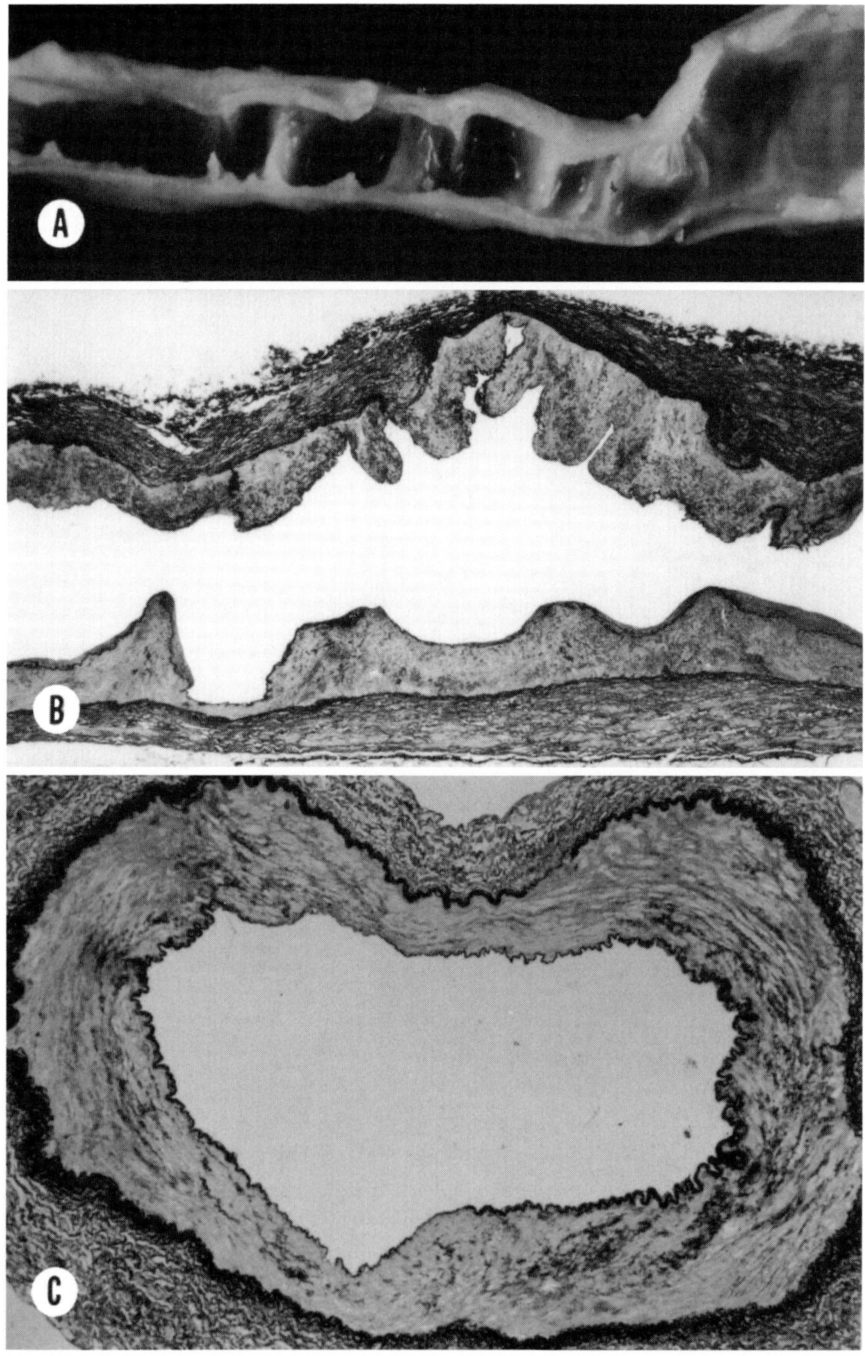

FIG. 6.7.   Correct preparation of arterial sample for the diagnosis of fibromuscular dysplasia is to section the artery longitudinally (*A*) to visualize and identify the corrugated dysplastic media (*B*); this diagnostic configuration is lost or becomes inapparent in a cross-section of the same artery (*C*). Magnification: *A,* ×4, *B,* ×16, *C,* ×160.

question well and have the right specimen to examine. A few selected illustrative examples are instructive.

BUERGER'S DISEASE

The vascular lesion in Buerger's disease is most diagnostic at the early acute phase, and when the vein is affected, readily recognizable clinically as in superficial thrombophlebitis. If such lesions are biopsied, they often show occlusive thrombosis of the vein with transmural inflammation and, within the organizing thrombus, one or more focal collections of polymorphonuclear cells with karyorrhexis ("microabscesses") and containing one or more multinucleated foreign-body–type giant cells (Fig. 6.8). The vascular lesions at the intermediate or subacute phase may be only suggestive of the disease. At the chronic phase or end stage of the disease, as would be seen in amputated specimens, the bland, fibrotic, occluded arteries and veins without any residual signs of inflammation are totally nondiagnostic.[5]

GIANT CELL ARTERITIS

Both temporal arteritis and Takayasu arteritis are giant cell arteritis. However, the granulomatous inflammation with a predominantly lymphoplasmacytic infiltrate is seen only in the active phase of both of these entities. Furthermore, the number of giant cells within the transmural inflammation is highly variable; the giant cells, when present, are focal and segmental in distribution. In an analysis of a large series of 535 patients with temporal arteritis,[13] less than 50% of all positive temporal artery biopsies have identifiable giant cells. In some of these positive biopsies the infiltrate in the vessel wall is entirely lymphomononuclear and the granuloma is in the adventitia (Fig. 6.9). Therefore, the identification or finding of giant cells is not a prerequisite for the diagnosis of giant cell arteritis in the appropriate histopathologic setting of arterial biopsies.[4,14]

POLYARTERITIS NODOSA

Polyarteritis nodosa is a necrotizing vasculitis affecting medium-sized and small arteries. Characteristically, it has an irregular distribution in the target organs; active and healed lesions often occur side by side, as may uninvolved and involved vessels. Polyarteritis nodosa is a systemic disease, but it can also occur in isolated organs, which are often clinically asymptomatic. The inflammatory infiltrate in small-vessel lesions may occasionally have a granulomatous character (Fig. 6.10). The veins, cerebral and pulmonary blood vessels are rarely affected, and there are no credible (with proper histologic documentation) known cases of polyarteritis involving the aorta, the aortic arch branches, and arteries in the limbs.[6]

WEGENER'S GRANULOMATOSIS

The histopathology of Wegener's granulomatosis is first and foremost a necrotizing granulomatous inflammation, and vasculitis is found in less than 50% of cases. The classic form involves the upper and lower respiratory tracts and the kidney, but virtually any organ may be affected. The so-called limited form of Wegener's granulomatosis has no overt renal involvement. Although

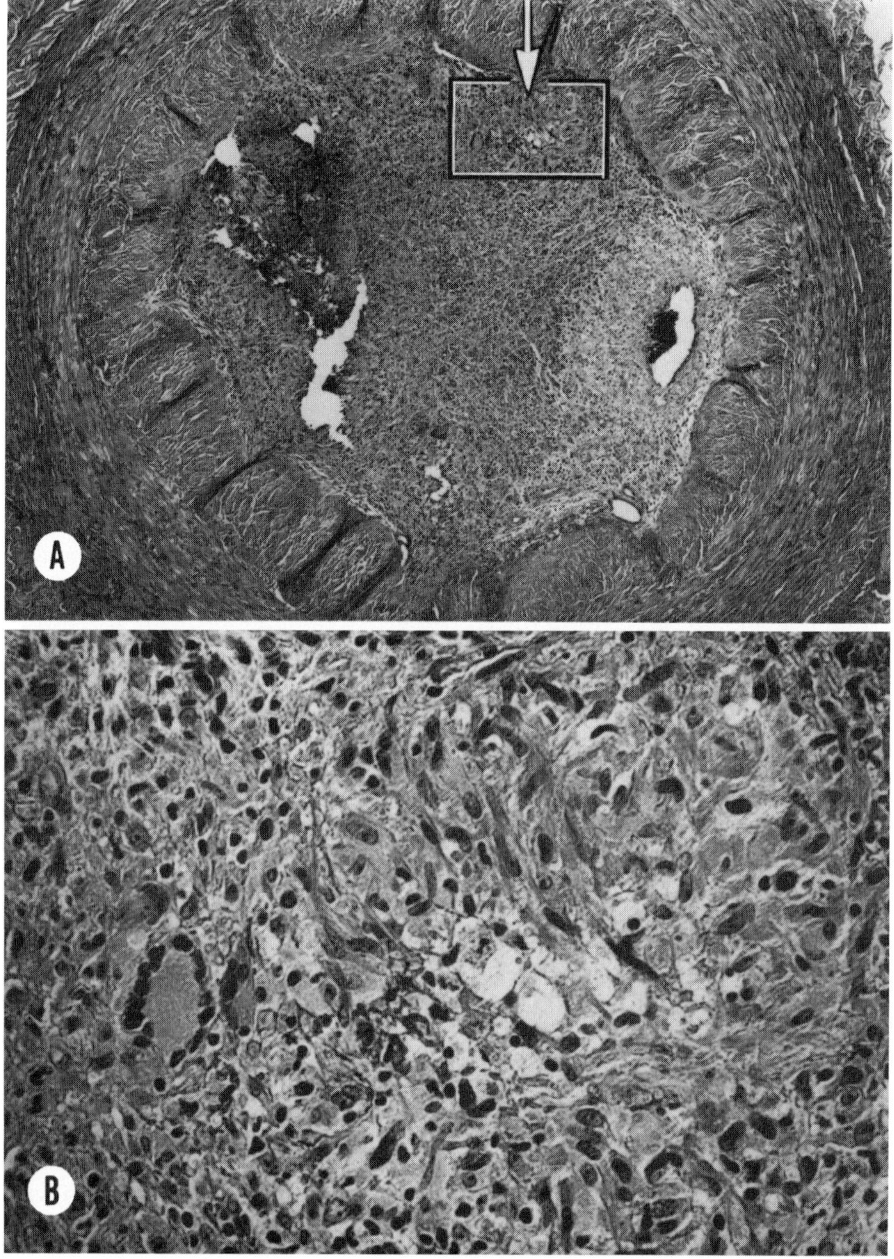

FIG. 6.8. Diagnostic histopathology of acute-phase Buerger's disease (*A*) is a peculiar form of thrombophlebitis with granulomatous inflammation of an organizing thrombus containing "microabscesses" (*arrow*), which is shown at higher magnification in *B* to show the giant cell. Magnification: *A,* ×64, *B,* ×400.

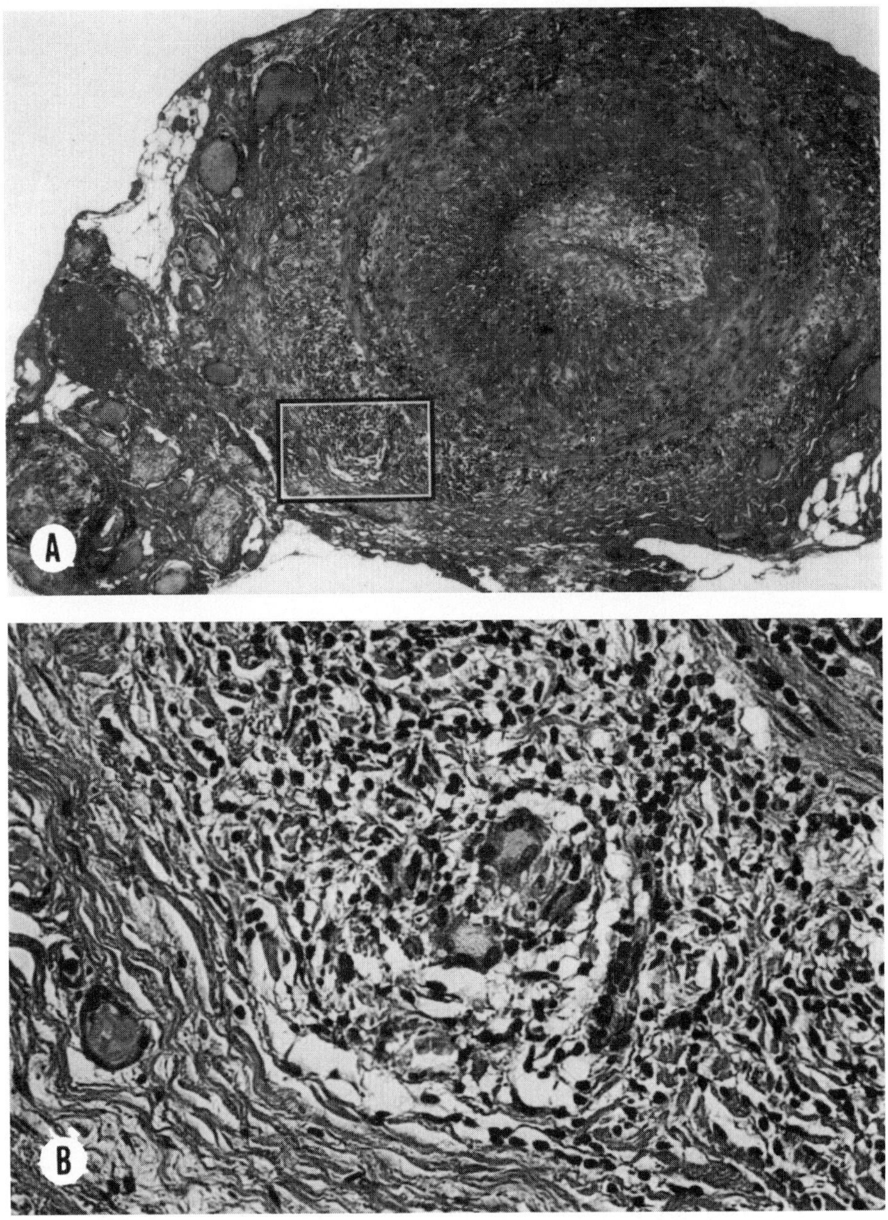

FIG. 6.9. A positive biopsy for temporal arteritis (*A*) with only lymphomononuclear infiltrate in the vessel wall and a granuloma with giant cells outside in the adventitia (*boxed area*), which is shown at higher magnification in *B*. Magnification: *A*, ×64; *B*, ×400.

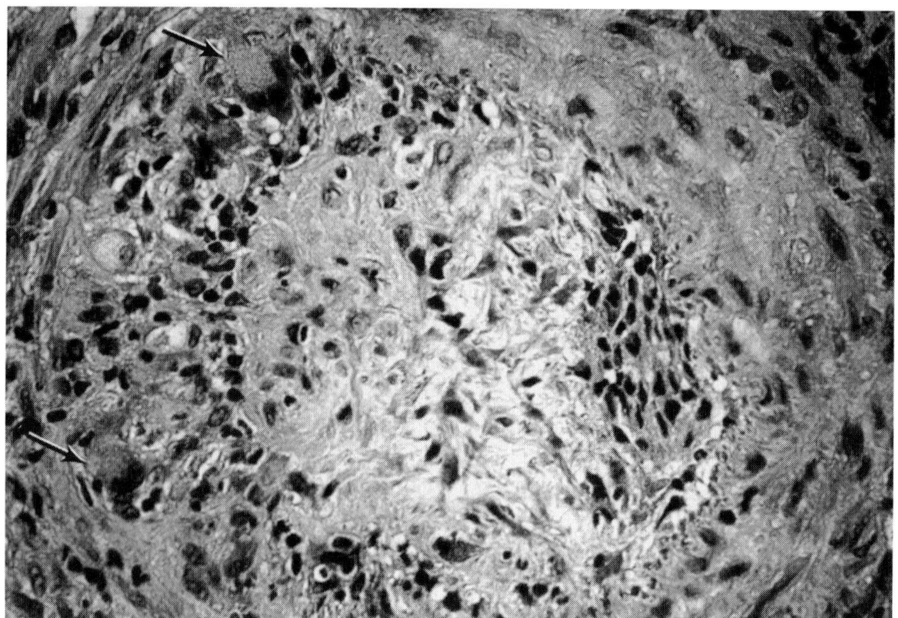

FIG. 6.10.   An uncommon granulomatous small-vessel vasculitis lesion of polyarteritis nodosa, with giant cells (*arrows*). Magnification: ×400.

the geographic-pattern tissue necrosis is the hallmark of the disease in the lung, extrapulmonary lesions are more variable. Vasculitis, when present, may be granulomatous or necrotizing in character, and are usually confined to small blood vessels.[6,7] About 30% of Wegener's granulomatosis may present as pulmonary capillaritis and the alveolar hemorrhage syndrome (Fig. 6.11).[15,16]

CHURG-STRAUSS SYNDROME

Originally known as allergic granulomatosis and angiitis, Churg-Strauss syndrome is a relatively uncommon form of systemic vasculitis with histologic features that overlap polyarteritis nodosa and Wegener's granulomatosis.[17] The classic form is characterized by the triad of pulmonary and systemic vasculitis and extravascular granulomas with prominent eosinophil infiltrate occurring almost exclusively in individuals with asthma or a history of allergy. A limited form of Churg-Strauss syndrome[18] is defined as eosinophilic vascular and extravascular lesions occurring only in isolated organs, most commonly in the gastrointestinal tract (Fig. 6.12).

WHAT ARE THE MIMICS AND SIMULATORS?

The manifestations of systemic vasculitis are characteristically diverse and unpredictable. Without pathognomonic clinical signs and symptoms, or specific laboratory tests, the diagnosis of vasculitis is essentially based on pattern recognition and analytical deduction of the overt clinical features and angiographic findings, and only infrequently on confirmatory biopsies of the affected tissue organs. However, a variety of common and uncommon nonvasculitic disorders may

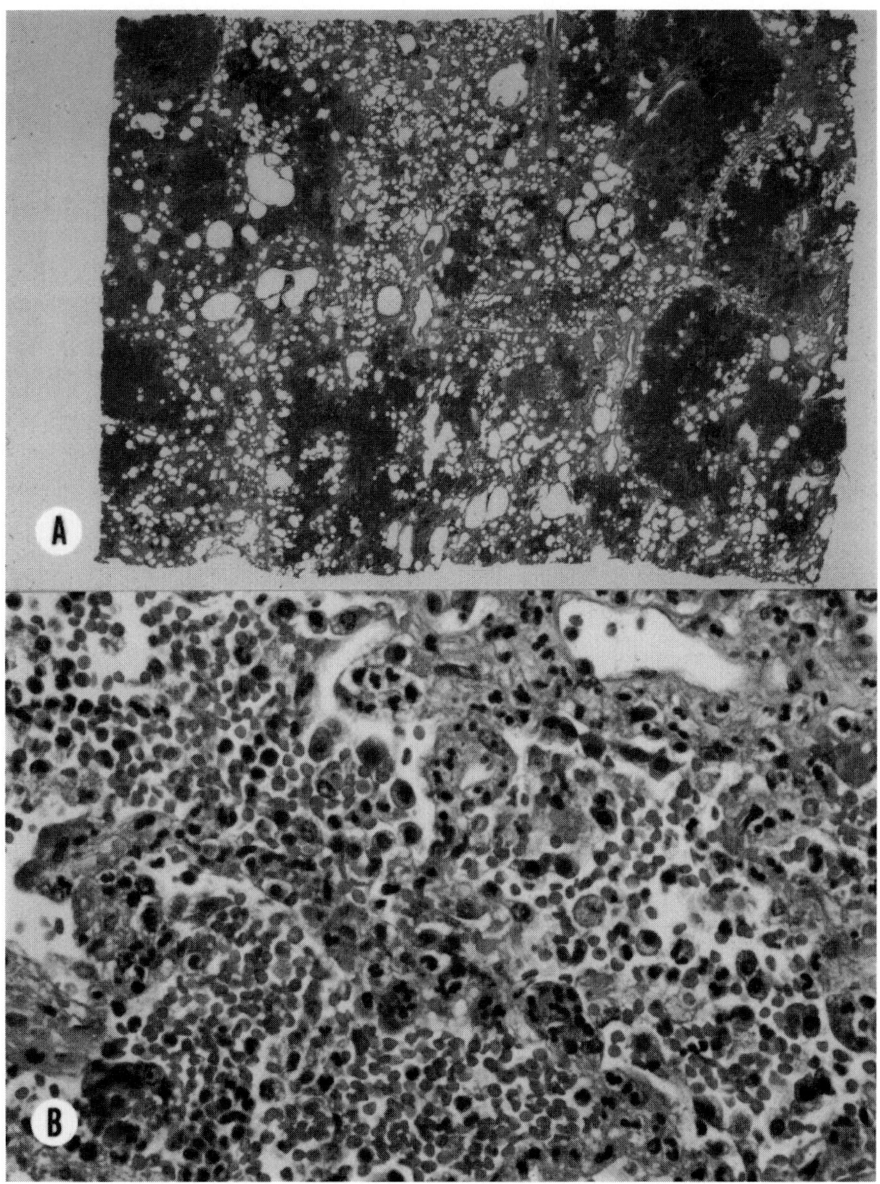

FIG. 6.11. Wegener's granulomatosis presenting as diffuse alveolar hemorrhage (*A*), clinically with hemoptysis. High magnification view of pulmonary capillaritis and alveolar hemorrhage (*B*). Magnification: *A,* ×4, *B,* ×400.

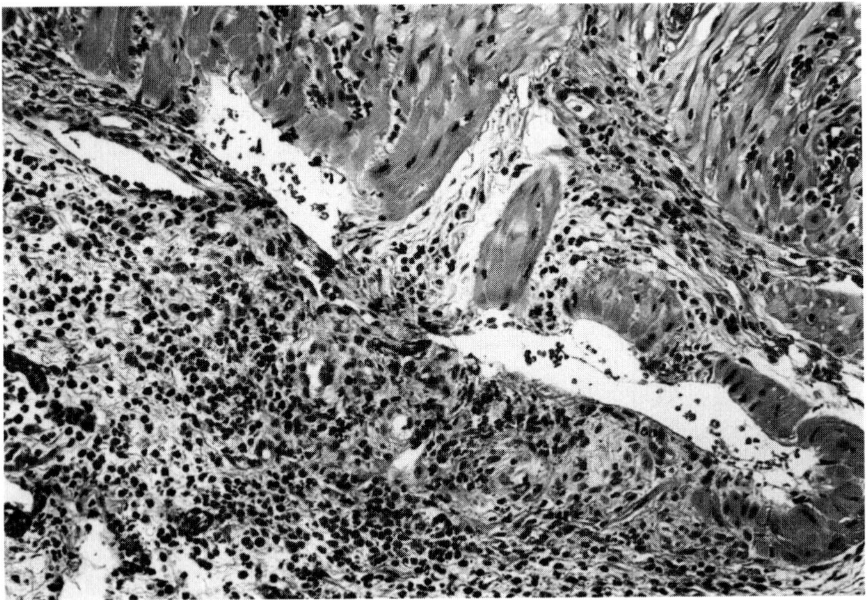

FIG. 6.12.　Limited form of Churg-Strauss syndrome manifesting as isolated granulomatous eosinophilic vasculitis of the gastrointestinal tract. Magnification: ×160.

TABLE 6.1.　VASCULITIS LOOK-ALIKES AND MIMICKERS

Cholesterol atheroembolism
Endocarditis embolism
Cardiac myxoma embolism
Arterial dysplasia, hypoplasia, or coarctation
Chronic ergotism
Radiation-induced arteriopathy
Vasculopathy of antiphospholipid syndromes
Vasculopathy of neurofibromatosis
Ehlers-Danlos syndrome
Köhlmeier-Degos disease
Sweet's syndrome (acute febrile neutrophilic dermatosis)
Malignant angioendotheliomatosis

mimic true vasculitis clinically, angiographically, or even histologically.[19,20] These vasculitis look-alikes are often unexpected and consist of a long list of miscellaneous conditions (Table 6.1). They often elude recognition unless there is a high index of clinical suspicion. It behooves the practicing pathologist to be on the alert to distinguish vasculitis simulators from true vasculitis to prevent exposing the patient to the unnecessary harmful effects of treatment with corticosteroids and cytotoxic agents, the mainstay of drug therapy of systemic vasculitis.

CONCLUSION

To be successful at diagnostic vascular pathology requires the intellectual faculty of careful observation and analytical deduction. To accomplish the task, one adopts the same principles as they have been applied to the strategic planning for a successful military campaign. These would include a thorough understanding of the enemy's strengths and weaknesses, familiarity with the terrain of the battleground, proper selection of the weaponry, and the ability to recognize allies from hostile forces and to act accordingly in an apparent confrontation.

REFERENCES

1. Lie JT. The structure of the normal vascular system and its reactive changes. In: Juergens JL, Spittell JA, Jr., Fairbairn JF, II, eds. *Allen-Barker-Hines peripheral vascular diseases*. 5th ed. Philadelphia: WB Saunders, 1980:51–81.
2. Lie JT, Brown AL Jr., Cater ET. Spectrum of aging changes in temporal arteries: Its significance in interpretation of biopsy of temporal artery. *Arch Pathol Lab Med* 1970;90:278–285.
3. Lie JT, Juergens JL. Degenerative arterial disease other than atherosclerosis. In: Juergens JL, Spittell JA, Jr., Fairbairn JF II, eds. *Allen-Barker-Hines Peripheral Vascular Diseases*, 5th ed. Philadelphia: WB Saunders, 1980:237–251.
4. Lie JT. The classification and diagnosis of vasculitis in large and medium-sized blood vessels. *Pathol Annu* 1987;22 (part 1):125–162.
5. Lie JT. Thromboangiitis obliterans (Buerger's disease) revisited. *Pathol Annu* 1988;23 (part 2):257–291.
6. Lie JT. Systemic and isolated vasculitis: A rational approach to diagnosis and pathologic diagnosis. *Pathol Annu* 1989;24 (part 1):25–114.
7. Lie JT. Classification of pulmonary angiitis and granulomatosis: Histopathologic perspectives. *Semin Respir Med* 1989;10:111–121.
8. Lie JT. Primary (granulomatous) angiitis of the central nervous system: a clinicopathologic analysis of 15 new cases and review of the literature. *Hum Pathol* 1992;23:164–171.
9. Lie JT. Pathology of angiodysplasia in Klippel-Trenaunay syndrome. *Pathol Res Pract* 1988;183:747–755.
10. Pennell RC, Hollier LH, Lie JT, et al. Inflammatory abdominal aortic aneurysms. *J Vasc Surg* 1985;2:859–869.
11. Lie JT. Inflammatory aneurysm of the aorta or chronic periaortitis: a nosologic quandary. *Cardiovasc Pathol* 1992;1:75–77.
12. Lüscher TF, Lie JT, Stanson AW, et al. Arterial fibromuscular dysplasia. *Mayo Clin Proc* 1987;62:931–952.
13. Achkar AA, Lie JT, Hunder GG, et al. Prior corticosteroid therapy on temporal artery biopsy results. *Arthritis Rheum* 1993;36 (Suppl):S95.
14. Lie JT. Diagnostic histopathology of major systemic and pulmonary vasculitic syndromes. *Rheum Dis Clin North Am* 1990;16:269–292.
15. Travis WD, Carpenter HA, Lie JT. Capillaritis and pulmonary hemorrhage in Wegener's granulomatosis. *Am J Surg Pathol* 1989;13:78–79.
16. Travis WD, Colby TV, Lombard C, Carpenter HA. A clinicopathologic study of 34 cases of diffuse pulmonary hemorrhage with lung biopsy confirmation. *Am J Surg Pathol* 1990;14:1112–1125.
17. Lie JT. The classification of vasculitis and a reappraisal of allergic granulomatosis and angiitis (Churg-Strauss syndrome). *Mount Sinai J Med* 1986;53:429–439.
18. Lie JT. The limited forms of Churg-Strauss syndrome. *Pathol Annu* 1993;28:199–220.
19. Lie JT. Vasculopathy in the antiphospholipid syndromes: thrombosis or vasculitis, or both? *J Rheumatol* 1989;16:713–715.
20. Lie JT. Vasculitis simulators and vasculitis look-alikes. *Curr Opin Rheumatol* 1992;4:47–55.

Chapter 7

New Insights into the Genetic Basis of Aortic Aneurysms

HARRY C. DIETZ

Rupture of aortic aneurysm represents a significant cause of mortality in industrialized countries, accounting for greater than 1% of all deaths in this population.[1] Conventional wisdom had maintained that aneurysm formation in the general population was largely a secondary event, manifesting the isolated or cumulative ravages of primary hypertension, atherosclerosis, or unspecified albeit "normal" age-dependent processes. The notable and exclusive exceptions were the heritable disorders of connective tissue that include aortic aneurysm as a component of a disease phenotype that involves a diversity of tissues, such as Marfan syndrome or the "arterial" variant of Ehlers-Danlos syndrome. This conventional wisdom has now been challenged, and largely abandoned. As outlined in this chapter, erosion of its foundation has occurred in progressive fashion. Evidence for major genetic determinants that influence the occurrence and progression of aneurysmal disease will be presented. Although selected abnormal gene products may exert their pathogenic influence through adverse modulation of homeostatic mechanisms such as blood pressure control or cholesterol clearance, it is clear that others have a primary effect on the structural integrity of the vascular wall. A discussion of pathogenesis will be provided for the subset of conditions for which a molecular etiology has been determined.

The first major breakthrough in the transition from the "old" era to the new was the appreciation that first-degree relatives of a propositus with aortic aneurysm were at greater risk for a concordant phenotype than were members of the general population. Although preceded by multiple anecdotal reports, Tilson and Seashore are credited with the first large prospective family study examining the recurrence risk of abdominal aortic aneurysm (AAA).[2] Fifty families were identified with AAA occurring in two or more first-degree relatives. Many subsequent studies have confirmed these findings. Ultrasonographic screening of the family members of an index case suggests a risk of approximately 14.5% for offspring and a risk ranging from 13 to 32% for siblings.[2–7] Considering a prevalence of AAA in the general population of approximately 2–5%,[8] it is clear that a family history represents a major risk factor.

Although most studies agree that male sex compounds the risk, the relative importance of smoking, hypertension, and arterial occlusive disease in familial cases remains controversial.[3,6,7] The report of a large pedigree segregating aortic aneurysm in the absence of any recognized systemic disorder of connective tissue, hypertension, or advanced atherosclerosis demonstrates that at least a subset of familial cases manifest primary pathology of the arterial wall.[9] It is also clear that people with familial aortic aneurysm can present in childhood or early adult life and in the absence of a history of systemic cardiovascular disease (reviewed in Ref. 10). The lesson: the disease is not manifesting the effects of extreme or chronic stress on a normal vascular wall, but rather a vascular wall that is extremely predisposed to dilate in the presence of physiologic levels of hemodynamic stress.

Although autosomal recessive inheritance has been suggested, a clear autosomal dominant mode of transmission has been documented in selected families (reviewed in Ref. 11). It has also been proposed that the male sex predominance in familial cases may be due to X-linked recessive inheritance.[12] Many factors including variable and often late age of onset of the phenotype and perhaps a multifactorial etiology or incomplete penetrance can cloud interpretation of familial segregation patterns. Nevertheless, such data clearly implicate a major genetic determinant of disease in a substantial subset of patients.

A common strategy for the identification of disease genes makes use of localized sites of normal sequence variation, termed polymorphic markers, that are scattered throughout the human genome. Such landmarks can be used to track the inheritance pattern of specific regions of DNA through families displaying a phenotype of interest. If the phenotype is consistently coinherited with a specific copy of a region of DNA, then it is likely that the disease gene is close by. Linkage analysis relies upon the propensity for recombination to occur between two fixed points in the genome. The greater the physical distance between loci, the greater the frequency of recombination and the greater the chance that the two markers will be separated during meiosis and therefore will not appear in the same offspring. Using large and well-characterized families, it can be reasoned that the identification of a polymorphic marker allele that shows cosegregation with the aneurysm phenotype will allow precise localization of the site of genetic defect. With a location in hand, two approaches could be taken to identify the disease gene. Either genes that had already been localized to the region could be scrutinized (candidate gene approach) or new genes with coincident map positions could be found (positional cloning).

This approach for the identification of genes responsible for aortic aneurysm has been frustrated by the need for DNA samples from many persons in large kindreds where the mode of inheritance and the phenotypic status has been clearly identified. In most families the number of affected members available for participation is low because of early mortality, late emergence of the disease phenotype, or unclear inheritance patterns. As an alternative, selected investigators have used a modification of this method. If there is a major genetic locus for a given phenotype, and if a predominant single ancient mutation accounts for most disease, then it is reasoned that a polymorphic marker that is

in close physical proximity and occurs on the same allele as the mutation will
be seen with greater frequency among affected persons than in the general
population. If such an observation is made, the marker allele is said to be in
linkage dysequilibrium. Using such techniques, weak evidence was found for
an aneurysm locus on the long arm of chromosome 16. Two candidate genes,
haptoglobin and cholesterol ester transfer protein, were known to map to the
region.[13] It was found that the haptoglobin α-1 allele was seen with greater frequency in apparently unrelated aneurysm patients than in control subjects. In
addition, a polymorphic marker at the cholesterol ester transfer protein locus
was also increased in aneurysm patients. The authors reasoned that because
haptoglobins containing the α-1 chain accelerated the degradation of aortic
elastin and defects in cholesterol ester transfer protein could promote atherosclerosis, these genes were likely sites of primary defects causing aneurysm.[13]
It must be stressed that artifactual associations can be seen when one fails to
correct for confounding variables. In addition, in the absence of demonstration
of mutations in these genes, the observed linkage dysequilibrium seen at these
2 loci might only suggest that a true disease gene has a map position close by.

In contrast, many investigators have turned to a pure candidate gene approach. It is reasoned that an understanding of the molecular anatomy,
histopathology, and natural history of the diseased aorta might suggest specific proteins or biofunctional pathways for focused scrutiny (Table 7.1). The
major matrix components of the vascular wall include types I and III collagens,

Table 7.1.   CANDIDATE GENES IN ISOLATED AORTIC ANEURYSM

Genes Encoding	Function of Proteins
Connective tissue Elements	
Collagens	Tensile strength
Type III, ? others	
Elastic fiber system	Elasticity, force modulation
Tropoelastin	
Lysyl oxidase	
Microfibrillar proteins	
Fibrillin-1	
Fibrillin-2	
Microfibrillar-associated glycoprotein	
Associated microfibrillar protein	
Proteolytic system elements	
Proteases	Healing, remodelling, turnover
Elastases	
Collagenases	
? others	
Protease inihibitors	Homeostasis, stability
TIMP	
α$_1$-antitrypsin	
? others	
Miscellaneous	
Haptoglobin	Hemoglobin metabolism, ? role in elastic fiber stability
Cholesterol ester transferase	Cholesterol metabolism

[a]TIMP, tissue inhibitor of metallaproteinases.

proteoglycans, and the elements of the elastin-microfibrillar array system, including tropoelastin and fibrillin. The fact that collagens are a major source of tensile strength and elastic fibers allow the vascular wall to accommodate systolic hemodynamic stress supports the candidacy of these matrix elements in the pathogenesis of aortic aneurysm. Other potential leads have stemmed from histopathologic study of aneurysm tissue. One nearly unifying finding is a deficiency and abnormal organization of elastic fibers and accumulation of acid mucopolysaccharide (reviewed in Ref. 14). This is a particularly prominent finding in Marfan syndrome and annuloaortic ectasia. In contrast, many patients with dissection of the distal thoracic and abdominal aorta also show zonal fibrosis and abnormal dilation of vessels in the aortic media.[14]

The finding of deficient or abnormal extracellular matrix components at the site of aneurysm raises certain interesting possibilities. First, a primary defect in the genes encoding these structural proteins could abolish their expression or greatly alter their structure and function. It must be considered, however, that these proteins have a fairly wide tissue distribution. The finding of apparently isolated tissue defects in focal regions of the vascular wall in a large subset of patients would seem to argue that this is not a unifying hypothesis. Second, primary mutations in these genes could lead to subtle alterations in protein structure and function. Although the defect would be present in a variety of tissues, only those regions exposed to a critical level and duration of environmental stress would manifest an abnormal phenotype. Finally, mutations in other genes, whose protein products control the regional synthesis, trafficking, or metabolism of matrix elements, could be involved.

Indeed, a series of recent studies have identified apparent abnormalities of proteolytic activity at the site of aortic aneurysm.[12,15–18] A pathogenic and primary increase in enzymatic function of collagenases, elastases or pancreatic proteases has been postulated.[15–17] Alternatively, others have proposed a deficiency of protease inhibitors including tissue inhibitor of metalloproteinases (TIMP) and α_1-antitrypsin.[12,18] These hypotheses were supported by the finding of increased elastinolytic activity in both the circulating neutrophils and aneurysm tissue of affected patients.[17] In 1991 Tilson and colleagues found reduced amounts of immunoreactive TIMP in aortic extracts from aneurysm patients than from unaffected control subjects.[12] A primary defect in the gene encoding TIMP has not been demonstrated. It has been reasoned that an increase in proteolytic activity for any reason might cause a secondary decrease in the amount of TIMP that can be assayed from affected tissues. In any event, a primary or secondary decrease in proteolytic inhibitors would lead to enhanced degradation of structural components of the vascular wall and would therefore contribute to progression of aortic dilation.

The association between aortic dilation and bicuspid aortic valve has been well documented.[19] It has been long postulated that hemodynamic alteration created by the bicuspid and often stenotic valve might predispose to secondary changes in the vascular wall. For example, an asymmetric high-velocity jet might cause extreme hemodynamic stress at the aortic root. In addition, any accompanying valvular regurgitation would increase stroke volume and hence systolic pressure in the ascending aorta. In contrast to these hypotheses, a recent study found no correlation between valve function and the occurrence or severity of aortic dilation.[20] The same degree and frequency of aortic dilation were seen with regurgitant, stenotic, and functionally normal bicuspid aortic valves. These data suggest that a common primary developmental defect might lead to both bicuspid aortic valve and aortic root dilatation. If this is so, then the clear genetic predisposition for bicuspid aortic valve and other forms of left heart obstructive disease would also pertain to the aneurysm phenotype.

As further and direct evidence for a genetic basis of aortic aneurysm, the precise sites of genetic defect in patients with systemic connective tissue disorders involving the aortic, such as Marfan syndrome and EDS IV, have been identified (Table 7.2).[21,22] As described below, emerging evidence suggests that some unknown proportion of patients with aortic aneurysms and either minimal or absent extravascular manifestations of these disorders may have primary defects in these same genes.

Type I collagen abnormalities are clearly the cause of various forms of osteogenesis imperfecta. Although mild aortic dilation can been seen, aneurysm formation is not a component of the phenotype. In contrast, a deficiency of type III collagen is associated with the vascular form of Ehlers-Danlos syndrome.[21] This disorder is characterized by the rupture of large vessels and hollow organs in conjunction with prominent skin abnormalities and small vessel fragility. The phenotypic overlap between this disorder and isolated aortic aneurysm

TABLE 7.2. CARDIOVASCULAR CONNECTIVE TISSUE AND ASSOCIATED DISORDERS

Protein	Disease	Cardiovascular Features	Systemic Features
Type I collagen	Osteogenesis imperfecta	? Aortic dilatation (mild)	Bone fragility Blue sclera
Type III collagen	Ehler-Danlos type IV	Vessel fragility Large-vessel rupture Mitral valve prolapse	Bruisability Joint laxity Skin abnormalities
Elastin	SVAS[a]	SVAS Peripheral vascular stenosis	

	Williams syndrome	SVAS
		Peripheral vascular
		  stenosis
			Abnormal facies
			Retardation
			Abnormal affect
			Abnormal calcium
			  homeostasis

Fibrillin-1	Marfan	Aortic dilation,
		  dissection
		Mitral valve prolapse
		Valve dysfunction
		Primary cardiomyo-
		  pathy (rare)
			Long bone overgrowth
			
			Ectopia lentis
			Joint laxity
			Striae distensae

	MASS	Aortic dilation (mild) Mitral valve prolapse	Long bone overgrowth Striae distensae

[a]SVAS, supravalvar aortic stenosis; MASS, mitral valve prolapse and mild aortic dilatation without dissection.

prompted Kuivaniemi *et al.* to undertake an ambitious screening project for type III procollagen defects in a panel of aortic aneurysm patients. Three mutations, including one splicing defect and two glycine substitutions in the triple helical domain have been identified.[23–25] Type III collagen is known to form fibrils, and the normal structure requires that three identical polypeptide chains form a stable triple helix. This structure, and hence the function of the protein, is exquisitely sensitive to proper alignment of monomers and the presence of glycine residues at every third position within "collagenous" domains. It is therefore clear that these mutations would result in peptides that would interrupt type III collagen fibrillogenesis. Interestingly, although aortic aneurysm was clearly the predominant feature of the disease phenotype, all three patients had features of a systemic disorder of connective tissue including easy bruisability, joint hypermobility, tissue fragility, and/or generalized fibromuscular dysplasia. Other investigators have demonstrated that 2 of 14 patients tested had apparent decreased stability of type III procollagen *in vitro* but these findings have not been correlated with precise genetic defects.[26] It remains unclear whether a subset of mutations in the gene encoding type III procollagen selectively manifest aortic disease out of proportion to systemic features in other tissues. Alternatively, if these identical mutations had occurred within a different genetic background, or if the patients had been exposed to different environments, then a more classic Ehlers-Danlos syndrome phenotype may have resulted. Nevertheless, comprehensive analysis of many patients with "isolated" aneurysms suggests that defects in type III collagen account for less than 2% of disease.[25]

The search for the site of primary defect in the Marfan syndrome was long and arduous. The pattern of tissue involvement in this disorder suggested a defect in the elastic fiber system. Indeed, an early histologic observation demonstrated decreased and disorganized elastic fibers in the aortic media of Marfan syndrome patients.[27] Linkage studies using anonymous polymorphic markers excluded the tropoelastin locus as the site of the Marfan gene, but rather localized the gene defect to the long arm of chromosome 15 in close proximity to marker D15S1.[28,29]

In 1986 Sakai and colleagues[30] first identified a 350-kD glycoprotein component of the extracellular microfibril termed fibrillin. The microfibril was known to be an abundant component of all elastic tissues, and localization of microfibrils to the maturing ends of amorphous elastic fibers suggested that they may play a regulatory role in organizing the deposition of tropoelastin molecules.[31] In addition, fibrillin was found to be expressed in all tissues altered in the Marfan phenotype, including the suspensory ligaments of the ocular lens and the vascular wall.[30] These observations made the fibrillin gene an attractive candidate for the site of primary defect in this disorder. Subsequent immunohistochemical analysis revealed an apparent deficiency of fibrillin in the tissues of patients with Marfan syndrome.[32] Cultured fibroblasts from affected patients demonstrated multiple abnormalities of fibrillin metabolism including decreased synthesis, delayed secretion, or diminished incorporation into the extracellular matrix.[33] These data clearly suggested that fibrillin was somehow involved in the pathogenesis of the Marfan syndrome. It remained to be determined whether the fibrillin gene was the site of primary defect. Alternatively, defects in another gene and protein could have a secondary effect on fibrillin processing.

Linkage analysis using intragenic fibrillin gene polymorphisms established a coincident map location for the fibrillin gene and the Marfan locus.[22,34] Simultaneous work by Magenis and colleagues[35] mapped the fibrillin gene to 15q21.1 using *in situ* hybridization methods. In addition, during identification of fibrillin clones, other fibrillinlike sequences were characterized and mapped to chromosome 5.[34] The gene on chromosome 15, now termed FBN1, was linked to the Marfan phenotype, and was subsequently shown to cosegregate with autosomal dominant ectopia lentis in large families. The related gene on chromosome 5 (FBN2) was genetically linked to the congenital contractural arachnodactyly phenotype, a disorder with significant clinical overlap with Marfan syndrome including all typical skeletal features but no ocular or aortic involvement.

In 1991, a causal relationship between mutations in the chromosome 15 gene encoding fibrillin (FBN1) and the Marfan phenotype was finally established.[22] Two unrelated patients with early onset of severe and classic disease were found to carry the identical mutation. In the absence of linkage evidence for genetic heterogeneity, it appears that FBN1 mutations are the predominant, if not the sole cause of this disorder.

Subsequently, over 30 mutations have been identified.[22,36–44] At this early stage of correlation of mutant genotype to phenotype, certain patterns are emerging. First, with the exception of the first mutation that was identified, all others have been specific to individual families. This likely manifests a high rate of new mutation and impairment of reproductive fitness in the Marfan syndrome due to early morbidity and mortality. Second, mutations have been found with approximately equal frequency along the length of the fibrillin gene. There is no apparent correlation between the position of the mutation and disease severity. Third, mutations appear to cluster at highly conserved residues within the repetitive epidermal growth factor-like motifs of the fibrillin gene.[36,38,40,42–44] These motifs encode 6 predictably spaced cysteine residues that dictate local folding patterns of the monomers.[45] In addition to substituting cysteine residues, naturally occurring mutations also substitute residues that are known to be crucial to calcium binding to epidermal growth factor-like domains.[46] Calcium binding is believed to influence the stability of secondary structure of the domains and may also influence protein-to-protein interactions and susceptibility of the peptide to the activity of proteases.

Recent data suggest a dominant negative pathogenesis for the Marfan syndrome. According to this model, the presence of abnormal protein, rather than a relative deficiency of the wild-type product, is central to the expression of the disease phenotype.[47] The first evidence for this pathogenic mechanism arose from the observation that a mutation in the fibrillin gene that was associated with a severe reduction in the level of mutant RNA, predicted to produce very low levels of mutant protein, occurred in a patient with an extremely mild phenotype.[42] Fibrillin monomers are known to multimerize via disulfide linkage in the formation of microfibrils.[48] If normal monomers are produced in great abundance relative to the amount of abnormal peptides, one would predict a preponderance of normal multimers, and hence mild disease (Fig. 7.1). More direct evidence has come from *in vitro* expression studies. It was found that the expression of a mutant fibrillin allele on a normal genetic background could reproduce the typical Marfan cellular phenotype (H.C. Dietz, unpublished data).

The medical significance of fibrillin may not be limited to its role in the pathogenesis of Marfan syndrome. In fact, the members of the fibrillin gene family have been genetically linked to a wide range of disorders[34,49] and a mutation has been found in a patient with the MASS phenotype,[42] which includes mitral valve prolapse and borderline aortic dilation without progression to dis-

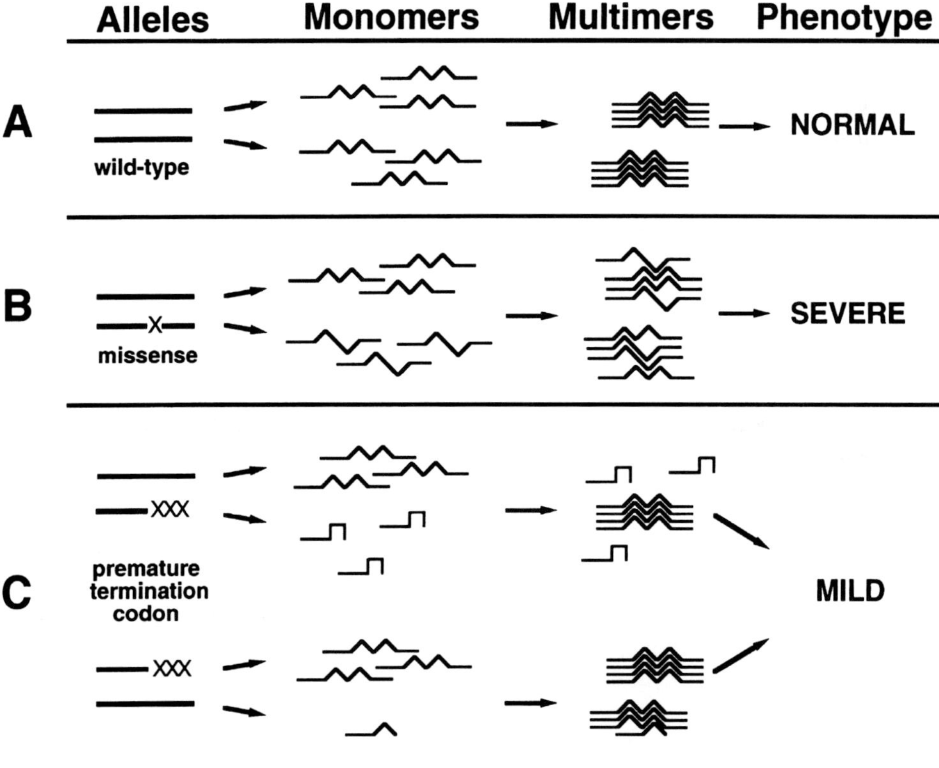

FIG. 7.1. The mild phenotype in a patient with Marfan syndrome explained by a dominant negative model of disease. *A.* Two normal alleles produce wild-type monomer and multimer and hence a normal phenotype. *B.* Heterozygosity for a missense mutation (*X*) produces equal populations of normal and mutant monomer, a homogeneous population of abnormal multimer, and hence a severe phenotype. *C.* A mutation that causes a premature signal for termination of translation (*XXX*) can predict a truncated monomer that no longer participates in multimer formation (*upper panel*). Alternatively, a reduction in mutant allele transcript will predict a relative abundance of normal monomer (*lower panel*). Either situation predicts a preponderance of wild-type multimer and hence a mild disease phenotype.

section. The 10-nm microfibril, largely composed of fibrillin, has been proposed to associate with many other components of the extracellular matrix. By virtue of these interactions, fibrillin abnormalities may impair the structural or functional integrity of a diversity of tissues with these proteins as constitutive elements. The observation that fibrillin is synthesized and secreted early in fetal life, that virtually all manifestations of the Marfan syndrome may be present at birth, and that the microfibril-rich extracellular matrix forms the ground over which cells migrate in the developing fetus all suggest that fibrillin may play an important role in normal (and hence aberrant) human growth and development. In addition, the fact that the microfibril is believed to regulate the organization of tropoelastin into maturing elastic fibers, and that tropoelastin gene defects have recently been demonstrated in supravalvar aortic stenosis and the Williams syndrome (reviewed in Ref. 50), underscores the vital role that the elastic fiber-microfibril array system plays in early patterning of the cardiovascular system.

It is reasonable to speculate that fibrillin gene defects may play an etiologic role in patients with isolated features of the Marfan phenotype. Although substitution of highly conserved residues appears to lead to the classic Marfan phenotype, it seems reasonable to speculate that more conservative substitutions might predispose the microfibril and hence elastic tissues to damage when exposed to a sufficient severity and duration of hemodynamic stress. A role for FBN1 gene defects in the evolution of isolated aortic aneurysm is supported on many levels. First, a subset of patients with Marfan syndrome develop aneurysms in the abdominal aorta, the most frequent site of pathology in patients with isolated aortic disease. Second, we have identified a fibrillin gene mutation in a patient with Marfan syndrome and multiple peripheral aneurysms involving the descending thoracic and abdominal aorta and the iliac, coronary, carotid, and subclavian arteries (H.C. Dietz, unpublished data). Third, diminished and disrupted elastic fibers, a consistent feature in isolated aneurysmal disease, are also a hallmark of the typical Marfan aorta. We are currently screening FBN1 cDNA from patients with isolated late-onset aortic aneurysm for disease-producing alterations.

Although the identification of FBN1 as the site of defect in Marfan syndrome only provides the precise etiology for a subset of patients with aneurysmal disease, it provides a first meaningful opportunity to study the factors influencing phenotypic expression and to provide presymptomatic risk assessment for a large body of patients. Allelic heterogeneity likely contributes to interfamilial variation in the Marfan phenotype, and intrafamilial clinical variability is also a hallmark of the Marfan syndrome. A previous study demonstrated that this variability can be seen among family members who carry the identical FBN1 mutation, and that the only two individuals with the identical phenotype were monozygotic twins.[36] These data predict the existence of genetic and/or environmental modifiers to phenotypic expression. We have recently identified a highly informative panel of intragenic FBN1 microsatellite polymorphisms and studied a number of families with variable manifestations by haplotype segregation analysis.[51] A second molecular explanation for intrafamilial variability is offered. Within given families, members manifesting the complete Marfan phenotype segregated the same FBN1 allele, whereas members with significant ocular, skeletal, or cardiovascular features, but no aortic dilation or ectopia lentis, all shared a different fibrillin allele. These data suggest that *de novo* FBN1 mutations causing Marfan syndrome have occurred upon the genetic background for a mild, albeit related, connective tissue disorder. It is also clear that all "affected" family members do not share the same risk for life-threatening cardiovascular manifestations. These methods can also be used for routine prenatal and presymptomatic diagnosis of Marfan syndrome and should aid reproductive and management decisions.

It is clear that aneurysmal dilation of the aorta has a genetically heterogeneous basis. It is also clear that the vascular wall does not have sufficient structural redundancy to make it immune to defects in any single gene. Therefore, the search for a predominant site of genetic defect is both approachable and on firm theoretical ground. A clear understanding of pathogenesis will provide a greater understanding of vascular biology in both health and disease and should optimize medical management of this common yet largely preventable cause of premature death.

REFERENCES

1. Collin BR. Screening for abdominal aortic aneurysms. *J Surg* 1985;72:851–852.
2. Tilson MD, Seashore MR. Human genetics of the abdominal aortic aneurysm. *Surg Gynecol Obstet* 1984;158:129–132.
3. Bengtsson H, Sonesson B, Lanne T, et al. Prevalence of abdominal aortic aneurysm in the offspring of patients dying from aneurysm rupture. *Br J Surg* 1992;79:1142–1143.
4. Johansen K, Koepsell T. Familial tendency for abdominal aortic aneurysms. *JAMA* 1986;256:1934–1936.
5. Powell JT, Greenhalgh RM. Multifactorial inheritance of abdominal aortic aneurysm. *Eur J Vasc Surg* 1987;1:29–31.
6. Bengtsson H, Norrgard O, Angquist KA, Ekberg O, Oberg L, Bergqvist D. Ultrasonographic screening of the abdominal aorta among siblings of patients with abdominal aortic aneurysms. *Br J Surg* 1989;76:589–591.
7. Adamson J, Powell JT, Greenhalgh RM. Selection for screening for familial aortic aneurysms. *Br J Surg* 1992;79:897–898.
8. Fine LG. Abdominal aortic aneurysm: report of a meeting of physicians and scientists, University College London Medical School. *Lancet* 1993;341:215–220.
9. Nicod P, Bloor C, Godfrey M, et al. Familial aortic dissecting aneurysm. *J Am Coll Cardiol* 1989;13:811–819.
10. Sarkar R, Cilley RE, Coran AG. Abdominal aneurysms in childhood: report of a case and review of the literature. *Surgery* 1991;109:143–147.
11. Majumder PP, St. Jean PL, Ferrell RE, Webster MW, Steed DL. On the inheritance of abdominal aortic aneurysm. *Am J Hum Genet* 1991;48:164–170.
12. Brophy CM, Sumpio B, Reilly JM, Tilson MD. Decreased tissue inhibitor of metalloproteinases (TIMP) in abdominal aortic aneurysm tissue: a preliminary report. *J Surg Res* 1991;50:653–657.
13. Powell JT, Bashir A, Dawson S, et al. Genetic variation on chromosome 16 is associated with abdominal aortic aneurysm. *Clin Sci* 1990;78:13–16.
14. Niitsuya M, Kuwao S, Sato B, Kameya T, Kikawada R. Histopathological study of aortic wall dissection. *J Cardiol* 1991;21:445–452.

15. Busuttil RW, Abou-Zamzam AM, Machleder HI. Collagenase activity of the human aorta: a comparison of patients with and without abdominal aortic aneurysms. *Arch Surg* 1980;115: 1373–1378.

16. Brophy CM, Sumpio I, Ratner L, Tilson MD. Electrophoretic characterization of protease expression in aneurysmal aorta: report of a unique 80kDa elastolytic activity. *Surg Res Commun* 1991;10:315–321.

17. Cannon D, Read R. Blood elastolytic activity in patients with aortic aneurysms. *Ann Thorac Surg* 1982;34:10–15.

18. Cohen JR, Sarfai I, Ratner L, Tilson MD. Alpha-1 antitrypsin phenotypes in patients with abdominal aortic aneurysms. *J Surg Res* 1990;49:319–321.

19. Lindsay J, Jr. Coarctation of the aorta, bicuspid aortic valve and abnormal ascending aortic wall. *Am J Cardiol* 1988;61:182–184.

20. Hahn RT, Roman MJ, Mogtader AH, Devereux RB. Association of aortic dilatation with regurgitant, stenotic and functionally normal bicuspid aortic valves. *J Am Coll Cardiol* 1992: 19:283–288.

21. Pope FM, Martin GR, Lichtenstein JR, et al. Patients with Ehlers-Danlos syndrome type IV lack type III collagen. *Proc Natl Acad Sci USA* 1975;72:1314–1316.

22. Dietz HC, Cutting GR, Pyeritz RE, et al. Marfan syndrome caused by a recurrent de novo missense mutation in the fibrillin gene. *Nature* 1991;352:337–339.

23. Kontusaari S, Tromp G, Kuivaniemi H, Ladda RL, Prockop DJ. Inheritance of an RNA splicing mutation (G$^{+1IVS20}$) in the type III procollagen gene (COL3A1) in a family with aortic aneurysms and easy bruisability. Phenotypic overlap between familial arterial aneurysms and the Ehlers-Danlos syndrome type IV. *Am J Hum Genet* 1990;47:112–120.

24. Kontusaari S, Tromp G, Kuivaniemi H, Romanic AM, Prockop DJ. A mutation in the gene for type III procollagen (COL3A1) in a family with aortic aneurysms. *J Clin Invest* 1990;86: 1465–1473.

25. Tromp G, Wu Y, Prockop DJ, et al. Sequencing of cDNA from 50 unrelated patients reveals that mutations in the triple-helical domain of type III procollagen are an infrequent cause of aortic aneurysms. *J Clin Invest* 1993;91:2539–2545.

26. Deak SB, Ricotta JJ, Mariani TJ, et al. Abnormalities of the biosynthesis of type III procollagen in cultured skin fibroblasts from two patients with multiple aneurysms. *Matrix* 1992;12:92–100.

27. Abraham PA, Perejda AJ, Carnes WH, Uitto J. Marfan syndrome. Demonstration of abnormal elastin in aorta. *J Clin Invest* 1982;70:1245–1252.

28. Kainulainen K, Pulkkinen L, Savolainen A, Kaitila I, Peltonen L. Location of chromosome 15 of the gene defect causing Marfan syndrome. *N Engl J Med* 1990;323:935–939.

29. Dietz HC, Pyeritz RE, Hall BD, et al. The Marfan syndrome locus: confirmation of assignment to chromosome 15 and identification of tightly linked markers at 15q15–q21.3. *Genomics* 1991;9:355–361.

30. Sakai LY, Keene DR, Engvall E. Fibrillin, a new 350-kD glycoprotein, is a component of extracellular microfibrils. *J Cell Biol* 1986;103:2499–2509.

31. Cleary EG, Gibson MA. Elastin-associated microfibrils and microfibrillar proteins. *Int Rev Connect Tissue Res* 1983;10:97–209.

32. Hollister DW, Godfrey M, Sakai LY, Pyeritz RE. Marfan syndrome:immunohistologic abnormalities of the elastin-associated microfibrillar fiber system. *N Engl J Med* 1990;323: 152–159.

33. McGookey-Milewicz D, Pyeritz RE, Crawford ES, Byers PH. Marfan syndrome:defective synthesis, secretion and extracellular matrix formation of fibrillin by cultured dermal fibroblasts. *J Clin Invest* 1992;89:79–86.

34. Lee B, Godfrey M, Vitale E, et al. Linkage of Marfan syndrome and a phenotypically related disorder to two fibrillin genes. *Nature* 1991;352:330–334.

35. Magenis RE, Maslen CL, Smith L, Allen L, Sakai LY. Localization of the fibrillin gene to chromosome 15, band 15q21.1. *Genomics* 1991;11:346–351.

36. Dietz HC, Pyeritz RE, Puffenberger EG, et al. Marfan phenotype variability in a family segregating a missense mutation in the EGF-like motif of the fibrillin gene. *J Clin Invest* 1992;89:1674–1680.

37. Kainulainen K, Sakai LY, Child A, et al. Two unique mutations in Marfan syndrome resulting in truncated polypeptide chains of fibrillin. *Proc Natl Acad Sci USA* 1992;88:5917–5921.

38. Dietz HC, Saraiva JM, Pyeritz RE, Cutting GR, Francomano CA. Clustering of fibrillin (FBN1) missense mutations in Marfan syndrome patients at cysteine residues in EFG-like domains. *Hum Mutation* 1992;1:366–374.

39. Dietz HC, Valle D, Francomano CA, Kendzior FJ, Pieritz RE, Cutting GR. The skipping of constitutive exons in vivo induced by nonsense mutations. *Science* 1993;254:680–683.

40. Hewett DR, Lynch JR, Smith R, Sykes B. Fibrillin mutation in the Marfan syndrome may disrupt calcium binding of the epidermal growth factor module. *Hum Mol Genet* 1993;2:475–477.

41. Godfrey M, Vandemark N, Wang M, et al. Prenatal diagnosis and a donor splice mutation in fibrillin in a family with Marfan syndrome. *Am J Hum Genet* 1993;53:472–480.

42. Dietz HC, McIntosh I, Sakai LY, et al. Four novel FBN1 mutations: significance for mutant transcript level and EGF-like domain calcium binding in the pathogenesis of Marfan syndrome. *Genomics* 1993;17:468–475.

43. Tynan K, Comeau K, Pearson M, et al. Mutation screening of complete fibrillin-1 coding sequence: report of five new mutations, including two in 8-cysteine domains. *Hum Mol Genet* 1993;2:1813–1821.

44. Kainulainen K, Karttunen L, Puhakka L, L. Mutations in the fibrillin gene responsible for dominant ectopia lentis and neonatal Marfan syndrome. *Nature Genet* 1994;6:64–69.

45. Cooke RM, Wilkinson AJ, Baron M, et al. The solution structure of human epidermal growth factor. *Nature* 1987;327:339–341.

46. Handford PA, Mayhew M, Baron M, Winship PR, Campbell ID, Brownlee GG. Key residues involved in calcium-binding motifs in EFG-like domains. *Nature* 1991;351:164–167.

47. Herskowitz I. Functional inactivation of genes by dominant negative mutations. *Nature* 1987;329:219–222.

48. Sakai LY, Keene DR, Glanville RW, Bachinger HP. Purification and partial characterization of fibrillin, a cysteine-rich structural component of connective tissue microfibril. *J Biol Chem* 1991;266:14763–14770.

49. Tsipouras P, Del Mastro R, Sarfarazi M, et al. Linkage of Marfan syndrome, dominant ectopia lentis and congenital contractural arachnodactyl to the fibrillin genes on chromosomes 15 and 5. *N Engl J Med* 1992;326:905–909.

50. Ewart EK, Morris CA, Atkinson D, et al. Hemizygosity at the elastin locus in a developmental disorder, Williams syndrome. *Nature Genet* 1993;5:11–16.

51. Pereira L, Levran O, Ramirez F, et al. A molecular approach to the stratification of cardiovascular risk in families with Marfan's Syndrome. *N Engl J Med* 1994;331:148–153.

Chapter 8

Update on the Pathobiology of Vasculitis

J. CHARLES JENNETTE AND RONALD J. FALK

The pathobiology of systemic vasculitides remains poorly understood. Over the past decade, however, there have been major advances in our knowledge of the inflammatory mechanisms and pathogenic processes that cause many forms of vasculitis. Our understanding of inflammatory injury in general, including that involved in vasculitis, has been improved by increased knowledge about the pathogenic roles of cytokines, cell adhesion molecules, growth factors, humoral mediator systems, proteases and oxygen metabolites. The identification of previously unrecognized etiologic agents, such as hepatitis C virus, and potentially pathogenic autoantibodies, such as antineutrophil cytoplasmic autoantibodies and antiendothelial antibodies, also has shed light on the pathogenesis of several types of vasculitis.

PATHOGENIC MECHANISMS

Table 8.1 categories vasculitides based on putative pathogenesis. Infection and immunologic injury are the major known pathogenic mechanisms for vasculitis.

Infection is an important cause for both localized and systemic vasculitides. In fact, syphilitic aortitis and tuberculous arteritis were the first types of vasculitis recognized by pathologists in the 16th century. Infections cause vascular inflammation by direct extension from an adjacent focus of infection, septic embolization, and hematogenous dissemination. Examples of the latter are Niesserial septicemia and Rickettsial diseases, such as Rocky Mountain spotted fever. *Niesseria* and *Rickettsia* attach to and penetrate endothelial cells and cause vascular necrosis, thrombosis, and inflammation (Fig. 8.1). In Niesserial and Rickettsial vasculitis, the etiologic microbes can be identified in leukocytes and endothelial cells at the site of injury (Fig. 8.2).[1,2]

When considering the pathogenesis of vasculitis, the possibility of an infectious etiology should always be considered and ruled out, if possible, before concluding that the patient has an idiopathic or immune-mediated disease. This is particularly important given the fact that many patients with presumed immune-mediated as well as idiopathic vasculitis are treated with immunosuppressive agents.

TABLE 8.1. TYPES OF VASCULITIS CATEGORIZED ON THE BASIS OF PROPOSED PATHOGENIC MECHANISMS

Direct infection of vessels
    Bacterial vasculitis (*e.g.,* Neisserial)
    Rickettsial vasculitis (*e.g.,* Rocky Mountain spotted fever)
    Spirochetal (*e.g.,* syphilitic)
    Fungal (*e.g.,* mucormycosis)
    Viral (*e.g.,* herpes zoster-varicella)
Immunologic Injury
    Immune complex-mediated
        Henoch-Schönlein purpura
        Cryoglobulinemic vasculitis
        Lupus and rheumatoid vasculitis
        Serum sickness vasculitis
        Infection-induced immune complex vasculitis
            Viral (*e.g.,* hepatitis B and C virus)
            Bacterial (*e.g.,* streptococcal)
        Some drug-induced vasculitis (*e.g.,* sulfonamide)
    Direct antibody attack-mediated
        Goodpasture's syndrome (antibasement membrane antibodies)
        Kawasaki disease (antiendothelial antibodies)
    Antineutrophil cytoplasmic autoantibody-mediated
        Wegener's granulomatosis
        Microscopic polyangiitis (microscopic polyarteritis)
        Churg-Strauss syndrome
        Some drug-induced vasculitis (*e.g.,* thiouracil)
    Cell-mediated
        Allograft cellular vascular rejection

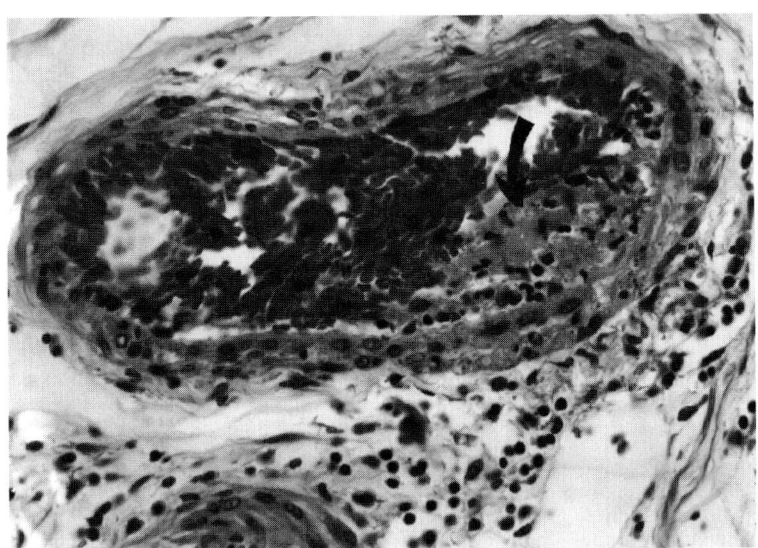

FIG. 8.1. Segmental inflammation in a small testicular artery of a patient with Rocky Mountain spotted fever. Note the thrombosis (*arrow*) overlying an area of endothelial necrosis and mural inflammation. Hematoxylin & eosin.

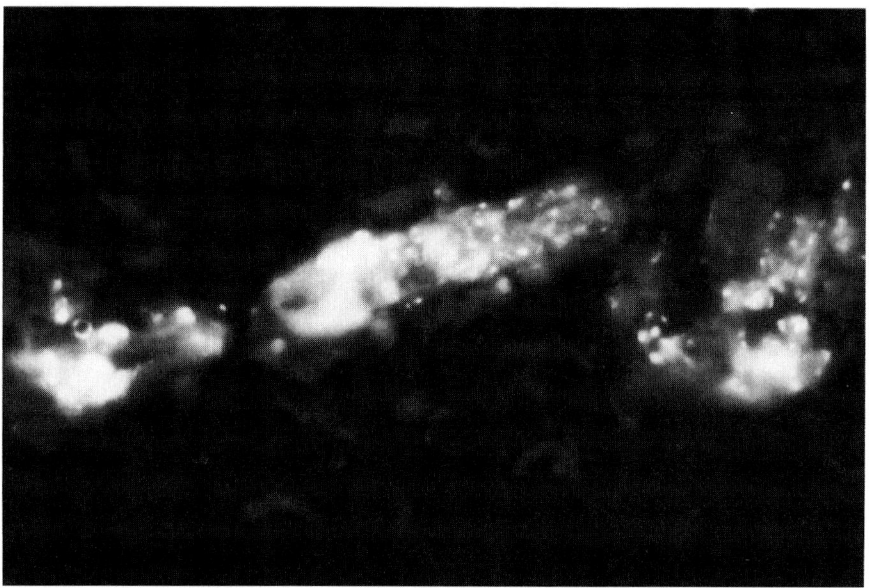

FIG. 8.2.   Direct immunofluorescence microscopy of a skin biopsy specimen from a patient with Rocky Mountain spotted fever. Note the Rickettsial organisms and antigenic debris in the small dermal vessels. Fluorescein isothiocyanate (FITC)-conjugated anti-*R. rickettsii*.

Although cellular immunity has been incriminated in the pathogenesis of many forms of vasculitis, the only form of noninfectious vasculitis with convincing evidence that this is the major mechanism is acute cellular vascular allograft rejection. In this process, there is T-lymphocyte and mononuclear leukocyte attack on vessel walls with resultant adhesion of leukocytes to vascular endothelium, and penetration into the intima and less commonly into the media of arteries (Fig. 8.3). There is no other type of noninfectious human vasculitis that has pathologic features similar to cellular rejection vasculitis. There are, however, other vasculitides that have a predominance of lymphocytes, including activated CD4 T-lymphocytes and macrophages involved in the inflammatory process, such as giant cell (temporal) arteritis and Takayasu's arteritis. However, there is no strong evidence that the inflammation is initiated by T-lymphocyte recognition of nonmicrobial antigens. The infiltrating T-lymphocytes may be present as a result of nonimmunologic activation of lymphocytes and mononuclear phagocytes as part of a chronic inflammatory response to tissue injury.

Antibody-mediated injury is well documented or strongly suspected to be the basis for a number of vasculitides (Table 8.1). This review will focus on vasculitides that are thought to be induced by (1) immune complexes, (2) antibodies specific for vessel wall constituents, and (3) antineutrophil cytoplasmic autoantibodies.

A variety of different etiologic agents and pathogenic events initiate a final common pathway of inflammation that results in acute vasculitis. A corollary to this is that clinically and histologically identical vasculitis can be produced by multi-

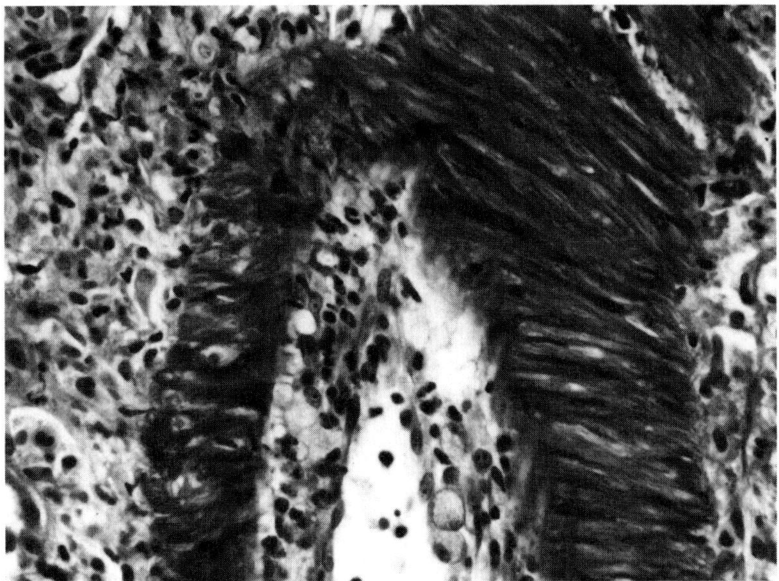

FIG. 8.3. Acute renal allograft rejection causing intimal inflammation in an arcuate artery. Note the intimal edema and infiltration by predominantly mononuclear leukocytes.

ple causes. In a patient with vasculitis, recognition of the initiating mechanism is useful for identifying the etiology and predicting the natural history (prognosis) and response to treatment. Effective strategies for recognizing initiating mechanisms take advantage of our knowledge of the pathobiology of vasculitis.

INITIATING MECHANISMS OF VASCULAR INFLAMMATION

In vasculitides that are characterized by acute inflammation and necrosis, the initial mediation of neutrophil and monocyte attack on vessels involves activation of the leukocytes as well as endothelial cells, followed by adhesion of leukocytes to endothelial cells, penetration into vessel walls, and release of injurious leukocyte products such as lytic enzymes and toxic oxygen metabolites, which may cause necrosis and thrombosis (Fig. 8.4). These events can be induced by multiple pathogenic processes, including infection and a variety of immune mechanisms. All of these initiating mechanisms feed into a common final pathway of vascular inflammation.

VASCULAR IMMUNE COMPLEX LOCALIZATION

Immune complexes can localize in vessel walls by deposition from the circulation, by *in situ* formation, or by a combination of both processes. Vascular immune complex localization can be detected immunohistologically as granular vessel wall staining for immunoglobulins and complement in some forms of vasculitis, such as Henoch-Schönlein purpura, cryoglobulinemic vasculitis, and serum sickness vasculitis (Fig. 8.5).

Many investigators, spearheaded by the seminal work of Dixon, Cochrane and their associates,[3,4] have elucidated the phlogogenic factors that contribute

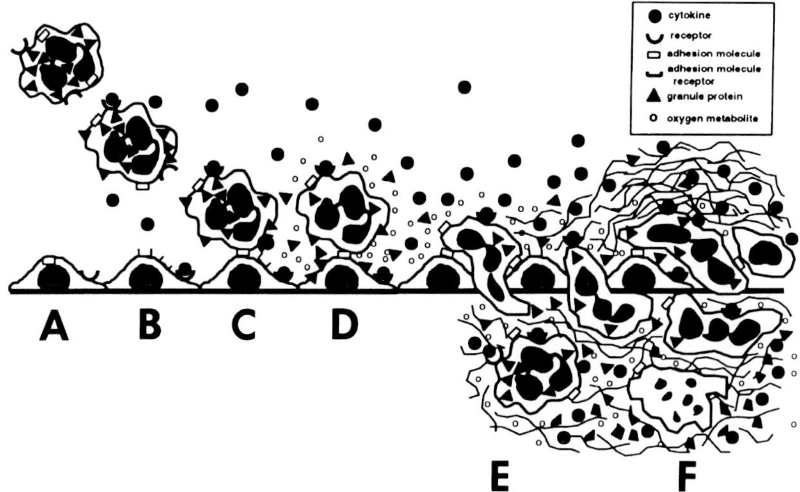

FIG. 8.4. Common pathway of acute vascular inflammation that can be initiated by multiple pathogenic mechanisms. *A.* Unstimulated leukocytes (neutrophils and monocytes) and endothelial cells constitutively express some receptors and have latent capabilities for expressing additional receptors. *B.* Stimulation (priming), with cytokines such as IL-1 or TNF, induces expression or activation of additional receptors, *e.g.,* E-selectin by endothelial cells and integrins on leukocytes. *C.* Primed leukocytes adhere to primed endothelial cells, initially by loose binding of selectins to carbohydrate ligands and subsequently by firm binding of integrins to IgCAMS. *D–F.* At sites of vasculitis, various pathogenic factors (e.g., microbes, immune complexes, autoantibodies attached to vessels, antineutrophil cytoplasmic autoantibodies) drive leukocytes to full activation before they exit the vessel wall. The leukocytes release injurious products, such as toxic oxygen metabolites and lytic enzymes. *F.* Activation of coagulation factors in the lumen causes thrombosis. Activation of coagulation factors that have exuded into the injured tissue produces fibrinoid necrosis.

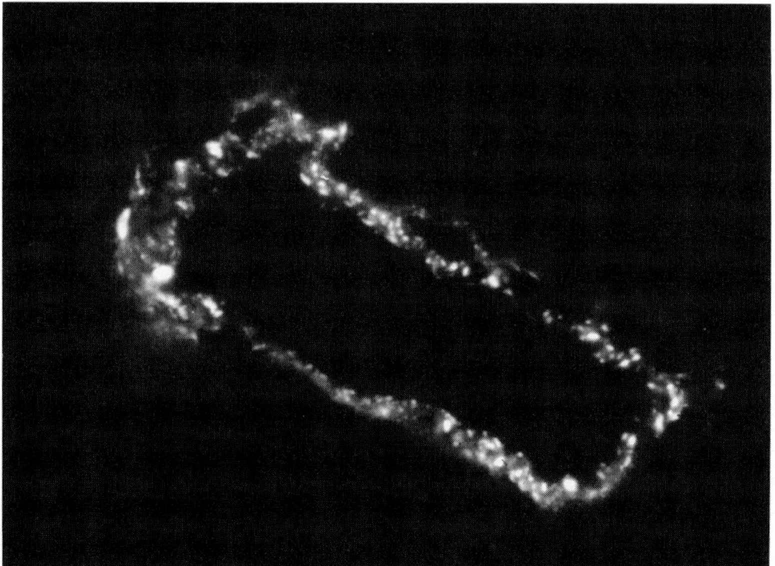

FIG. 8.5. Direct immunofluorescence microscopy demonstrating granular staining of a vessel wall that is indicative of immune complex localization. FITC-conjugated anti-C3.

to immune complex-mediated vasculitis. Cellular as well as humoral mediator systems are involved. Platelets, neutrophils, monocytes, and endothelial cells are all active participants, along with the complement, coagulation, kinin and plasminogen systems.[5] Activation of complement is particularly important. C2a and C3a have kininlike and anaphylatoxin activity that mediate changes in vascular permeability and induce granulocyte degranulation, C5a is a strong chemoattractant and activator for neutrophils and monocytes, and C5b-9, the membrane attack complex, is cytotoxic. In addition, engagement of immune-complexed IgG and IgM Fc regions by Fc receptors on neutrophils and mononuclear phagocytes results in leukocyte localization and activation. Engagement of Fc and complement receptors on neutrophils and monocytes stimulates them to produce and release additional proinflammatory products, such as interleukin-8 (IL-8), leukotriene B_4 and monocyte chemotactic peptide-1 (MCP-1). These factors recruit more neutrophils and monocytes, thus amplifying the inflammation.

The antigens that comprise immune complexes can be autoantigens, such as DNA in lupus vasculitis and IgG in type II cryoglobulinemia, or heterologous antigens, such as viral proteins in hepatitis B-associated vasculitis,[6] injected foreign proteins such as streptokinase,[7] and drugs, such as sulfonamides.[8] Recent evidence indicates that a major etiologic factor in the development of cryoglobulinemic vasculitis is hepatitis C infection.[9,10]

DIRECT ANTIBODY BINDING TO VESSEL WALLS

Direct antibody binding to autoantigens in vessel walls, such as antigens on endothelial cells, smooth muscle cells, or basement membranes, is in essence a form of *in situ* immune complex formation. As such, it would be expected to mediate acute inflammation by the same phlogistic pathways used by other types of immune complex-mediated inflammation, including complement activation and leukocyte Fc receptor engagement.

The first recognized example of this mechanism of vascular injury was Goodpasture's syndrome,[11] which is caused by autoantibodies against type IV collagen that bind to capillary basement membranes in pulmonary alveolar capillaries and glomerular capillaries, resulting in necrotizing inflammation. Antibasement membrane antibodies can be detected in biopsy specimens by immunohistology as linear staining of basement membranes with fluorescenated or enzyme-labeled antibodies specific for human IgG.

Recently, there has been an increasing interest in the possibility that antibodies with specificity for antigens on the lumenal surfaces of endothelial cells can cause vasculitis.[12–14] Detection of antiendothelial antibodies (AECAs) requires more sensitive methods than direct or indirect immunohistochemistry, such as enzyme-linked immunosorbent assay, and may be directed against inducible endothelial antigens that are expressed on endothelial cells only after stimulation, *e.g.,* by cytokines such as interleukin-1 (IL-1) or tumor necrosis factor (TNF). AECAs have been implicated in the pathogenesis of a number of vasculitides, most notably Kawasaki disease. In patients with Kawasaki disease, Leung and associates[13] have detected AECAs that are directed against cytokine-induced endothelial antigens, and have proposed that these may be involved in the initiation of vascular inflammation. AECAs also may occur in patients with microscopic polyangiitis (microscopic polyarteritis) and Wegener's granulomatosis, but their pathogenic significance in these diseases is unclear.

ACTIVATION OF LEUKOCYTES BY ANTINEUTROPHIL CYTOPLASMIC AUTOANTIBODIES

Antineutrophil Cytoplasmic Autoantibody (ANCA)-associated vasculitides, such as microscopic polyangiitis, Wegener's granulomatosus, and Churg-Strauss syndrome, have necrotizing vasculitis (Fig. 8.6) affecting vessels ranging in size from capillaries to medium-sized arteries (Fig. 8.7). Most patients have involvement predominantly of small vessels. ANCAs are a useful diagnostic serologic marker for these diseases and also may be involved in their pathogenesis.[15]

ANCAs are specific for proteins in the cytoplasm of neutrophils and monocytes. When alcohol-fixed normal human neutrophils are used as substrate for indirect immunofluorescence detection of ANCAs, two major subtypes are identified: C-ANCAs, producing cytoplasmic staining, and P-ANCAs, producing perinuclear staining (Fig. 8.8). The latter pattern results from diffusion of the antigen from the cytoplasm to the nucleus during substrate preparation. In patients with vasculitis, most C-ANCAs are specific for proteinase 3 (PR3-ANCA) and most P-ANCA for myeloperoxidase (MPO-ANCA). Both PR3 and MPO are in the primary granules of neutrophils and the peroxidase-positive lysosomes of monocytes. Therefore, if ANCAs are capable of activating leukocytes, they can activate both neutrophils and monocytes.

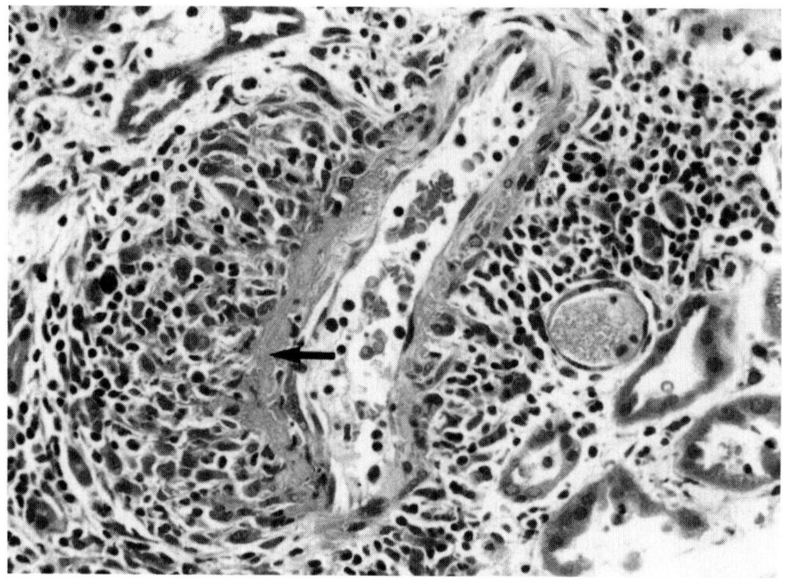

FIG. 8.6. ANCA-associated vasculitis affecting a small artery. Note the segmental fibrinoid necrosis (*arrow*) with adjacent leukocyte infiltration. Hematoxylin & eosin. (From Ref. 23, with permission.)

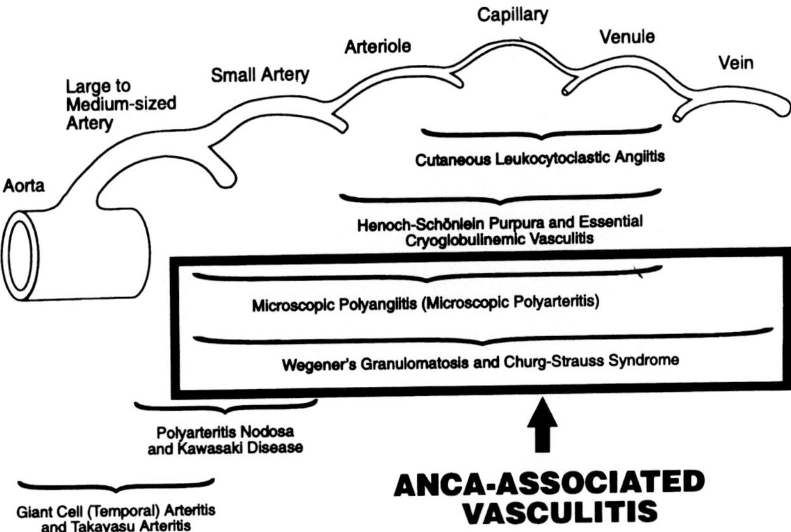

FIG. 8.7. Diagram demonstrating the types of vessels predominantly affected by certain types of vasculitis. Note that the ANCA-associated vasculitides can affect a variety of vessels, ranging in size from medium-sized arteries to capillaries. Also note that there is substantial overlap among vasculitides with respect to the types of vessels involved. (Modified from Jennette JC, Falk RJ, Andrassy K, et al. *Arthritis Rheum* 1994;37:187–192.)

If ANCAs are pathogenic, they must be able to interact with PR3 and MPO *in vivo*. One hypothesis for mediation of vasculitis by ANCAs proposes that ANCAs react with antigens released at the surface of primed neutrophils and monocytes, resulting in activation of the leukocytes.[15] This would lead to adhesion to endothelium, degranulation, respiratory burst, and induction of vascular inflammation and necrosis (Fig. 8.9). Most of the support for ANCA-mediated injury comes from *in vitro* observations of ANCA-induced neutrophil activation.[15]

In vitro, neutrophils release small amounts of ANCA target antigens at their surfaces after exposure to priming doses of cytokines (*e.g.,* TNF and IL-1) or certain microbial products (*e.g.,* formyl tripeptides or lipopolysaccharides). Incubation of primed neutrophils with isolated ANCA IgG, or with heterologous anti-MPO or anti-PR3, results in degranulation and respiratory burst. When cytokine-primed neutrophils are incubated with ANCA IgG in the presence of an endothelial monolayer, the ANCA-activated neutrophils adhere to and kill endothelial cells. This requires β_2-integrin-mediated adhesion.

The mechanism(s) by which ANCAs activate neutrophils is unknown. Both Fc-dependent and Fc-independent mechanisms have been proposed.[15] The Fc-independent hypotheses suggest that leukocyte activation is initiated by binding of ANCAs to ANCA target antigens at the cell surface of primed neutrophils and monocytes. One Fc-dependent hypothesis suggests that immune complexes composed of ANCA and ANCA target antigens form in the microenvironment adjacent to primed neutrophils and monocytes, and that these

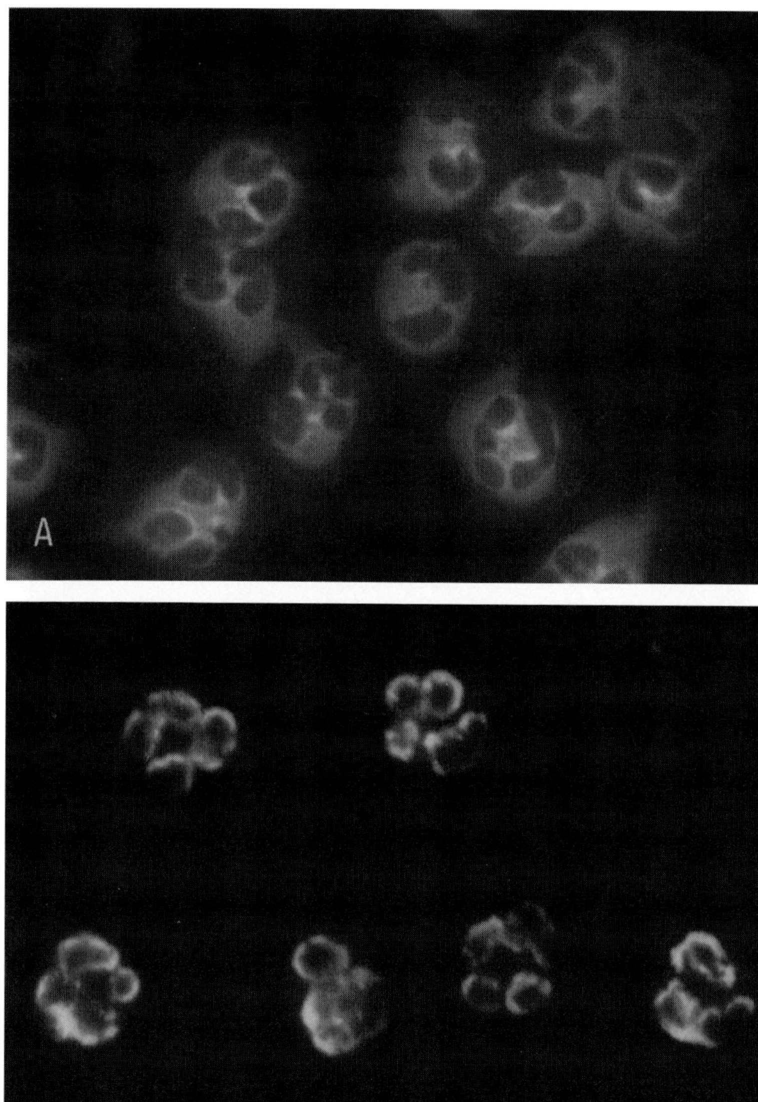

FIG. 8.8.   Indirect immunofluorescence microscopy demonstrating the staining of alcohol-fixed normal human neutrophils by *A,* C-ANCA (PR3-ANCA) and *B,* P-ANCA (MPO-ANCA). FITC-conjugated anti-human IgG secondary antibody.

immune complexes then engage Fc receptors, thus driving the leukocytes to full activation. Yet another hypothesis proposes that ANCA target antigens bind passively to endothelial cell surfaces, or are actively expressed by endothelial cells, and function as targets for injurious binding of ANCAs to endothelial cells. There are *in vitro* data supporting each of these scenarios, and it is possible that ANCA-induced leukocyte activation is multifactorial.

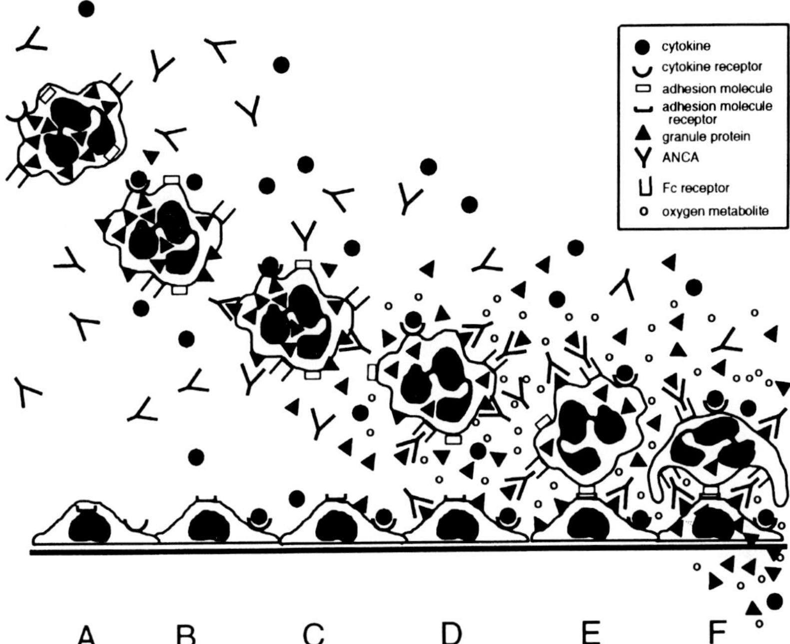

FIG. 8.9. Diagram of a putative ANCA-mediated pathogenesis. *A.* Unstimulated neutrophils (and monocytes not shown) contain ANCA target antigens (*e.g.,* PR3 and MPO) within the cytoplasm where they are not accessible to interact with ANCA. *B.* Stimulation (priming) of neutrophils, for example with cytokines (*e.g.,* IL-1 or TNF) or microbial products (*e.g.,* formyl tripeptides), releases small amounts of target antigens at the cell surface. *C* and *D.* ANCAs bind to target antigens and stimulate respiratory burst with release of toxic oxygen radicals, and degranulation with release of lytic enzymes. ANCA-induced neutrophil activation occurs by both Fc-independent and Fc-dependent mechanisms, with the latter involving Fc receptor engagement. *E* and *F.* Up-regulated adhesion molecules cause attachment of neutrophils to endothelial cells. Additional attraction and activation of neutrophils is caused by absorption of target antigens to vessel walls followed by ANCA binding. Toxic oxygen radicals and lytic enzymes injure vessel walls and perivascular tissue.

There is no unequivocal animal model of ANCA-mediated vasculitis. ANCAs have been detected in mice with polyclonal B cell activation, such as MRL mice and mercury-treated mice, that have glomerulonephritis and vasculitis, but their pathogenic significance in this setting is confounded by the presence of many other autoantibodies. A potential animal model of ANCA-mediated disease is being evaluated by Kinjoh et al.[16] These investigators have bred mice derived from (BXSB/MpxMRL/Mp-lpr/lpr)F1 that have severe crescentic glomerulonephritis and a high incidence of necrotizing small vessel vasculitis, which resemble ANCA-associated glomerulonephritis and vasculitis in humans.[16] Preliminary observations suggest that these animals have ANCAs (personal communication).

FINAL COMMON PATHWAY OF VASCULAR INFLAMMATION

All of these antibody-mediated initiating mechanisms result in a final common pathway of necrotizing vascular inflammation. This involves a rather stereotypical sequence of events that begins with leukocyte and endothelial activation, leads to leukocyte adhesion to endothelial cells, and culminates in vessel wall invasion and injury by leukocytes (Fig. 8.4). This is followed by an equally stereotypical repair process that involves mesenchymal remodeling, which is orchestrated by cytokines and other growth factors and often results in fibrosis.

PRIMING AND ACTIVATION OF LEUKOCYTES AND ENDOTHELIAL CELLS

The resting state for leukocytes and endothelial cells is characterized by constitutive expression of receptors that will transduce priming and activating signals when contacted by appropriate ligands, as well as latent capabilities for expressing additional receptors and secreting proinflammatory factors after activation.[5,17–22]

Primed neutrophils and monocytes express small amounts of granule contents, such as proteases, adhesion molecules, and myeloperoxidase, at the cell surface, but have not yet undergone full degranulation or respiratory burst. Cytokines, such as IL-1, TNF-α, and γ-interferon, play a major role in leukocyte and endothelial priming and activation. Other factors can play a role in particular vasculitides, such as microbial products, for example formyl peptides and lipopolysaccharides. Primed leukocytes are more receptive to many forms of immune-mediated activation, and thus priming events, such as infections, may synergize with immune mechanisms in causing vasculitis. This could explain the observed "flulike illness" that often precedes the initial onset and subsequent exacerbations of several types of systemic vasculitis, including Wegener's granulomatosis, microscopic polyangiitis (microscopic polyarteritis), and Goodpasture's syndrome.

Endothelial cells are not passive bystanders or innocent victims at sites of vasculitis, but rather contribute to the mediation of the inflammatory process by producing many of the same mediators that are produced by activated leukocytes.[17–22] Activated endothelial cells produce a number of proinflammatory cytokines, including IL-1, IL-6, and IL-8, which promotes chemotaxis and degranulation of neutrophils. Activated endothelial cells also produce proteins that attract and activate macrophages, such as MCP-1 and macrophage inflammatory protein-1 α. Endothelial lipid metabolites, such as leukotrienes, prostaglandins, and platelet activating factor, also are important early in vascular inflammation.

Fully activated neutrophils and monocytes release not only directly injurious products, such as oxygen metabolites and lytic enzymes, but also mediator molecules that amplify the inflammatory process by autocrine and paracrine influences on leukocytes and endothelial cells. Once monocytes transform into macrophage, they become particularly efficient secretors of proinflammatory cytokines, including a wide spectrum of interleukins.

ADHESION OF LEUKOCYTES TO ENDOTHELIAL CELLS

Adhesion of leukocytes to endothelial cells is the initial event in many types of vasculitis. This is a complex and dynamic process that involves reciprocal receptor-ligand binding between leukocytes and endothelial cells.[17–22]

Selectins act during the early phase of leukocyte-endothelial attachment. The rapid association and dissociation rate between selectins and their ligands leads to rolling of leukocytes along the endothelial surface as these adhesion molecules grab and release their ligands. Selectins have an N-terminal lectin domain, which binds to carbohydrate ligands, such as sialyl-Lewis x and similar sialylated molecules. Leukocytes constitutively express L-selectin. E-selectin and P-selectin are expressed by stimulated but not unstimulated endothelial cells. Expression of E-selectin is induced by many of the same factors that prime leukocytes, such as IL-1, TNF, and lipopolysaccharides. Expression of P-selectin is induced by a variety of inflammatory mediators, such as histamine and thrombin. P-selectin also is expressed on the surface of activated platelets.

Tight adhesion of neutrophils and monocytes to endothelial cells is mediated by β_1-integrins, such as VLA-4 (CD49b/CD29), and especially β_2-integrins, such as LFA-1 (CD11a/CD18), Mac-1 (CD11b/CD18), and p150,95 (CD11c/CD18). Increased expression and avidity of leukocyte integrins are induced by many inflammatory mediators, including IL-8, TNF, platelet activating factor, leukotriene β_4, MCP-1, and C5a. Integrins bind to endothelial immunoglobulin family cell adhesion molecules (IgCAMs), such as ICAM-1, ICAM-2, ICAM-3 and VCAM-1. IgCAM expression is up-regulated by cytokines, such as IL-1 and TNF.

Adhesion molecule-ligand interactions also are involved in leukocyte diapedesis, but this is a multifactoral process that is poorly understood. The immunoglobulin superfamily molecule PECAM-1, which is expressed at endothelial tight junctions, may be important for diapedesis.

Vascular Inflammation and Necrosis

Neutrophils and monocytes adhere to and penetrate vessel walls, primarily the walls of postcapillary venules, at sites of inflammation where no vasculitis is occurring. This is part of the normal trafficking of inflammatory cells to appropriate sites of inflammation. The leukocytes must be stimulated (primed) to up-regulate their adhesion molecules and to release small amounts of lytic enzymes that allow diapedesis and migration into the tissue. The leukocytes follow chemoattractant gradients until they reach a zone of adequate stimulation for full activation. At sites of nonvasculitic inflammation, this occurs only after leukocytes exit the vessel wall. At sites of vasculitis, the leukocytes are driven to full activation while still in the vessel wall. This "premature" activation is caused by one of the initiating mechanisms discussed earlier, *i.e.,* vascular infection, immune complex localization, direct antibody binding, or ANCAs.

At sites of vasculitis, activated neutrophils and monocytes penetrate through the endothelium into the mural and perivascular tissues, where they cause necrotizing injury by releasing the toxic products and by activating humoral mediator systems. Activated neutrophils and monocytes produce oxygen metabolites, such as hydrogen peroxide, which interacts with myeloperoxidase to cause toxic halogenation. Activated neutrophils and monocytes also release enzymes, such as elastase, cathepsin G, and proteinase 3, which can degrade tissue. In infectious vasculitides, the effects of these autologous injurious agents are augmented by toxic products from pathogens.

Neutrophils and monocytes have receptors for matrix proteins, including collagen, laminin, fibronectin, and vitronectin. These matrix receptors facilitate diapedesis of leukocytes into the vascular and perivascular tissues. Even during physiologic diapedesis at sites where leukocytes are exiting the circulation to participate in "normal" inflammatory responses, there is release of small amounts of lytic enzymes, such as elastase and cathepsin G, which lyse basement membrane and matrix to allow passage of the leukocytes. At sites of vasculitis, neutrophils and monocytes are driven to full activation within vessel walls, resulting in pathologic degrees of vascular lysis. In very small vessels, such as capillaries and venules, this often causes rupture and hemorrhage; whereas in larger vessels, such as arteries, this results in insudation of plasma proteins into the necrotic vessel wall, where they are transformed into fibrinoid material.

Humoral protease cascades, such as the complement, coagulation, kinin, and fibronolytic systems, contribute to lesion development. The inflammatory process is modulated by both active proteases, such as complement proteases, thrombin, kallikrein, plasmin, and protein split products, such as C3a, C4a, C5a, fibronectin peptides, and fibrinopeptides. The fibrinoid material so characteristic of necrotizing vasculitis (Fig. 8.10) is largely fibrin (Fig. 8.11) generated by the extravasation of coagulation proteins into the thrombogenic focus of necrosis. The coagulation cascade is activated, resulting in conversion of fibronogen to fibrin.

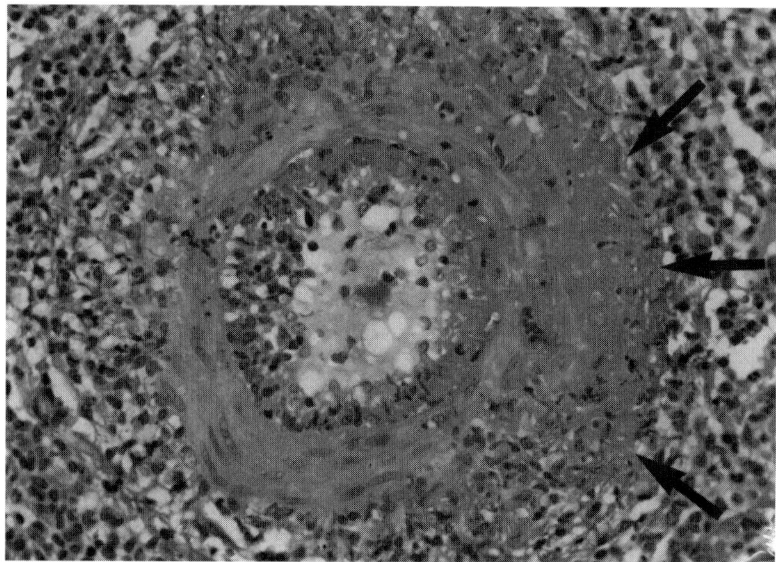

FIG. 8.10.   Necrotizing vasculitis affecting a small artery in a skeletal muscle biopsy. Note the segmental fibrinoid necrosis (*arrows*). Hematoxylin & eosin.

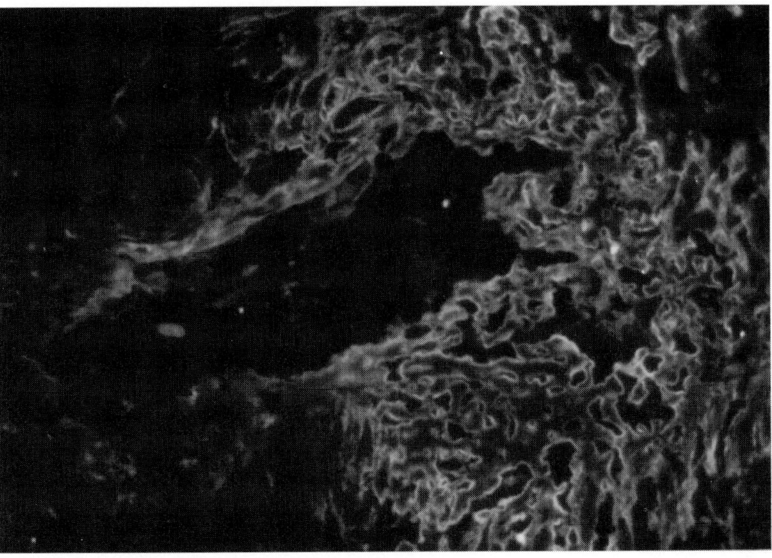

FIG. 8.11.   Direct immunofluorescence microscopy of fibrin in an area of fibrinoid necrosis in a small artery affected by necrotizing vasculitis. FITC-conjugated antifibrin.

INFLUENCE OF SHARED PATHOGENIC PATHWAYS ON DIFFERENTIAL DIAGNOSIS

Because of the shared final common pathway of acute vascular inflammation, many etiologically different vasculitides share a common histology that is characterized by leukocyte infiltration, leukocytoclasia and fibrinoid necrosis. A corollary to this is that histology alone is inadequate for pathologic diagnostic categorization of vasculitides, and must be supplemented with serology, immunohistology, or other methods for identifying the pathogenic initiating factors.

For example, histologic demonstration of leukocytoclastic angiitis in the skin of a patient with purpura doesn't add much to the understanding of the patient's disease, but immunohistologic demonstration of IgA-dominant immune complexes indicates Henoch-Schönlein purpura; demonstration of IgM and IgG immune deposits along with serum cryoglobulins indicates cryoglobulinemic vasculitis and raises the possibility of hepatitis C infection; and lack of immune deposits and serologic identification of ANCA, suggest Wegener's granulomatosis, Churg-Strauss syndrome, or microscopic polyangiitis (microscopic polyarteritis).

Immunopathologic categorization of vasculitis is important for patient management because appropriate treatment is different for different categories of vasculitis. For example, Henoch-Schönlein purpura usually can be managed with supportive care alone, hepatitis C-induced cryoglobulinemic vasculitis may respond to α-interferon treatment, and ANCA-associated vasculitis often requires aggressive immunosuppression to avoid substantial morbidity and mortality.

Correlation of pathogenic mechanisms with clinicopathologic expressions of disease reveals that the same pathogenic mechanism can produce multiple patterns of disease; for example, ANCA-associated disease can manifest as Wegener's granulomatosis, Churg-Strauss syndrome, or microscopic polyangiitis (microscopic polyarteritis).[23] In addition, the same clinicopathologic expression of vasculitis can be caused by multiple pathogenic mechanisms; for example, pulmonary-renal vasculitic syndrome can be caused by immune complexes, ANCA, or anti-glomerular basement membrane antibodies (Fig. 8.12). And to further complicate matters, in a minority of patients with vasculitis, there is evidence for the presence of more than one immunopathogenic process; for example, ANCA-associated disease superimposed on immune complex or antibasement membrane disease.

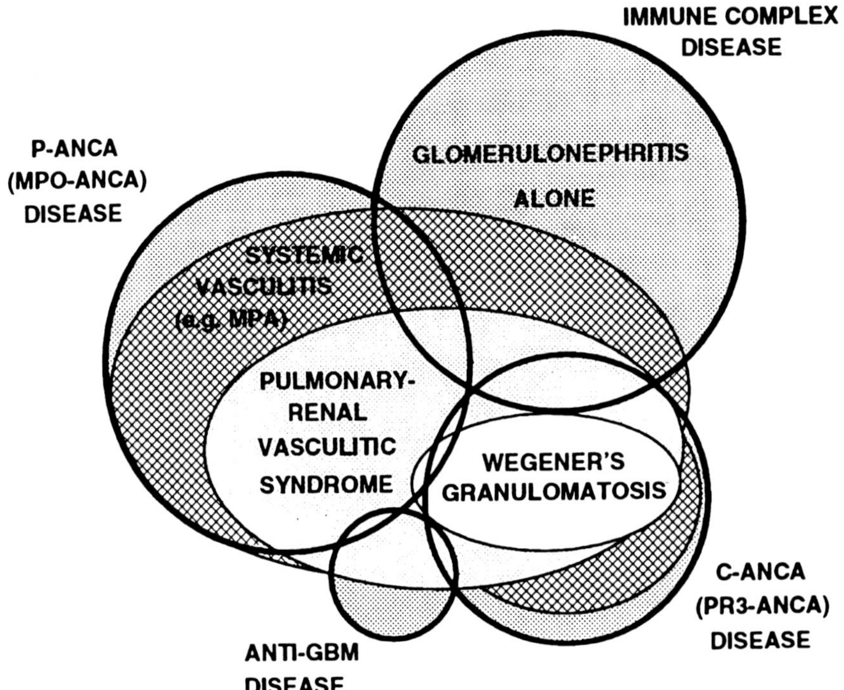

FIG. 8.12. Diagram correlating different immunopathologic categories of vasculitis (*circles*) with clinicopathologic expressions of vasculitis (*shaded oval areas*) based on their frequencies among patients with severe (crescentic) glomerulonephritis. Note that some clinical expressions of vasculitis, such as pulmonary-renal vasculitic syndrome, are caused by many different immunopathologic processes, which overlap in a minority of patients. Also note that a particular immunopathologic category includes multiple clinicopathologic expressions of disease. For example, patients with P-ANCA (MPO-ANCA) and glomerulonephritis can have glomerulonephritis alone, glomerulonephritis with systemic necrotizing small-vessel vasculitis without pulmonary involvement (*i.e.,* microscopic polyangiitis), or glomerulonephritis with systemic necrotizing small-vessel vasculitis causing pulmonary capillaritis (*i.e.,* pulmonary-renal vasculitic syndrome caused by microscopic polyangiitis). (From Ref. 23, with permission.)

IMPACT OF PATHOBIOLOGY ON TREATMENT STRATEGIES

Current therapy of immune-mediated vasculitides relies on crude immunosuppressive treatment with corticosteroids, cytotoxic drugs, and plasmapheresis. More effective treatment approaches should result from a better understanding of the pathobiology of vasculitis. This understanding will allow specific targeting of critical pathogenic events. There already is experimental evidence that vasculitis can be abrogated or ameliorated by agents that interfere with cell adhesion (*e.g.*, antibodies against selectins and integrins, and ligand mimics), cytokine signaling (*e.g.*, soluble cytokine receptors, anticytokine antibodies and pharmacologic agents that inhibit cytokine production), protease injury (*e.g.*, cloned and synthetic protease inhibitors), oxygen metabolite injury (*e.g.*, oxygen metabolite scavengers, catalase), pathogenic antibodies (*e.g.*, antiidiotypic therapy), and etiologic agents (*e.g.*, interferon treatment for hepatitis C-induced vasculitis).

REFERENCES

1. Kingston ME, Mackey D. Skin clues in the diagnosis of life-threatening infections. *Rev Infect Dis* 1986;8:1–11.
2. Walker DH, Cain BG, Olmstead PM. Laboratory diagnosis of Rocky Mountain spotted fever by immunofluorescent demonstration of Rickettsia rickettsii in cutaneous lesions. *Am J Clin Pathol* 1978;69:619–623.
3. Dixon FJ, Vazquez JJ, Weigle WO, Cochrane CG. Pathogenesis of serum sickness. *Arch Pathol* 1958;65:18–28.
4. Cochrane CG, Koffler D. Immune complex disease in experimental animals and man. *Adv Immunol* 1973;16:185–264.
5. Jennette JC, Charles LA, Falk RJ. The neutrophil and its role in systemic vasculitis. In: LeRoy EC, ed. *The biologic basis of systemic vasculitis.* New York: Marcel Dekker, 1992:65–92.
6. Sergent JS, Lockshin MD, Christian CL, Gocke DJ. Vasculitis with hepatitis B antigenemia: long-term observations in nine patients. *Medicine* 1976;55:1–18.
7. Patel A, Prussick R, Buchanan WW, Sauder DN. Serum sickness-like illness and leukocytoclastic vasculitis after intravenous streptokinase. *J Am Acad Dermatol* 1991;24:652–653.
8. Giger U, Werner LL, Millichamp NJ, et al. Sulfadiazine-induced allergy in six Doberman pinchers. *J Am Vet Med Assoc* 1985;86:479–484.
9. Agnello V, Chung RT, Kaplan LM. A role for hepatitis C virus infection in type II cryoglobulinemia. *N Engl J Med* 1992;327:1490–1495.
10. Marcellin P, Descamps V, Martinot-Peignoux M, et al. Cryoglobulinemia with vasculitis associated with hepatitis C virus infection. *Gastroenterology* 1993;104:272–277.
11. Lerner RA, Glassock RJ, Dixon FJ. The role of anti-glomerular basement membrane antibody in the pathogenesis of human glomerulonephritis. *J Exp Med* 1967;126:989–1004.
12. Meroni PL, Papa ND, Conforti G, Barcellini W, Borghi MO, Gambini D. Antibodies to endothelial cells in systemic vasculitis. In: Cervera R, Khamashta MA, Hughes GR, eds. *Antibodies to endothelial cells and vascular damage.* Boca Raton, FL: CRC Press, 1994:121–133.
13. Leung DYM, Collins T, Lapierre LA, Geha RS, Pober JS. Immunoglobulin M antibodies present in the acute phase of Kawasaki syndrome lyse cultured vascular endothelial cells stimulated by gamma interferon. *J Clin Invest* 1986;77:1428–1435.
14. Chan TM, Frampton G, Jayne DR, Perry GJ, Lockwood CM, Cameron JS. Clinical significance of anti-endothelial cell antibodies in systemic vasculitis: a longitudinal study comparing anti-endothelial cell antibodies and anti-neutrophil cytoplasmic antibodies. *Am J Kidney Dis* 1993;22:387–392.
15. Jennette JC, Falk RJ. Pathogenic potential of anti-neutrophil cytoplasmic autoantibodies. *Lab Invest* 1994;70:135–137.

16. Kinjoh K, Kyogoku M, Good RA. Genetic selection for crescent formation yields mouse strain with rapidly progressive glomerulonephritis and small vessel vasculitis. *Proc Natl Acad Sci USA* 1993;90:3413–3417.

17. Bevilacqua MP. Endothelial-leukocyte adhesion molecules. *Annu Rev Immunol* 1993;11:767–804.

18. Cotran RS, Pober JS. Cytokine-endothelial interactions in inflammation, immunity, and vascular injury. *J Am Soc Nephrol* 1990;1:225–235.

19. Swerlick RA, Lawley TJ. Role of microvascular endothelial cells in inflammation. *J Invest Dermatol* 1993;100:111S–15S.

20. Lasky LA. Selectins: interpreters of cell-specific carbohydrate information during inflammation. *Science* 1992;258:964–969.

21. Williams TJ, Hellewell PG. Endothelial cell biology. Adhesion molecules involved in the microvascular inflammatory response. *Am Rev Respir Dis* 1992;146:S45–S50

22. Springer TA. Traffic signals for lymphocyte recirculation and leukocyte emigration: the multistep paradigm. *Cell* 1994;76:301–314

23. Jennette JC. Antineutrophil cytoplasmic autoantibody-associated diseases: a pathologist's perspective. *Am J Kidney Dis* 1991;18:164–170.

Chapter 9

Problems in Forensic Cardiovascular Pathology

RENU VIRMANI, ALLEN P. BURKE, ANDREW FARB, AND JOHN SMIALEK

Most cases of cardiac death that are seen by the forensic pathologist are sudden cardiac deaths. By definition, sudden cardiac death (SCD) must be natural, rapid, and unexpected. SCD has been variously defined as death occurring instantaneously or within 1, 2, 6, 12, or 24 hours after onset of symptoms. Clinicians usually use death within 1 hour of the onset of acute symptoms for defining SCD.[1] The World Health Organization has defined SCD as death occurring within 24 hours of onset of symptoms. The forensic pathologist is often confronted with unwitnessed death and will at best be told when the patient was last seen alive. In such cases there is no way of knowing the duration of symptoms before death or if any symptoms occurred. Therefore, from the forensic pathologist's view, SCD must be natural, unexpected, and without extracardiac cause; the exact duration of symptoms is often irrelevant.

FREQUENCY

Most studies in the United States indicate that there are 300,000 SCDs annually, a figure that represents 50% of all cardiovascular deaths in this country.[1] Some estimates place the frequency even higher, at 400,000 annually,[1] depending on the definition of sudden death. If the time interval between onset of symptoms to death is 1 or 2 hours, 12–13% of all natural deaths are sudden, 88% of which are due to coronary heart disease (CHD). If the 24-hour definition is used, 32% of natural deaths are sudden, 75% of which are due to CHD.[2,3] Fifty-six percent of sudden deaths occur among persons aged 35–74 years and the proportion of these deaths that are due to CHD decreases with advancing age.[1] Data from several studies indicate that 76% of CHD deaths in men and women 20–39 years of age are sudden; this proportion decreases with advancing age (62% for 45–54-year-olds, 58% for 55–64-year-olds, and 42% for 65–74-year-olds).[4,5] The incidence of SCD in women is only one-third that of men[6,7]; women lag behind men by 20 years.[6] Although controversial, SCD is probably more frequent in blacks than in whites.

CAUSES OF SUDDEN CARDIAC DEATH

Causes of SCD include atherosclerosis, cardiomyopathies, hypertensive heart disease, valvular heart disease, myocarditis, nonatherosclerotic coronary artery disease, congenital heart disease, and pathologic changes of the conduction system (Table 9.1). We reviewed our files at the AFIP for cases referred from the state of Maryland between January 1, 1990 and December 31, 1993 from people more than 14 years old with SCD. Almost all subjects 15–45 years old dying suddenly in Maryland are autopsied, and this forms a database from which to determine the frequency of the various causes of SCD. Atherosclerotic heart disease was excluded for this analysis because autopsies are often not performed on older people with a history of coronary heart disease. A total of 166 cases of sudden cardiac death were reviewed and are tabulated in Table 9.2 and Figure 9.1.

In this review, only important causes of SCD will be addressed. Because coronary heart disease accounts for 80% of all sudden death in the western world, it will be discussed in detail. An overview of cardiomyopathy and SCD will follow, with explanations of the definition of cardiomyopathy and the role of cardiac hypertrophy in the etiology of ventricular arrhythmias. Among the various valvular diseases that may result in SCD, mitral valve prolapse (MVP) and aortic stenosis will be reviewed briefly. Aortic stenosis is a well-known cause of SCD; MVP has a high prevalence in the general population, and the differen-

TABLE 9.1   ETIOLOGY OF SUDDEN CARDIAC DEATH[a]

I. Coronary artery abnormalities
    Coronary artery atherosclerosis
    Anomalous coronary artery origin
    Hypoplastic coronary artery
    Coronary embolism
    Coronary artery dissection
    Coronary arteritis
    Small-artery disease
    Functional obstruction-coronary spasm, myocardial bridges
II. Myocardial disease
    Hypertrophic cardiomyopathy, idiopathic left ventricular hypertrophy (LVH), LVH
        with systemic hypertension
    Idiopathic dilated cardiomyopathy
    Infiltrative disease: sarcoidosis, myocarditis, amyloidosis
    Right ventricular dysplasia (Uhl's anomaly)
III. Valvular diseases
    Aortic stenosis, mitral valve prolapse
    Prosthetic valve dysfunction
    Infective endocarditis
    Myxoma
IV. Conduction system
    Sinoatrial node: small-vessel disease, hemorrhage, fibrosis
    Atrioventricular node: mesothelioma, fibrosis, dystrophic calcification
    His bundle: congenital or acquired anatomic discontinuity
    Accessory pathways
    Prolonged Q-T interval

[a]Modified from Ref. 33.

TABLE 9.2. MODE OF CARDIAC DEATH IN 242 AUTOPSY CASES[a]

	All Deaths	Sudden Deaths (%)		NSCD (%)		Exercise (%)	
I. Anomalous origin of one or more CA from PT							
LMCA or LAD from PT	37	14	(38)	23	(62)	2	(14)
Both CAs from PT	3	3	(100)	0	(0)	0	(0)
RCA from PT	1	0	(0)	1	(100)	0	(0)
II. Anomalous origin of one or more CA from aorta							
LMCA and RCA from R sinus	49	28	(57)	8	(16)	18	(64)
RCA and LMCA from L sinus	52	13	(25)	2	(4)	6	(46)
LCx and RCA from R sinus	21	2	(10)	6	(29)	0	(0)
LCA and/or LMCA from P sinus	17	5	(29)	4	(24)	2	(40)
RCA and LAD from R sinus	1	1	(100)	0	(0)	0	(0)
III. Single CA ostium from aorta							
Single RCA ostium	22	4	(18)	5	(23)	2	(50)
Single LCA ostium	22	2	(9)	8	(36)	1	(50)
IV. Hypoplastic CAs	13	5	(38)	4	(31)	3	(60)
V. CA fistula	4	1	(25)	3	(75)	0	(0)
Total	242	78	(32)	64	(26)	34	(44)

[a]Exercise-related sudden deaths are expressed as percentage of sudden deaths. Patients not accounted for in totals died from noncardiac causes. NSCD, nonsudden cardiac death; CA, coronary artery; L, left; LAD, left anterior descending coronary artery; LCA, left coronary artery; LCx, left circumflex coronary artery; LMCA, left main coronary artery; R, right; P, posterior; RCA, right coronary artery; PT, pulmonary trunk. Reproduced with permission from Ref. 27.

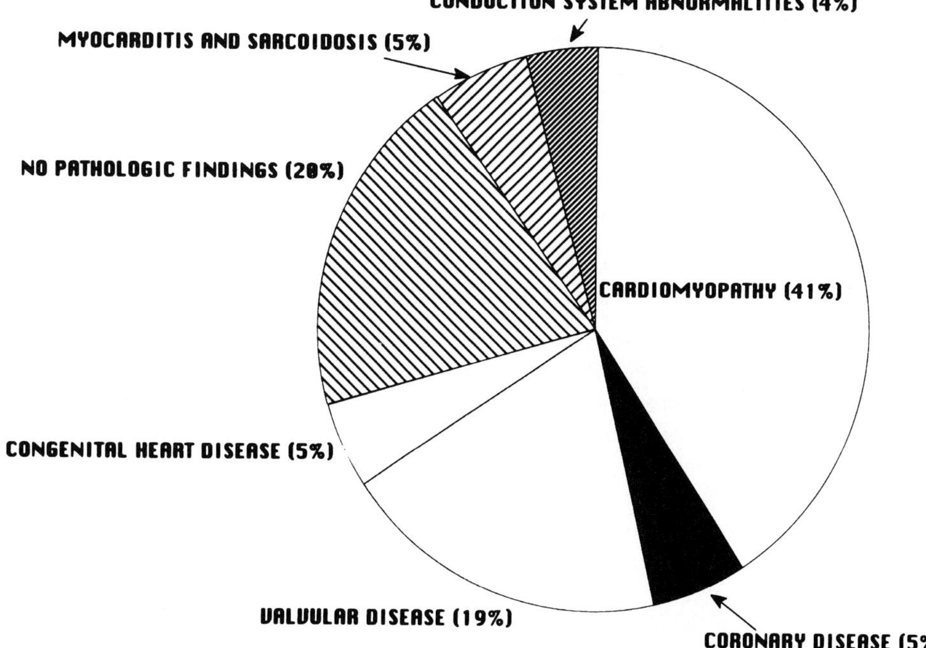

FIG. 9.1. Distribution of cause of death in 166 people in the State of Maryland who died suddenly, excluding cases with severe coronary atherosclerotic heart disease from January 1, 1990 to December 31, 1993.

tial pathologic features in incidental MVP *versus* sudden death associated with MVP are not widely known. Finally, the "normal heart" and SCD will be discussed. A relatively large group of SCDs will have no cardiac structural abnormality to account for death, and the forensic pathologist relies on the circumstances of death and toxicologic analysis to rule out noncardiac causes of death.

MECHANISM OF SUDDEN CARDIAC DEATH

Sudden death is usually arrhythmic in origin and is the leading cause of death in patients with coronary heart disease. However, the mechanism of sudden death and the nature of the terminal arrhythmia in SCD cases are often unclear. Review of available data shows that chest pain as a prodromal symptom is infrequent (11–35%), whereas fatigue and dyspnea are the most common symptoms experienced by SCD victims.[8] At least one-third of patients who suffer SCD due to coronary disease have consulted a family physician within 4 weeks before death.[8] Sudden death occurs more frequently during physical activity, standing, sitting, and less frequently, during sleep.[9]

Electrophysiologic events during sudden cardiac death have been obtained from continuous electrocardiographic monitoring in coronary care units or by mobile resuscitation teams. Emergency rescue electrocardiographic tracings were recorded in Miami in people with witnessed prehospital cardiac arrest between 1975 and 1978. Sixty-two percent demonstrated ventricular fibrillation, 7% sustained ventricular tachycardia, and 31% bradyarrhythmias of various types or asystole.[10] The number of patients successfully resuscitated and discharged from the hospital was highest in patients with ventricular tachycardia and hypotension (67%). The worst prognosis was observed in the bradyarrhythmic group (0%). Those patients with ventricular fibrillation had an intermediate prognosis (23%). In this group of resuscitated patients, coronary heart disease was the most common diagnosis (79%), followed by congestive cardiomyopathy (10%), conduction system disease (7%), valvular heart disease (5%), and hypertensive heart disease (5%). Subsequent studies have shown improvement in the outcome of ventricular fibrillation.[11]

PATHOLOGY OF SUDDEN DEATH CAUSED BY CORONARY HEART DISEASE

Severe coronary atherosclerosis is the most frequent pathologic finding in SCD. Because some degree of atherosclerosis is ubiquitous in the coronary arteries of people living in industrialized countries,[12] an established definition of the degree of coronary atherosclerosis that can be regarded as a direct cause of death is needed. The vast majority of people who die suddenly have more than 75% cross-sectional area luminal narrowing by atherosclerotic plaque; this figure is often used as the minimum degree of narrowing to account for SCD.[13–15] Developing strict pathologic criteria is difficult, however, because oxygen demand varies with myocardial mass, heart rate, contractibility, and myocardial tension. We believe that after forensic examination has ruled out other natural and unnatural causes of death, coronary narrowing of at least 65% by an atherosclerotic plaque in one or more arteries is sufficient as a cause of death.

The incidence of severe disease (>75% stenosis) in 3 or 4 major coronary arteries ranges from 52 to 61% in most series of SCD.[13,14,16] The sex and race of the person appear to play a role in the proportion of SCD cases with severe 3-vessel coronary artery disease. In one study,[16] 70% of white men had 3- or 4-vessel disease compared with only 34% of white women and 58% of black men and women. In a recent series of SCD, we have found, in contrast to most reports, that only 15% of patients had 3-vessel disease, and that 71% had 1- or 2-vessel disease.[15] The low incidence of 3-vessel disease in our study may be because our patient population was young and had a higher proportion of Blacks and women than did other studies.

Coronary atherosclerosis as a cause of sudden cardiac death is nearly incontestable when a thrombus is present in the coronary artery; unfortunately, in cases of sudden cardiac death, thrombi are not always encountered. The incidence of thrombosis, which varies widely from 15 to 74%, depends on the time interval between onset of symptoms and death. We have found that incidence of acute thrombus in SCD due to atherosclerosis is 89% in patients with acute myocardial infarction, 63% in patients with acute or healed myocardial infarction, 40% in patients without acute myocardial infarction, and 39% in the absence of infarction.[15] Davies *et al* reported a 73% incidence of mural and occlusive coronary thrombi in patients dying suddenly with 6 hours onset of symptoms; the patients in his study had a high incidence of recent chest pain and/or acute myocardial infarction (69%) and healed myocardial infarct (78%).[13] Warnes and Roberts reported only a 19% incidence of thrombosis; 46% of the people in this study had either a history of angina pectoris or had a previous myocardial infarction, and the incidence of thrombosis was similar in patients with or without infarction.[14] It is evident that further study is necessary to determine the factors that affect the incidence of coronary thrombosis in patients with SCD due to coronary artery disease.

The underlying plaque morphology may play an important role in the understanding of thrombosis. Angiographic studies of patients with subsequent coronary occlusive thrombosis have shown that two-thirds of patients have mild to moderate coronary disease (<50% angiographic diameter stenosis or <75% cross-sectional area luminal narrowing) at the site of occlusive thrombus.[17] However, an autopsy study[18] has shown that most thrombi are superimposed on severely narrowed plaque. Davies *et al.*[13] found that 19% of cases of atherosclerosis-related thrombi lacked underlying severe lesions; 13% of the occlusive thrombi in our study had 65–74% cross-sectional area luminal narrowing. Plaque fissures, or rupture, have been implicated in the formation of occlusive thrombi, although the mechanism of plaque rupture is poorly understood. Constantinides[19] suggested that plaque rupture occurs from the lumen into the plaque, whereas Barger *et al.*[20] proposed that rupture occurs from the plaque into the lumen, based on the presence of a large number of vasa vasorum in atherosclerotic plaques. We have observed plaque fissures and/or acute thrombosis in 69% and plaque fissures in 54% of patients with acute or healed myocardial infarction, indicating that plaque fissure is not always observed in cases of coronary thrombosis. In addition, we have observed intimal fibrin deposition in arteries without plaque hemorrhage that are often narrowed less than 75% of the cross-sectional area lumen (Fig. 9.2).

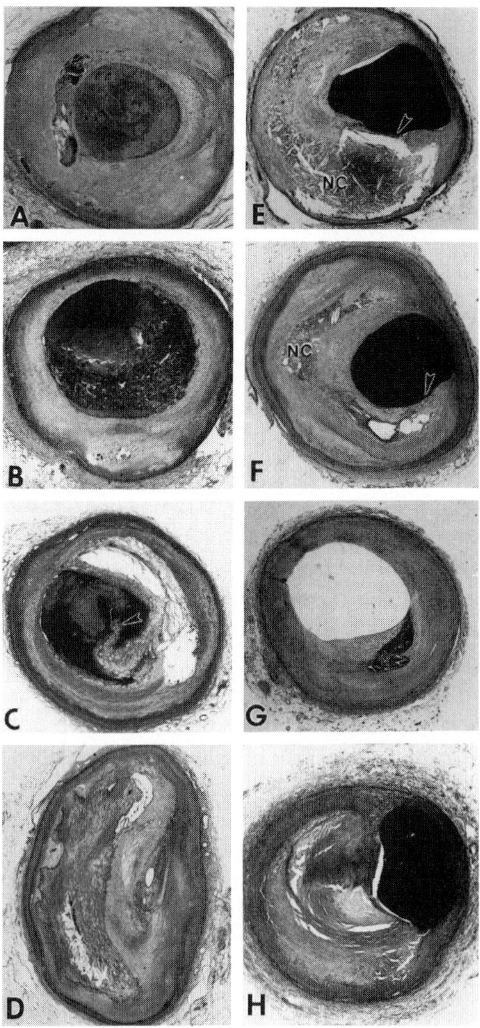

FIG. 9.2.   Photomicrographs from patients with sudden cardiac death and moderate to severe coronary artery disease at autopsy. *A–C.* Microscopic sections of coronary arteries from patients with acute myocardial infarction at autopsy. *A* shows characteristic changes of occlusive luminal thrombus with hemorrhage into a plaque and plaque rupture in a patient with acute myocardial infarction. *B.* An occlusive thrombus with underlying moderate atherosclerosis (51–75% cross-sectional area luminal narrowing) and no plaque hemorrhage, but there is mild intimal fibrin deposition. *C.* A typical plaque rupture (*arrowhead*) and nonocclusive thrombus in a man who died suddenly and had an acute myocardial infarct at autopsy. *D.* A total occlusion with organized thrombus (*arrowhead*) in a man with sudden cardiac death and healed myocardial infarction at autopsy. *E* and *F.* Sections from two different patients with varying degrees of luminal narrowing and plaque hemorrhage. In *E,* the overlying fibrous cap is markedly thin (*arrowhead*) with a large underlying necrotic core (*NC*) but there is no overlying thrombus; in *F* the necrotic core (*NC*) is small and the fibrous cap is thick and there is hemorrhage into a plaque and only in one area is the fibrous cap thinned (*arrowhead*) and contains foam cells. *G.* Plaque hemorrhage and fissure in an artery with 60% cross-sectional area luminal narrowing without luminal thrombus. The adjoining section of the artery (not shown) showed a 70% cross-sectional area luminal narrowing but there was no plaque hemorrhage or fissure. *H.* Fibrous plaque with no necrotic core or plaque hemorrhage in a patient with SCD and a 70% cross-sectional area luminal narrowing.

CORONARY ARTERY ANOMALIES

Coronary artery anomalies are found in approximately 1% of all patients undergoing coronary angiography and in approximately 0.3% of patients undergoing autopsy.[21,22] Although coronary anomalies can be an incidental autopsy finding, they are also a well-known cause of sudden death[23-27] and are found relatively more frequently in young persons who die during exercise.[26,27] We have reported recently on the frequency and mechanism of sudden death in patients with isolated or congenital coronary artery anomalies not associated with a congenital anomaly of the heart and great vessels. The most frequent anomalies were left main coronary artery or left anterior descending coronary artery from pulmonary trunk (n=37), left main and right coronary artery from right aortic sinus (n=49), right and left main from left aortic sinus (n=52), single coronary ostium from aorta (n=44), and hypoplastic coronary arteries (n=13) (Table 9.2). The highest frequency of sudden death was seen in patients with left main and right coronary origin from the right aortic sinus (57%) (Table 9.2) and in 64% death was exercise-related. Sudden death occurred infrequently when right and left main coronary arteries arose from the left aortic sinus (25%) or where there was a single coronary ostium from the aorta (14%) (Fig. 9.3).

Anomalous coronary arteries are believed to result in sudden death from several different mechanisms. Cheitlin *et al.*[23] first described the importance of a slitlike orifice in anomalous origin of the right coronary artery from the right aortic sinus. Acute-angle take-off and intramural (within the aortic wall) coronary segments have been observed in anomalous origin of coronary arteries, as well as in normal origin of coronary arteries.[28] We have found evidence that acute angle take-off of an intramural coronary segment is more frequently seen in patients dying suddenly with left or right coronary arteries arising from the contralateral coronary sinus or when the anomalous coronary artery is coursing between the pulmonary trunk and aorta.[27] The risk was particularly great for origin of the left coronary artery from the right coronary sinus; 84% of such patients died suddenly when the anomalous artery coursed between pulmonary trunk and aorta. Compression of the coronary artery occurs at the onset of diastole with aortic root distention. This take-off compression may explain the increased frequency of sudden death when the left coronary artery courses between the aorta and the pulmonary trunk and originates from two ostia as opposed to a single ostium.

We recently analyzed the differences between congenital coronary artery anomalies in patients less than 30 years of age and those older than 30 years.[27] We excluded patients with origin of left main artery from the pulmonary trunk, both coronary arteries from the pulmonary trunk, and coronary artery fistulas because all patients in these groups were younger than 30 years. The majority of cases of origin of the left main coronary from the right coronary sinus were observed in young patients; otherwise, anomalies were evenly distributed among patients younger than and older than 30 years. Patients younger than 30 years had higher rates of sudden death (62%) compared with patients older than 30 years (12%; *p* .00001) and a higher percent were exer-

     Cardiovascular Pathology

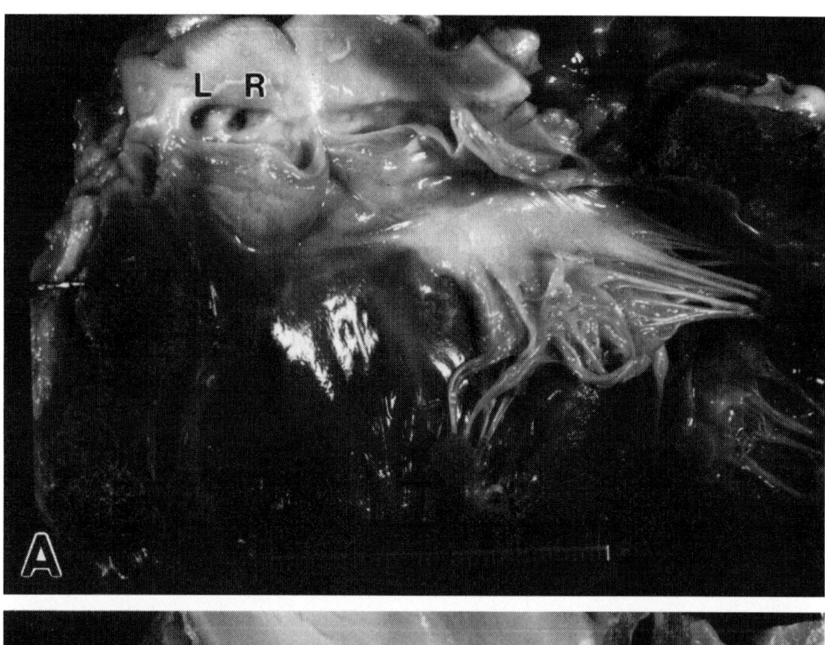

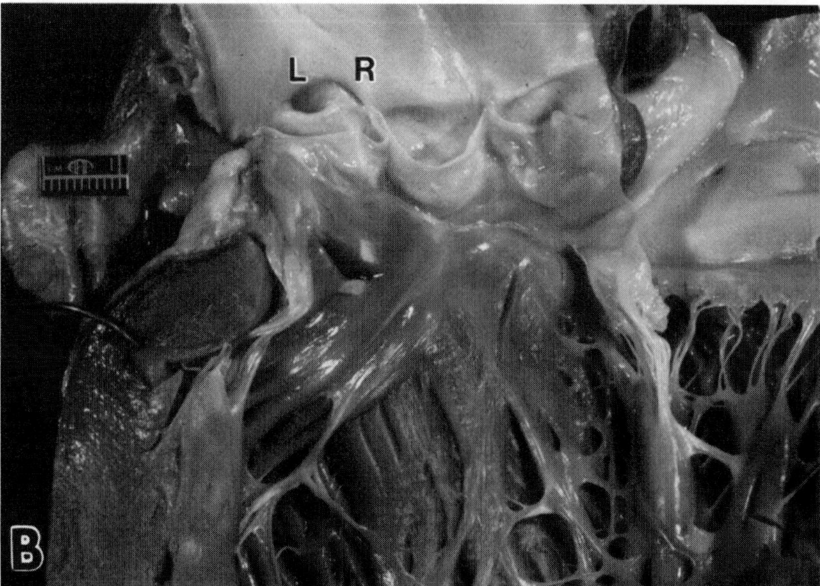

FIG. 9.3.   *A.* View of left ventricular outflow tract and aorta showing left (*L*) and right (*R*) coronary ostia arising in the right coronary sinus of a 14-year-old boy who died suddenly while playing soccer. *B.* View of left ventricular outflow tract and aorta showing left (*L*) and right (*R*) coronary arteries arising from the left coronary sinus in a 19-year-old man who died during exercise. (Reproduced with permission from Ref. 27.)

cise related (40% *vs.* 2%; *p* .00001). As expected, younger patients had a lower rate of atherosclerotic coronary artery disease. Only one patient younger than 30 years had significant coronary atherosclerosis, compared with 40% of patients older than 30 years. The single young patient with coronary atherosclerosis had origin of the right coronary artery from the left coronary sinus; autopsy showed acute myocardial infarction with left main coronary artery thrombosis. Because younger patients are at a high risk of sudden death with isolated coronary artery anomaly, a greater effort for early detection and surgical repair of these lesions is warranted; in older patients, the development of coronary atherosclerosis is a significant complication of coronary anomalies.

CARDIOMYOPATHY

Cardiac hypertrophy should be defined with population-derived criteria based on body weight and height.[29,30] Cardiac hypertrophy, in the absence of valvular, ischemic, or congenital heart disease, should be divided into five main categories, assessed by either cross-sections (breadloafing) of the myocardium (Fig. 9.4) cut parallel to the posterior atrioventricular sulcus, or by long axis sections along the left ventricular outflow tract or four-chamber view of the heart. Each of the five types of cardiomyopathy is a cause of SCD in the absence of other cardiac and noncardiac causes. In hypertrophic cardiomyopathy, there is asymmetric septal hypertrophy (the septum is 1.5 times thicker than the left ventricular free wall), left atrial dilatation, small or normal-sized left ventricular cavity, and microscopic fibromuscular disarray (Fig. 9.5) involving a significant portion of the ventricular septum.[31] Concentric idiopathic hypertrophy is defined by concentric left ventricular hypertrophy without ventricular dilation, fibromuscular disarray, or a history of hypertension. This category likely includes some patients with undiagnosed hypertension and some patients with concentric hypertrophic cardiomyopathy in the absence of myofiber disarray. The latter entity is poorly defined; however, in patients with concentric left ventricular hypertrophy, a family history of hypertrophic cardiomyopathy is sufficient to make a diagnosis of hypertrophic cardiomyopathy without asymmetry. Concentric hypertrophy with systemic hypertension requires a clinical diagnosis of hypertension or definite changes of arteriolonephrosclerosis in the absence of glomerular disease.[32] Idiopathic dilated cardiomyopathy is defined by cardiomegaly with four-chamber dilation, ventricular hypertrophy,[33,34] and a left ventricular cavity diameter greater than 4 cm at the level of the papillary muscles. The extent of ventricular dilatation is generally greater than atrial dilation, and microscopic examination is helpful in ruling out infiltrative and inflammatory disease. Lastly, arrhythmogenic right ventricular dysplasia, also referred to as right ventricular cardiomyopathy, consists of partial or complete replacement of right ventricle muscle by fat and/or fibrous tissue with or without entrapment of myocytes,[34] (Fig. 9.6). It may be associated with ventricular tachyarrhythmias of right ventricular origin and can cause sudden death, often with exercise in people usually less than 30 years of age.[35] Uhl's anomaly, a related condition, is characterized by hypoplasia of the right ventricular myocardium, with apposition of endocardial

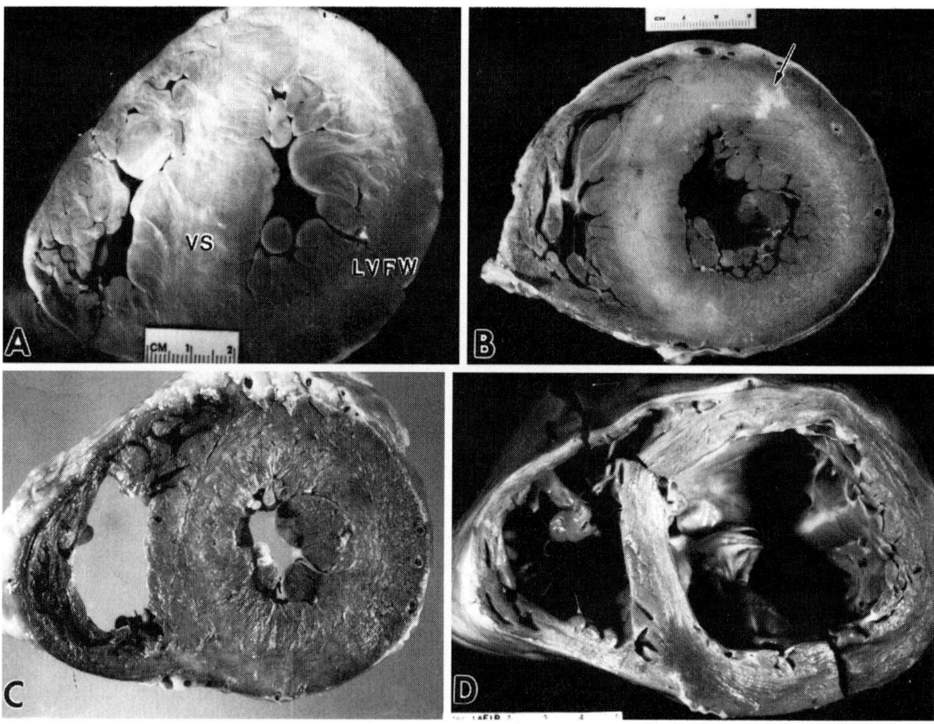

FIG. 9.4.   Left and right ventricular slices of hearts cut parallel to the posterior atrioventricular sulcus. Each slice shows characteristic changes of four types of cardiomyopathy. *A*. Heart of a
young patient who died suddenly after playing soccer. Note markedly thickened ventricular septum (*VS*) as compared with left ventricular free wall (*LVFW*). The right and left ventricular cavi-
ties are small and there is also right ventricular hypertrophy. *B*. Ventricular slice from a young
man who was found dead in bed, showing concentric left ventricular hypertrophy without left ventricular dilatation. Note there is focal scar in the anterior wall (*arrow*). *C*. Left ventricular slice
from a patient with known systemic hypertension who died suddenly. Note concentric left ventricular hypertrophy without cavity dilatation or any scarring. *D*. Heart of a 45-year-old man with
a history of drug abuse found dead, no known medical history. At autopsy, the heart weight was
575 g, and there was marked left and right ventricular dilatation. Microscopic examination
showed myocyte hypertrophy with rare foci of interstitial fibrosis.

and epicardial surfaces and is often associated with decreased contractility
and right-sided heart failure.[36] Although descriptively the two entities appear
distinct, morphologically there is considerable overlap.[34,36]

Few data are available regarding the incidence of various cardiomyopathies
in series of SCD. Of the 166 cases of SCD excluding those due to atherosclerotic coronary disease in Maryland, the diagnosis was cardiomyopathy in 68
(41%), with a mean age of 37 years (Table 9.3). Idiopathic dilated cardiomyopathy was the most frequent type (37%), followed by idiopathic concentric left
ventricular hypertrophy (34%), hypertensive heart disease (13%) and hypertrophic cardiomyopathy (10%), and right ventricular dysplasia (6%) (Fig. 9.7).
The mean age in all five types of cardiomyopathy ranged from 29 to 43 years.

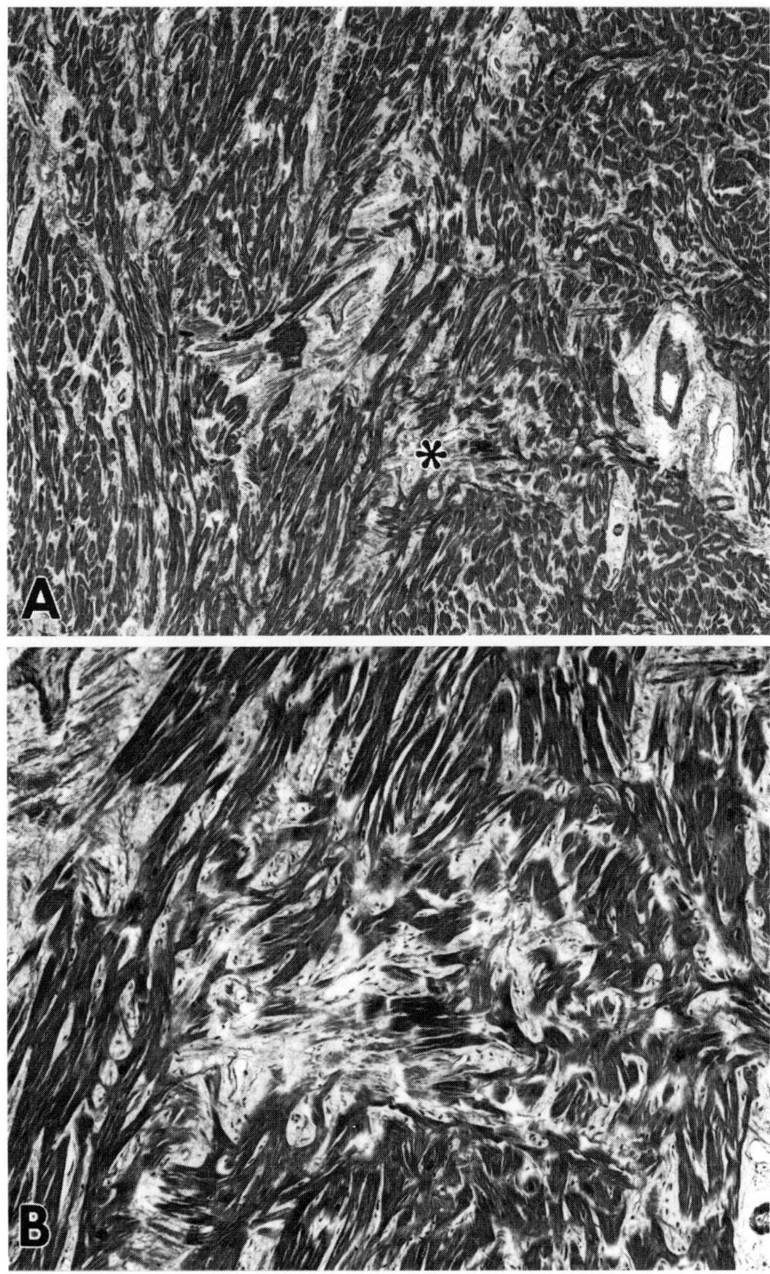

FIG. 9.5. Microscopic sections of the ventricular septum cut transversely from a patient with hypertrophic cardiomyopathy. Note marked fibromuscular disarray at low power in *A* and high-power view of the area marked with asterisk is seen in *B*. Note focal fibrous scarring.

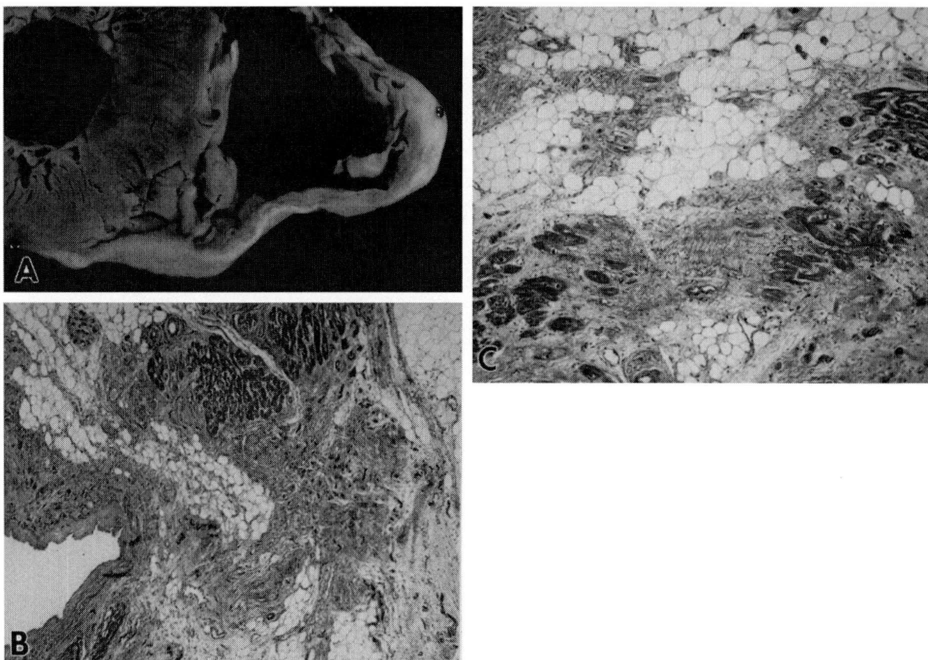

FIG. 9.6. A 24-year-old man who died suddenly while playing basketball. He had episodes of palpitations and had a brother with a history of ventricular tachycardia. There is marked dilation of the right ventricle, as well as thinning of the wall, indicative of right ventricular dysplasia (*A*). *B* shows full-thickness section of right ventricle showing myocyte loss and intermingling of fat, fibrous tissue, and myocytes. *C*. High-power view showing fat, fibrous tissue, and myocytes.

Patients with right ventricular dysplasia were the youngest (Table 9.3) and had the lowest mean heart weight (427 g). Hypertensive heart disease was associated with the greatest degree of cardiomegaly (mean weight, 715 g), even surpassing hypertrophic cardiomyopathy.

A detailed discussion of hypertrophic, hypertensive, and dilated cardiomyopathy is beyond the scope of this review. However, from our data it appears to be a surprisingly frequent cause of unexpected SCD, even in the absence of apparent congestive heart failure. In contrast, hypertrophic cardiomyopathy is a well-known cause of sudden death, and, unlike dilated cardiomyopathy, nearly 50% of cases present with sudden death. Factors predictive of sudden death in patients with known hypertrophic cardiomyopathy include age less than 30 years at diagnosis, family history of SCD due to hypertrophic cardiomyopathy, history of syncope, especially in children, and the presence of nonsustained ventricular tachycardia. However, sudden death also occurs in asymptomatic patients and those patients with stable disease.[37,38] Echocardiographic and clinical data from patients with essential hypertension have shown that mortality is 24% in those patients with concentric left ventricular hypertrophy and increased relative wall thickness, compared with 1% in patients with normal geometry.[39]

TABLE 9.3. CAUSES OF SUDDEN CARDIAC DEATH, EXCLUDING ATHEROSCLEROSIS, STATE OF MARYLAND, 1990–1993, AGE > 14 YEARS, n = 166

Diagnosis[a]	n (%)	M:F	Mean Age, yr, ± SD	Mean Heart Weight, g, ± SD
Cardiomyopathy	68 (41%)	54:14	36.8 ± 8.0	627 ± 148
Dilated	25	18:7	33.3 ± 8.9	657 ± 161
Concentric LVH	23	20:3	38.0 ± 8.2	570 ± 102
Hypertensive	9	8:1	42.8 ± 6.3	715 ± 162
Hypertrophic	7	5:2	42.1 ± 6.0	689 ± 93
RVD	4	3:1	28.8 ± 9.0	427 ± 71
No diagnosis	33 (20%)	21:12	31.4 ± 9.1	364 ± 68
Valvular disease	32 (19%)	23:9	42.2 ± 12.2	578 ± 154
MVP	11	5:6	37.1 ± 8.6	466 ± 91
HVP[b]	9	8:1	50.9 ± 13.9	655 ± 156
AS	5	5:0	39.6 ± 12.1	673 ± 161
IE	3	2:1	32.0 ± 9.5	515 ± 41
MS	2	1:1	49.5 ± 0.7	410 ± 14
AI	2	2:0	45.5 ± 10.6	695 ± 121
Myocarditis	9 (5%)	8:1	27.0 ± 6.4	422 ± 86
Lymphocytic	3	3:0	29.3 ± 0.6	414 ± 31
Idiopathic scar	3	2:1	26.7 ± 8.0	397 ± 67
Sarcoidosis	2	2:0	29.0 ± 8.4	470 ± 194
Acute RF	1	1:0	17.0	330
Coronary disease	9 (5%)	6:3	32.0 ± 2.4	387 ± 54
Congenital	4	2:2	32.3 ± 1.5	383 ± 57
Thrombosis	3	2:1	33.7 ± 2.5	363 ± 64
Vasculitis	2	2:0	29.0 ± 1.4	430 ± 28
Congenital disease[c]	8 (5%)	7:1	29.0 ± 9.0	632 ± 174
Conduction disease	7 (4%)	7:0	31.4 ± 17.5	418 ± 38
AVNA dysplasia	5	5:0	30.0 ± 17.5	433 ± 33
Lev's disease	2	2:0	35.0 ± 5.7	381 ± 13

[a]LVH, left ventricular hypertrophy; RVD, right ventricular dysplasia; MVP, mitral valve prolapse; HVP, heart valve prosthesis; AS, aortic stenosis; IE, infectious endocarditis; MS, mitral stenosis; AI, aortic insufficiency; RF, rheumatic fever; AVNA, atrioventricular nodal artery.
[b]cause of death presumed related to valve disease
[c]excluding isolated coronary anomalies

There are a number of risk factors for the development cardiomyopathy, only one of which will be discussed here. In our series, extreme obesity was seen in nearly 14% of cases of SCD due to dilated cardiomyopathy and idiopathic left ventricular hypertrophy. Although there are few data concerning the relationship of obesity, cardiomyopathy, and SCD, obesity has been associated with cardiac enlargement during life and at autopsy.[40,41] Massive obesity is accompanied by marked increase in blood volume and cardiac output, which are proportional to the excessive body weight and duration of obesity.[42] The increased cardiac output is secondary to increased end-diastolic left ventricular volume and stroke volume.[42] Gross examination of hearts reveals increased heart weight, left ventricular dilation, and eccentric hypertrophy with or without right ventricular hypertrophy.[41] Although marked obesity has been linked to sudden death due to sleep apnea, these data suggest that obesity may also be

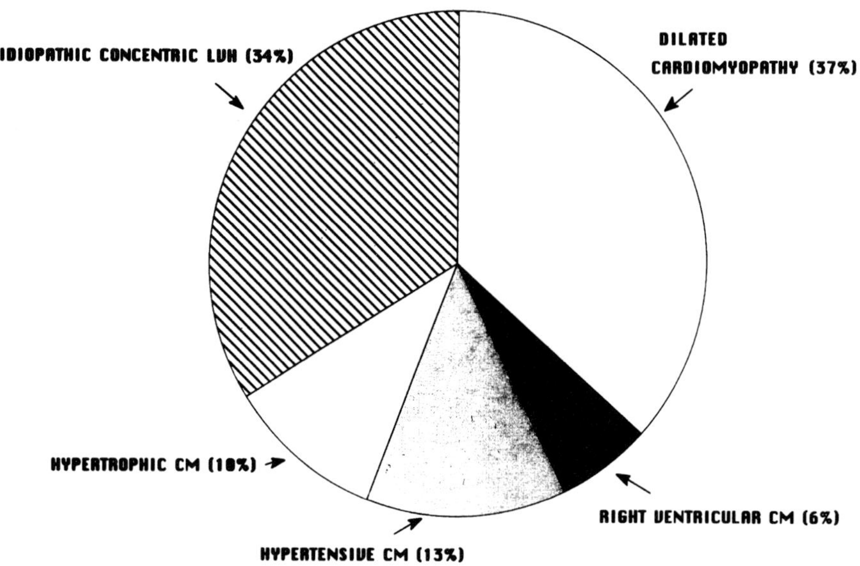

FIG. 9.7.   Distribution of the types of cardiomyopathies seen in 68 patients who died suddenly and for whom diagnosis of cardiomyopathy was made at autopsy.

a cause of cardiomyopathy, which may represent a mechanism in addition to viral and hereditary factors.

The fact that exercise causes cardiac hypertrophy is well known and may confound the evaluation of SCD in athletes. Although mild degrees of septal asymmetry may occur after prolonged conditioning, criteria for hypertrophic cardiomyopathy as defined above are valid, in our opinion, for athletes as well as other people. In addition, if population-derived guidelines for normal cardiac weights based on body size are followed,[29,30] cardiac hypertrophy is indicative of nonexercise-related pathology even in athletes.

The foregoing discussion has highlighted some of the problems in classification and some of the difficulties in the elucidating mechanisms of SCD in patients with cardiomyopathy. Unfortunately, the forensic pathologist often lumps all hypertrophy of the heart under the general heading "cardiomyopathy" once other causes of death, cardiac and noncardiac, have been excluded. For epidemiological studies, this is not a good practice, especially if we are to learn more about the underlying etiology of SCD in cardiac hypertrophy with or without hypertension.

VALVULAR HEART DISEASE

Valvular heart disease (Fig. 9.8) as a cause of sudden cardiac death is not as frequent as cardiomyopathy, accounting for 19% of nonatherosclerotic SCDs. In our series of 166 SCDs, 32 were from valvular heart disease and, of these, 11 (34%) had MVP as the only anatomic abnormality present, with no other

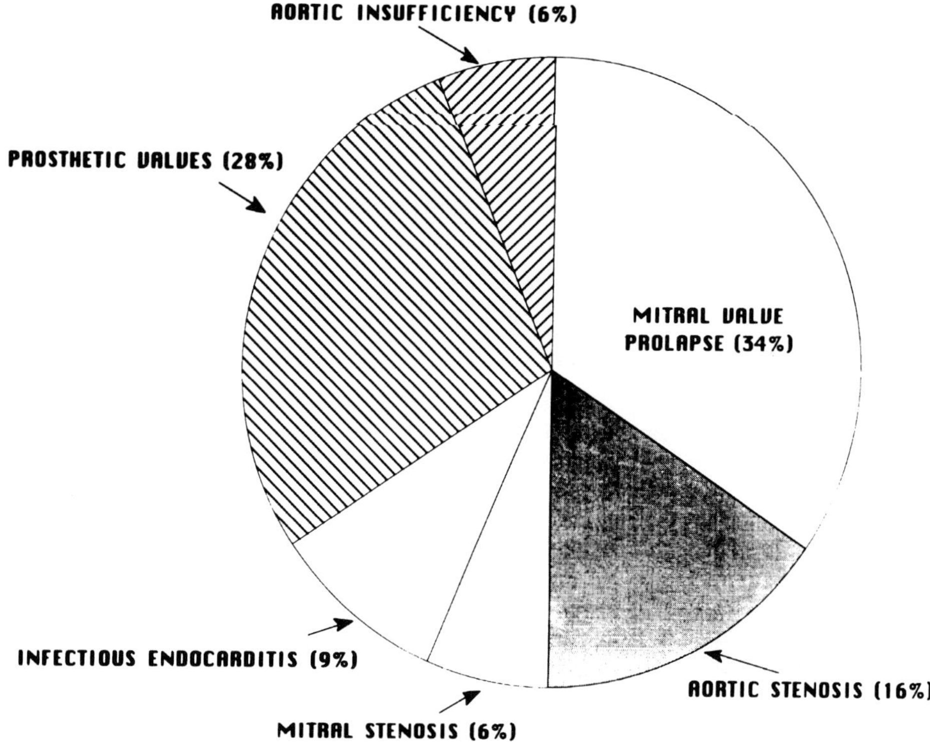

FIG. 9.8.   Distribution of the different types of valvular heart disease seen in 32 patients with sudden cardiac death and valvular heart disease.

cardiac or noncardiac condition present at autopsy that could explain the sudden death. Other valvular abnormalities found were the presence of a prosthetic valve in 9 (28%), aortic stenosis in 5 (16%), infective endocarditis in 3 (9%), and 2 each (6%) with mitral stenosis and aortic incompetence. Of these, the most controversial is the association of MVP with sudden cardiac death.

MITRAL VALVE PROLAPSE

MVP is present in approximately 4% of the general population and is most prevalent in young women.[43] Most patients with MVP are asymptomatic or only mildly symptomatic throughout their lives.[43] In contrast, approximately 15% of patients will develop mitral regurgitation and congestive heart failure; these patients require medical or surgical treatment.[43–45] A small group of patients (1.9–40/10,000 patients with MVP) will die suddenly and at autopsy MVP is the only significant pathologic finding.

In a recent study, we compared the anatomic features of MVP in three clinical settings: MVP as an incidental finding, MVP with severe mitral regurgitation, and MVP as a cause of SCD.[46] Mitral valve annular circumference (12.3 ± 1.9 cm *vs.* 9.9 ± 1.6 cm, $p<.001$), anterior (2.6 ± 0.4 *vs.* 2.2 ± 0.4 cm, $p > .5$) and posterior (2.3 ± 0.4 *vs.* 1.8 ± 0.6 cm, $p < .05$) mitral leaflet lengths, posterior mitral valve thickness, and incidence and extent of endocardial plaque were significantly greater in hearts from patients with SCD than in hearts from patients with incidental MVP (Fig. 9.9). Patients with MVP and SCD were younger than patients with MVP and mitral regurgitation and patients with incidental MVP. As expected, heart weights from patients with MVP and mitral regurgitation were significantly greater than hearts from patients with incidental MVP and MVP with SCD, and atrial and left ventricular cavity size were also greater. These anatomic differences are useful in establishing whether the patient death was caused by MVP.[46]

The mechanism of sudden cardiac death in patients with isolated MVP is uncertain but is presumed to involve the generation of malignant ventricular tachyarrhythmias. Endomycardial friction lesions are present in greater frequency and severity in cases of MVP and SCD compared with incidental cases of MVP. The clinical significance of friction lesions is conjectural, but the myocardium adjacent to these friction lesions may serve as an arrhythmogenic focus.

PROSTHETIC VALVES

Mechanical and bioprosthetic valves have improved longevity in patients with significant native valve disease; however, no prosthesis is totally free of complications. Approximately 7–38% of patients with prosthetic valves die suddenly[47]; the estimated annual risk for sudden death ranges from 0.2 to 0.9.[48–51] In hospital-based autopsies in patients dying with valve prosthesis, 25–50% of the deaths are related to valve dysfunction.[52–54] We have recently reviewed 37 hearts of patients who had valve replacement more than 1 month before sudden death.[55] Sudden death was defined as death within 6 hours after onset of symptoms. Causes of death in 15 of 37 (41%) were valve related and consisted of valve thrombosis (n=4), endocarditis (n=3), embolization of valve thrombi (n=2), strut fracture (n-2), anticoagulation-related hemorrhage (n-2), paravalvular leak (n=1), and left ventricular outflow obstruction (n=1). In 22 of 37 (59%), sudden cardiac death was not related to the valve prosthesis and the underlying etiology was arrhythmia with underlying cardiomegaly (n=10), arrhythmia with underlying coronary artery disease (no myocardial infarction) (n=4), acute myocardial infarction (n=6), and aortic rupture in two patients. The heart weight was significantly less (550 g) in patients dying from prosthesis complications *versus* cardiac death unrelated to prosthesis (735 g, p=.002). Therefore, in this series it appears that more than half the cases of sudden death with heart valve prosthesis were due to left ventricular hypertrophy with or without coronary atherosclerosis.[55]

In a more recent separate series of 32 cases of sudden cardiac death from valvular abnormalities reviewed at our institution, 9 had valvular prosthesis. Of these, 8 had mechanical valves and only 1 had bioprosthesis; 5 were in the mitral position and 4 in the aortic position. In 4 (44%), death was related to prosthetic valve complications, 3 had thrombosis, and 1 had obstruction of the left ventricle outflow; in 5 (56%), death was secondary to left ventricular hypertrophy and in 3 it was associated with coronary atherosclerosis. In the pre-

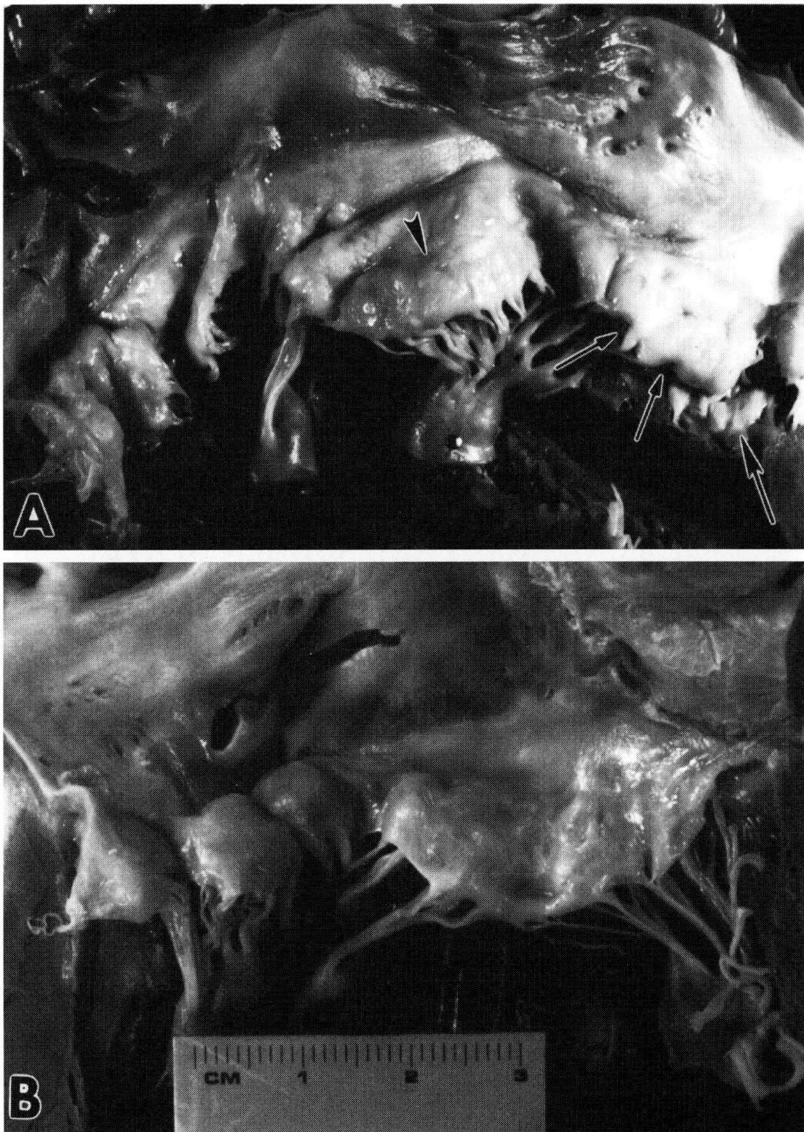

FIG. 9.9. *A.* Mitral valve prolapse. A 32-year-old man died suddenly and had mitral valve prolapse involving a portion of the anterior leaflet (*arrowhead*) and the posterior scallop of the posterior leaflet (*small arrows*). There is also subendocardial thickening seen in the posterior wall of the left ventricle (*large arrow*). *B.* An 18-year-old white woman who died in a motor vehicle accident of multiple injuries was found to have incidental mitral valve prolapse at autopsy. There is mild hooding and elongation of the intermediate and medial scallop of the posterior leaflet.

sent series, as well as prior series[55] it appears that nearly 60% of sudden deaths with prosthetic valves are not valve-related and the most frequent underlying etiology is left ventricular hypertrophy with or without coronary atherosclerosis. Our incidence of valve dysfunction is higher than the previous study by Lindblom,[56] who reported a 17% incidence. However, in the latter study, hearts were not available for review, and the incidence was derived from retrospective inspection of autopsy reports. Our experience indicates that heart valve prosthesis dysfunction as a cause of sudden death in patients with prosthetic valves is higher than 17% and closer to 40%.

AORTIC STENOSIS

Patients with aortic stenosis, in contrast to patients with mitral stenosis, may be asymptomatic for many years despite the presence of a severe outflow gradient. Sudden death is a well-known complication of aortic stenosis, and usually occurs in symptomatic patients. Of patients with asymptomatic aortis stenosis, only 4% die suddenly.[57] The mechanism of sudden death in patients with severe aortic stenosis is cerebral hypoperfusion, which is followed by cardiac arrhythmia.[58]

NORMAL HEART AND SUDDEN DEATH

There are a substantial number of cases of sudden death in which no pathologic abnormality is found in the heart at autopsy.[24] The incidence of terminal arrhythmias without a structural defect varies widely and can be as high as 50% in children[59] and as low as 3% in a retrospective study of adults.[60] In our series, 33 hearts (20%) from people who died were found at autopsy to be normal (Fig. 9.2, Table 9.3). The age was $31 \pm$ years and the heart weight was 364 ± 68 g. In each case, the heart weight was considered normal for the height and weight of the person, and pathologic studies of the conduction system were considered normal. In our experience, the examination of the conduction system is rarely fruitful in the evaluation of sudden cardiac death, in the absence of a documented history of arrhythmias, or conduction abnormalities.

Two conditions that may account for SCD that we have observed in the conduction system in otherwise normal hearts are atrioventricular nodal artery dysplasia[61] and premature sclerosis of the conduction system. Although we have reported a higher incidence of atrioventricular nodal artery dysplasia in SCD victims compared with control traumatic deaths, the clinical significance of these diseases is difficult to prove without a history of arrhythmias.

SUMMARY

Do we have a magic yardstick that will establish whether SCD of the patient is definitely caused by the presence of an underlying abnormality? We are afraid that in most cases of cardiac disease the cause of death is at best probable, or even presumed. It has always been that circumstantial evidence has helped us establish that the cause of death is related to the anatomic abnormality. Even the presence of severe coronary artery disease in a patient who dies suddenly, especially in the absence of a thrombus, cannot be stated categorically to be the cause and effect. With the knowledge we have today, establishing cause and effect are difficult in most cases of SCD.

REFERENCES

1. Myerburg RJ, Castellanos A. Cardiac arrest and sudden cardiac death. In: Braunwald, E, ed. *Heart disease. A textbook of cardiovascular medicine.* Philadelphia: WB Saunders, 1992:756–789.
2. Schatzkin A, Cupples A, Heeren T, Morelock S, Kannel WB. Sudden death in the Framingham heart study. Differences in incidence and risk factors by sex and coronary disease status. *Am J Epidemiol* 1984;120:888–899.
3. Kuller L, Lilienfeld A, Fisher R. An epidemiological study of sudden and unexpected deaths in adults. *Medicine* 1967;46:341–361.
4. Kuller L, Cooper M, Perper J. Epidemiology of sudden death. *Arch Intern Med* 1972;129: 714–719.
5. Kannel WB, Schatzkin A. Sudden death: lessons from subsets in population studies. *J Am Coll Cardiol* 1985;5:141B–149B.
6. Kannel WB, Thomas HE, Jr. Sudden coronary death. The Framingham Study. *Ann N Y Acad Sci* 1982;382:3–21.
7. Kannel WB, McGee DL. Epidemiology of sudden death: Insights from the Framingham Study. In: Josephson ME, ed. *Sudden cardiac death.* Philadelphia: FA Davis, 1985:93–105.
8. Feinleib M, Simon AB, Gillium JR, Margolis JR. Prodromal symptoms and signs of sudden death. *Circulation* 1975;52(Suppl 3):155–159.
9. Kala R, Romo M, Siltanen P, et al. Physical activity and sudden death. *Adv Cardiol* 1978;25:27–34.
10. Myerburg RJ, Conde CA, Sung RJ, et al. Clinical electropysiologic and hemodynamic profile of patients resuscitated from prehospital cardiac arrest. *Am J Med* 1980;68:568–576.
11. Myerburg RJ, Zaman L, Luceri RM, et al. Clinical characteristics of sudden death: implications for survival. In: Josephson ME, ed. *Sudden cardiac death.* Philadelphia: FA Davis, 1985:107–117.
12. Virmani R, Robinowitz M, Geer JC, McAllister HA, JR. Coronary artery atherosclerosis revisited in Korean war combat casualties. *Arch Pathol Lab Med* 1987;11:972–976.
13. Davies MJ, Bland JM, Hangartner JRW, Angelini A, Thomas AC. Factors influencing the presence or absence of acute coronary artery thrombi in sudden ischaemic death. *Eur Heart J* 1989;10:203–208.
14. Warnes CA, Roberts WC. Sudden coronary death: comparison of patients with to those without coronary thrombus at necropsy. *Am J Cardiol* 1984;54:1206–1211.
15. Farb A, Sessums L, Tang AL, Burke AP, Smialek J, Virmani R. Coronary artery morphology in sudden death due to atherosclerosis. *J Am Coll Cardiol* 1994;172A:Volume 1A (abstract).
16. Perper JA, Kuller LH, Cooper M. Atherosclerosis of coronary arteries in sudden, unexpected deaths. *Circulation* 1975;52(Suppl 3):27–33.
17. Little WL, Constantinescu M, Applegate RJ, et al. Can coronary angiography predict the site of a subsequent myocardial infarction in patients with mild to moderate coronary artery disease? *Circulation* 1988;78:1157–1166.
18. Qiao JH, Fishbein MC. The severity of coronary atherosclerosis at sites of plaque rupture with occlusive thrombosis. *J Am Coll Cardiol* 1991;17:1138–1142.
19. Constantinides P. Plaque fissure in human coronary thrombosis. *J Atheroscler Res* 1966;1: 1–17.
20. Barger AC, Beeuwkes R, Lainesy LL, Silverman KJ. Hypothesis: vasa vasorum and neovascularization of human coronary arteries. *N Engl J Med* 1984;310:175–177.
21. Hobbs RE, Millit HD, Raghaven PV, Moodie DS, Sheldon WC. Congenital coronary anomalies: clinical and therapeutic implications. *Cardiovasc Clin* 1981;12:43–58.

22. Alexander RW, Griffith GC. Anomalies of the coronary arteries and their clinical significance. *Circulation* 1956;14:800–805.

23. Cheitlin MD, DeCastro CM, McAllister HA. Sudden death as a complication of anomalous left coronary origin from the anterior sinus of Valsalva. *Circulation* 1974;50:780–787.

24. Roberts WC. Major anomalies of coronary arterial origin seen in childhood. *Am Heart J* 1986;111:941–963.

25. Barch CW III, Roberts WC. Left main coronary artery originating from the right sinus of Valsalva and coursing between the aorta and pulmonary trunk. *J Am Coll Cardiol* 1986;7:366–373.

26. Burke AP, Farb A, Virmani R, Goodin J, Smialek JE. Sports-related and non-sports-related sudden cardiac death in young adults. *Am Heart J* 1991;121:568–575.

27. Taylor AJ, Rogan KM, Virmani R. Sudden cardiac death associated with isolated congenital coronary artery anomalies. *J Am Coll Cardiol* 1992;20:640–647.

28. Virmani R, Chun PKC, Goldstein RE, Robinowitz M, McAllister HA. Acute takeoffs of the coronary arteries along the aortic wall and congenital coronary ostial valve-like ridges: association with sudden death. *J Am Coll Cardiol* 1984;3:766–771.

29. Kitzman DW, Scholz DG, Hagan PT, Ilstrup DM, Edwards WD. Age-related changes in normal human hearts during the first 10 decades of life. Part II (Maturity). A quantitative anatomic study of 765 specimens from subjects 20 to 99 years old. *Mayo Clin Proc* 1988;66:137–146.

30. Scholz DG, Kitzman DW, Hagen PT, Ilstrup DM, Edwards WD. Age-related changes in normal human hearts during the first 10 decades of life. Part I (Growth). A quantitative anatomic study of 200 specimens from subjects from birth to 19 years old. *Mayo Clin Proc* 1988;63:126–136.

31. Maron BJ, Epstein SE, Roberts WC. Causes of sudden death in competitive athletes. *J Am Coll Cardiol* 1986;7:204–214.

32. Burke AP, Farb A, Virmani R. Sports-related and non-sports-related sudden cardiac death in young adults. *Am Heart J* 1991;121:568–575.

33. Virmani R, Roberts WC. Sudden cardiac death. *Hum Pathol* 1987;18:485–492.

34. Burke AP, Farb A, Virmani R. Causes of sudden death in athletes. In: Maron BJ. *Cardiology clinics. The athlete's heart.* Philadelphia: WB Saunders, 1992;303–317.

35. Goodin J, Farb A, Smialek JE, Fields F, Virmani R. Right ventricular dysplasia associated with sudden death in young adults. *Mod Pathol* 1991;4:702–706.

36. Virmani R, Robinowitz M, Clark MA, McAllister HA. Sudden death and partial absence of the right ventricular myocardium: a report of three cases and a review of the literature. *Arch Pathol Lab Med* 1982;106:163–167.

37. Ventura HO, Messerli FH, Dunn FG, Frohlich ED. Left ventricular hypertrophy in obesity: discrepancy between echo and electrocardiogram. *J Am Coll Cardiol* 1983;1:682–687.

38. Warnes CA, Roberts WC. The heart in massive (more than 300 pounds or 136 kilograms) obesity: Analysis of 12 patients studied at necropsy. *Am J Cardiol* 1984;54:1087–1091.

39. Egan B, Fitzpatrick MA, Juni J, et al. Importance of overweight in studies of left ventricular hypertrophy and diastolic function in mild systemic hypertension. *Am J Cardiol* 1989;64:752–755.

40. Koren MJ, Casale PN, Savage DD, Laragh JH, Devereux RB. Left ventricular geometry and cardiac risk factors define high and low risk subgroups among essential hypertensives. *J Am Coll Cardiol* 1990;15:111A.

41. Aron LA, Hertzeanu HL, Fisman EZ, et al. Prognosis of non-obstructive hypertrophic cardiomyopathy. *Am J Cardiol* 1991;67:215.

42. McKenna WJ. The natural history of hypertrophic cardiomyopathy. *Cardiovasc Clin* 1988;19:135–148.

43. Procacci PM, Savran SV, Schreiter SL, Bryson AL. Prevalence of clinical mitral valve prolapse in 1169 young women. *N Engl J Med* 1976;294:1086–1088.

44. Mills P, Rose J, Hollingsworth J, Amara I, Craige E. Long-term prognosis of mitral valve prolapse. *N Engl J Med* 1977;297:13–18.

45. Duren DR, Becker AE, Dunning AJ. Long-term follow-up of idiopathic mitral valve prolapse in 300 patients: a prospective study. *J Am Coll Cardiol* 1988;11:42–47.

46. Farb A, Tang AL, Atkinson JB, McCarthy WF, Virmani R. Comparison of cardiac findings in patients with mitral valve prolapse who die suddenly to those who have congestive heart failure from mitral regurgitation and to those with fatal noncardiac conditions. *Am J Cardiol* 1992;70:234–239.
47. Santinga JT, Kirsh MM, Flora JD, Brylmer JF. Factors relating to late sudden death in patients having aortic valve replacement. *Ann Thorac Surg* 1980;29:249–253.
48. Baudet EM, Oca CC, Roques XF, et al. A 5 1/2 year experience with the St. Jude Medical cardiac valve prosthesis. *J Thorac Cardiovasc Surg* 1985;90:137–144.
49. Gohlke-Barwolf C, Peters K, Peterson J, et al. Influence of aortic valve replacement of sudden death in patients with pure aortic stenosis. *Eur Heart J* 1988;9:139–141.
50. Brudon RA, Miller DC, Oyer PE, et al. Durability of porcine valves at fifteen years in a representative North American patient population. *J Thorac Cardiovasc Surg* 1992;103:238–251.
51. Mikaeloff P, Jegaden O, Ferrini M, Coll-Mazzei J, Bonnefoy JY, Rumolo A. Prospective randomized study of St. Jude Medical versus Bjork-Shiley or Starr Edwards 6120 valve prosthesis in the mitral position. *J Cardiovasc Surg* 1989;30:966–975.
52. Ishibashi-Ueda H, Imakita M, Katsuragi M, Fujita H, Hao H, Yutani C. An analysis of autopsy findings in 108 patients who died after valve replacement. *Virchows Arch Pathol Anat Histopathol* 1993;422:397–403.
53. Joassin A, Edwards JE. Late causes of death after mitral valve replacement. Analysis of 36 cases. *J Thorac Cardiovasc Surg* 1973;65:255–263.
54. Schoen FJ, Titus JL, Lawrie GM. Autopsy-determined causes of death after cardiac valve replacement. *JAMA* 1983;249:899–902.
55. Burke AP, Farb A, Sessums L, Virmani R. Causes of sudden cardiac death in patients with replacement valves: an autopsy study. *J Heart Valve Dis* 1994;3:10–16.
56. Lindblom D. Long-term clinical results after mitral valve replacement with the Bjork-Shiley prosthesis. *J Thorac Cardiovasc Surg* 1988;95:321–333.
57. Pellikka PA, Nishimura RA, Bailey KR, Tajik AJ. The natural history of adults with asymptomatic hemodynamically significant aortic stenosis. *J Am Coll Cardiol* 1990;15:1012–1017.
58. Chizner MA, Pearle DL, deLeon AC, Jr. The natural history of aortic stenosis in adults. *Am Heart J* 1980;99:419–24.
59. Niimura I, Maki T. Sudden cardiac death in childhood. *Jpn Circ J* 1989;53:1571.
60. Maron BJ, Roberts WC, McAllister HA, et al. Sudden death in young athletes. *Circulation* 1980;62:218–229.
61. Burke A, Subramanian R, Virmani R, Smialek J. Non-atherosclerotic narrowing of atrioventricular nodal artery and sudden death. *J Am Coll Cardiol* 1993;21:117–122.

Chapter 10

Pathologic Considerations in Replacement Heart Valves and Other Cardiovascular Prosthetic Devices

FREDERICK J. SCHOEN

Biomaterials are synthetic or biological materials (including polymers, metals, ceramics, carbons, collagen, blood vessels, heart valves, and pericardium) that are used as *grafts* and *prosthetic devices* to augment or replace abnormal body structures and functions. Surgical implantation of prostheses is now common in cardiovascular, orthopedic, dental, ophthalmological, and reconstructive surgery. Cardiovascular prostheses, in particular, are used widely and at rates that have increased markedly during the past decade (Fig. 10–1). Data compiled by the National Center for Health Statistics and the American Heart Association suggest that approximately 1.5 million people now receive an artificial valve, vascular graft, pacemaker, or other cardiac or vascular device each year in the United States.

Most cardiovascular prostheses serve their recipients well for extended periods by correcting serious conditions. However, complications related to cardiovascular prostheses frequently necessitate reoperation, or cause death or serious disability.[1] Nearly all complications of cardiovascular medical devices, irrespective of specific anatomic site of implantation, can be grouped into six major categories: (1) thrombosis, thromboembolism, and anticoagulation-related hemorrhage; (2) infection; (3) exuberant or defective healing; (4) degeneration, fracture, or other biomaterials failure; (5) adverse local tissue interactions, such as excessive inflammation or toxicity; and (6) adverse systemic effects, such as distant migration of biomaterials or hypersensitivity. Complications are largely a consequence of biomaterials-tissue interactions, which all implants have with their environment. Effects of both the implant on the host tissues and the host on the implant are important in mediating complications and device failure.

Pathological examination of retrieved medical devices provides valuable information.[2,3] Determination of a cause of failure frequently contributes to management of individual patients. On a broader front, explant analysis elucidates the efficacy and safety of medical devices to an extent beyond that obtainable by *in vitro* tests of durability and biocompatibility or preclinical ani-

In thousands per year /USA

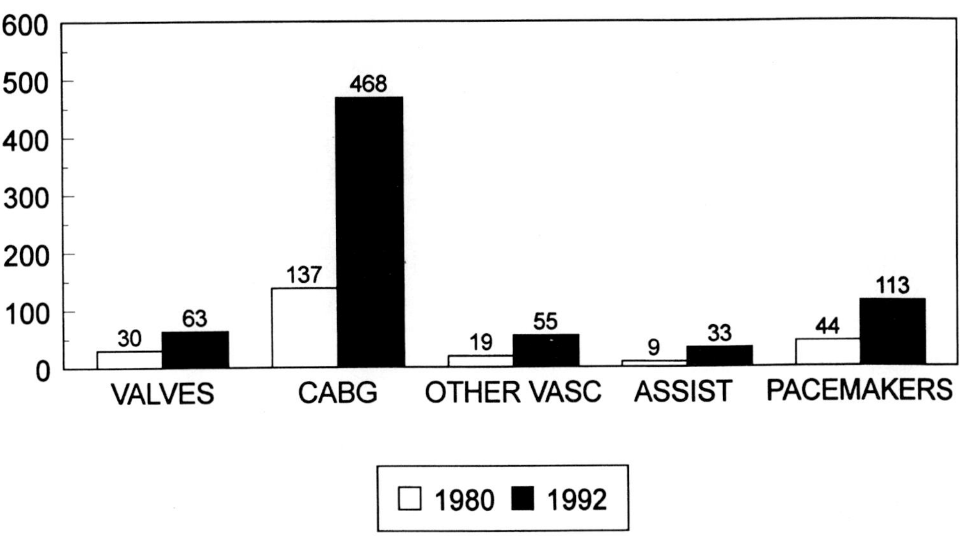

FIG. 10.1. Growth in utilization of major cardiovascular prostheses and devices from 1980 to 1992. VALVES, substitute cardiac valves; CABG, coronary artery bypass graft surgery; OTHER VASC, other vascular grafts; ASSIST, cardiac assist devices; PACEMAKERS, pacemaker implantations. (Data compiled by the American Heart Association and the National Center for Health Statistics).

mal investigations of new or modified designs. Moreover, enhanced understanding or biomaterials-tissue and patient-prosthesis interactions is fostered by careful and sophisticated analysis of removed prostheses that are functioning properly and have not failed. Information on mechanisms of device-patient interactions and failure modes derived from implant retrieval studies also contributes to enhanced clinical recognition of complications and can be used to guide future efforts to develop not only methods for failure detection but also improved prosthetic devices. In view of the above objectives in explant analysis, pathologists are typically involved in medical device studies at three levels: (1) evaluation of human explants as surgical pathology or autopsy specimens; (2) evaluation of explants of implant configurations in animal systems (such as rabbits, dogs, or sheep) in preclinical studies; and (3) experimental tissues and biomaterials derived from basic investigations of the pathophysiology of biomaterials-tissue interactions.

Practicing pathologists also have an important regulatory role in recognizing clinical prosthesis-associated complications. This responsibility is a key element of the Federal Safe Medical Devices Act of 1990 (PL 101–629)[4,5]; the first major amendment to the Federal Food, Drug and Cosmetic Act since the Medical Device Amendments of 1976. Under the "user reporting" requirements of this legislation, health care personnel and hospitals must report all device-related deaths, serious illnesses and injuries to the Food and Drug Administration, manufacturers, or both. Thus, a pathologist who provides the initial discovery of harm or death due to a malfunctioning cardiovascular device is required to initiate the reporting process (through his or her institution).

This paper summarizes pathological considerations in cardiovascular prostheses, with emphasis on the complications and approaches to pathological evaluation of substitute heart valves. These devices have been studied extensively and serve to illustrate many of the most pertinent issues. In particular, the major complications of heart valve replacements, including thrombosis and thromboembolism, infection, and durability limitations, occur to some degree with nearly all devices implanted into the cardiovascular system. Special considerations related to vascular grafts, cardiac-assist devices, pacemakers, stents, and other devices will also be discussed.

SUBSTITUTE HEART VALVES

TYPES OF VALVULAR PROSTHESES

The following discussion focuses on those aspects of replacement heart valves deemed to be most useful to pathologists. For more detailed information on historical development of prosthetic valves, as well as materials, design considerations, testing, and new developments, the reader is referred elsewhere.[6–9]

Heart valve prostheses are of two types—mechanical and tissue (illustrated in Fig. 10.2)[10] Both types respond passively to hemodynamic stimuli manifested as pressure gradients and flow changes. *Mechanical valves,* composed of nonphysiologic biomaterials, have three essential components: (1) the rigid, mobile occluder (also called a poppet), (2) the cagelike superstructure that guides and restricts poppet motion, and (3) the valve body or base.[11,12] Mechanical valves that have been widely used include the Starr-Edwards caged-ball valve, Bjork-Shiley and Medtronic-Hall tilting disk valves, and the St. Jude Medical bileaflet tilting-disk valve prosthesis (the latter used in approximately one-half of all valve replacements done today and thus the most widely used valve model). Several models of caged-disk valves were also used several decades ago. Mechanical valve cages are constructed of nearly pure titanium (*e.g.,* Medtronic-Hall valve) or cobalt-chromium alloy (*e.g.,* Starr-Edwards and Bjork-Shiley valves). Although the original but still occasionally implanted Starr-Edwards valve has a silicone poppet, tilting-disk valve occluders available today are composed of pyrolytic carbon, a thromboresistant, strong and rigid material, highly resistant to wear and fatigue. In some designs, both disks and supports are fabricated from carbon (*e.g.,* St. Jude valve). Because blood flow through mechanical valve prosthesis must course around the poppet, mechanical valves usually have areas of stasis distal to the orifice.[13,14] Because the combination of stasis and nonphysiological surfaces promotes thrombus formation, patients with mechanical valve receive chronic anticoagulation therapy (that induces a risk of hemorrhage; see below).

In contrast, *tissue valves* have a more natural configuration, with cusps that are composed of animal or human tissue. Tissue valves comprise hetero-

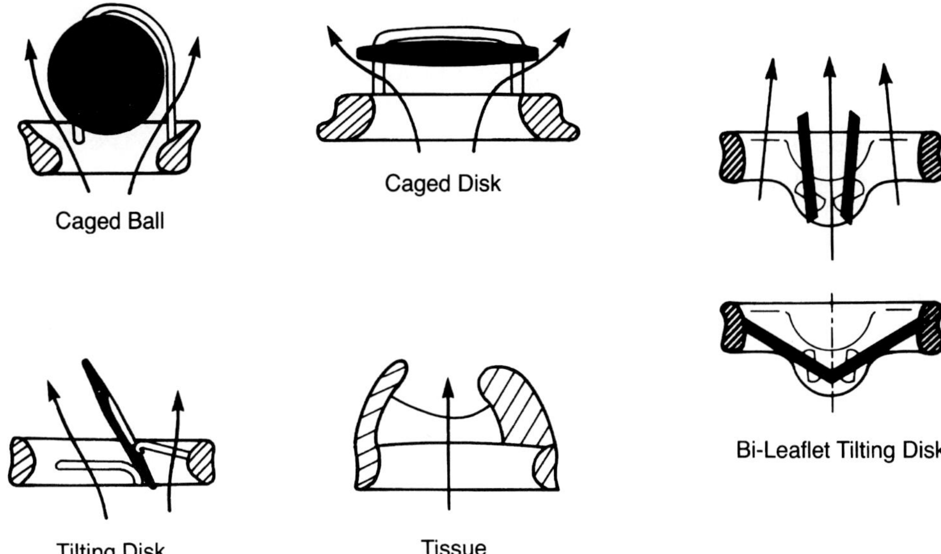

FIG. 10.2. Designs and flow patterns of major types of prosthetic heart valves, including mechanical valves (caged-ball, caged-disk, single leaflet tilting disk and bi-leaflet tilting disk valves) and tissue valves, here represented by a stent-mounted porcine bioprosthetic valve. Flow through mechanical valves must course along both sides of an occluder, but bioprostheses and other tissue valves have a central flow pattern. (Reproduced by permission from Schoen FJ, et al. *Ann Biomed Eng* 1982;10:97, and Schoen FJ. In: Morse D Steiner RM, Fernandez J, eds. *Guide to prosthetic heart valves,* New York: Springer Verlag 1985:209).

grafts/xenografts (*e.g.,* porcine aortic valve or bovine pericardial bioprostheses), homografts/allografts (*e.g.,* aortic [or pulmonic] valves primarily from human cadavers, with or without an aortic [or pulmonary arterial] sleeve as a conduit), or autografts (*e.g.,* composed of fascia lata, pericardium, or the patient's own pulmonary valve transplanted to the aortic root[15]). As the most frequently used tissue valve type, *bioprosthetic valves* are fabricated from chemically preserved (usually cross-linked) animal tissue, mounted on a prosthetic frame (called a stent). Stent-mounted porcine aortic valve bioprostheses are used in approximately one-third of all valve replacements currently done. Each is fabricated from a pig aortic valve preserved in glutaraldehyde (0.2% for the Hancock type and 0.6% for the Carpentier-Edwards). Pericardial tissue valves have also been used; each cusp is an individual piece of glutaralde hyde-treated parietal pericardium (usually of bovine origin) that is attached to the frame. Detailed descriptions of these valves, including the histologic architecture of porcine aortic valve and bovine pericardium, are available.[16,17] The other important tissue valve type is the *human aortic valve allograft,* today usually derived from cadavers and cryopreserved but not cross-linked, that is implanted directly into the aortic root without a stent. Despite the lack of preservation of the endothelium of both porcine valves[18] and allografts, flexible, trileaflet, tissue valves generally have biological blood-contacting surfaces and a central orifice analogous to natural valves. This generally yields hemodynamic efficiency and thromboresistance superior to those of mechanical valves. Consequently, most patients with bioprosthetic valves and virtually all of those with allografts are free of chronic anticoagulation.

Surrounding the base of both mechanical and tissue prostheses is a fabric sewing cuff (usually Dacron) into which sutures are placed that anchor the device into the surgically prepared annulus. In most cases, organized thrombus or fibrous tissue derived from the adjacent endothelium or myocardium or aortic wall ultimately covers the rough cloth surface. Sewing cuff configurations differ slightly for semilunar and atrioventricular valve sites, but most mechanical and bioprosthetic valves can otherwise be used in either site.

OVERVIEW OF CLINICAL PERFORMANCE AND VALVE-RELATED COMPLICATIONS

Despite considerable improvement in the technology of heart valve prostheses since the first successful use of these devices more than 30 years ago, no substitute valve approximates the natural valves with respect to hemodynamic function and freedom from complications. All types of contemporary cardiac valve substitutes (including mechanical, bioprosthetic, and allograft valves) suffer deficiencies and complications that limit their success. Thus, prosthesis-associated pathology is a major determinant of the prognosis of the patients who have had valve replacement. Autopsy studies and clinical analyses show that the immediate cause of death is device-related in 25–61% of patients.[19–21] Sudden death occurs in approximately one-fifth or more of valve recipients; in a recent autopsy study, 40% of valve recipients who died suddenly had a valve-related cause.[22] However, it must not be overlooked that the outcome after cardiac valve replacement is also critically dependent on both irreversible cardiac pathology secondary to the valvular disease (especially left ventricular myocardial hypertrophic and degenerative changes) and coronary arterial atherosclerotic occlusions.

It is useful to categorize valve-related complications as thromboembolism and related problems, infection, structural dysfunction, and nonstructural dysfunction, as summarized in Table 10.1.[23] Within 10 years postoperatively, clinical investigation of individual valve types and randomized studies consistently show that one or more of these problems necessitates reoperation or causes death in approximately 50–60% of patients with substitute valves.[24–26] Although overall rates of valve-related complications are similar for mechanical prostheses and bioprostheses, the frequency and nature of specific valve-

TABLE 10.1 COMPLICATIONS OF PROSTHETIC HEART VALVES

Thrombosis/thromboembolism/anticoagulant-related hemorrhage
Prosthetic valve endocarditis
Structural deterioration (intrinsic failure): *wear, fracture, poppet escape, cuspal tear, calcification*
Nonstructural dysfunction: *pannus overgrowth, suture/tissue entrapment, paravalvular leak, hemolytic anemia, noise*

related complications vary with the prosthesis type, model, site of implantation, and patient characteristics (such as ventricular function and cardiac index).

For example, although contemporary mechanical valves are thrombogenic (as discussed above), except for a very few notable exceptions they are durable. In contrast, tissue valves yield a relatively low rate of thromboembolism without anticoagulant therapy, but they have limited durability, almost exclusively because of cuspal degeneration (primary tissue failure). In particular, glutaraldehyde-pretreated porcine aortic valves suffer progressive calcification with secondary tearing as the major failure mode.[9,16,17]

The concepts summarized above are supported by data on the relative frequencies of specific causes of prosthesis-related death or reoperation. For example, in our autopsy study that largely comprised mechanical valve patients, thrombosis caused 28% of 46 late valve-related deaths, whereas thromboembolism and anticoagulant-associated hemorrhage caused an additional 24%. Thus, more than half of all valve-related deaths (and nearly one-quarter of all postoperative valve replacement deaths) were related to prosthesis thrombogenicity. In addition, our study of 45 mechanical valves and 112 bioprostheses, consecutively obtained in the surgical pathology laboratory at the Brigham and Women's Hospital over a 5 1/2 year period, showed modes of failure that included degenerative dysfunction (53%), endocarditis (16%), paravalvular leak (11%), thrombosis (9%), and tissue overgrowth (5%).[27,28] However, as summarized in Fig. 10.3, thromboembolic complications were a major cause of mechanical valve dysfunction (18% of failures), but were infrequent with bioprostheses. In contrast, sterile primary tissue failure necessitated 74% of bioprosthetic valve removals. Sterile paravalvular leak and device-associated infective endocarditis were encountered with approximately equal frequency in mechanical and bioprosthetic valves, consistent with clinical data that suggest that rates of these problems do not vary according to prosthesis type. Cryopreserved aortic valvular allografts have a comparable or slightly lower rate of failure than contemporary mechanical or bioprosthetic valves; they undergo progressive degeneration, leading to cuspal tearing, sagging, retraction, and/or calcification (in the cusps or aortic walls)[29,30] in many patients.

THROMBOEMBOLIC COMPLICATIONS

Thromboembolic complications include (1) thrombosis that impairs occluder opening or closing; (2) thromboemboli to distal arterial beds; and (3) anticoagulation-related hemorrhage. Thrombosis of a tilting disk mechanical valve is illustrated in Fig. 10.4. Thrombotic occlusion and thromboemboli occur with all currently available types of prostheses at rates of 1–4% per patient-year; actuarially determined freedom from thrombosis or thromboembolism at 10 years for patients with either porcine bioprostheses (usually used without chronic oral anticoagulation) or tilting disk prosthetic valves (with anticoagulation) is typically 70–80%.[31] Under these circumstances (*i.e.,* mechanical valves with anticoagulation, bioprostheses without), the risk of thromboembolism does not differ appreciably among a spectrum of widely used mechani-

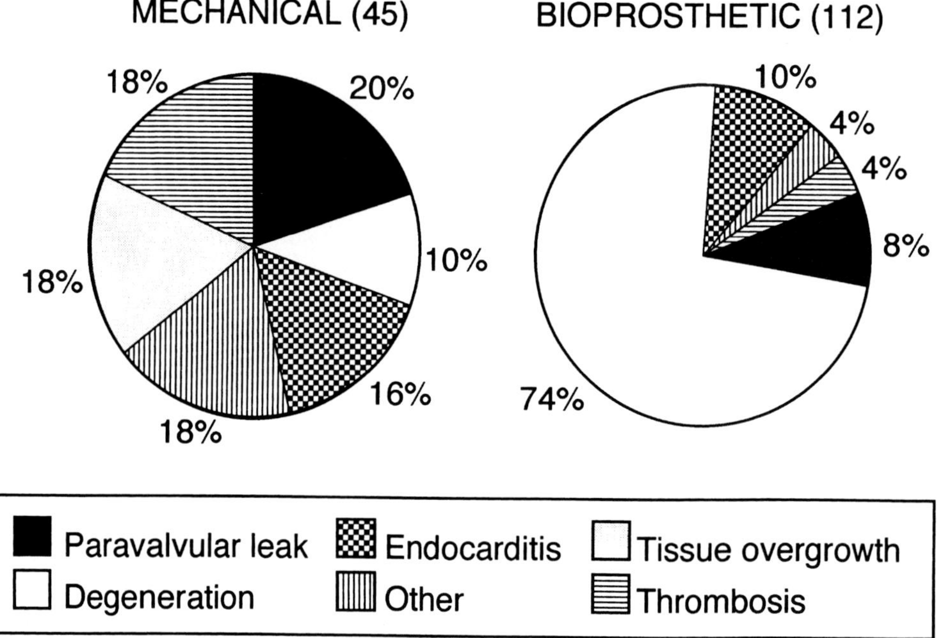

FIG. 10.3. Causes of failure of mechanical prosthetic valves (various types) and porcine aortic bioprosthetic heart valves removed at operation, 1980 to 1985. Failure modes of mechanical valves are diverse. In contrast, bioprosthetic valves fail most frequently by degenerative processes. Data from Ref. 28, with permission.

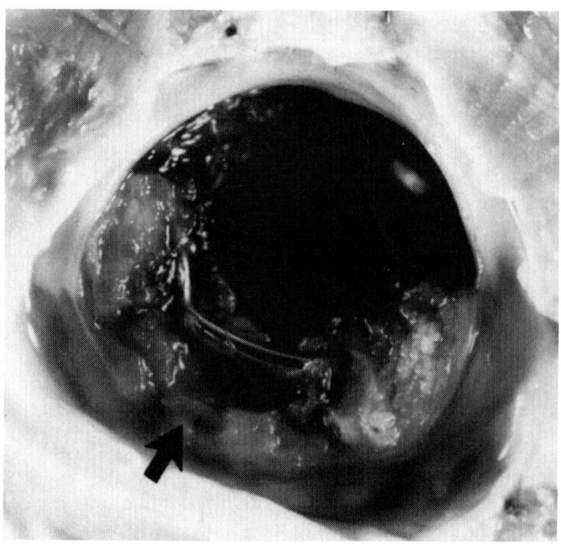

FIG. 10.4. Prosthetic valve thrombosis, exemplified on an aortic Bjork-Shiley tilting disk valve prosthesis, viewed from the distal (outflow aspect). Thrombus is localized to outflow strut near minor orifice, a major site of flow stasis (*arrow*). Reproduced from Ref. 38 with permission.

cal and bioprosthetic valves. Indeed, there is more variability among different studies of a specific valve type than among different models of prostheses. However, the risk of thromboembolism depends on the adequacy of anticoagulation (particularly high in poorly anticoagulated patients with mechanical valves), cardiac rhythm (increases with atrial fibrillation), and anatomic site of valve replaced (mitral > aortic). Local valve dysfunction due to thrombosis, on the other hand, is much more likely with mechanical than bioprosthetic valves, particularly for those implanted into the mitral position. Moreover, chronic oral anticoagulation induces a risk of hemorrhage, particularly retroperitoneal, gastrointestinal, or cerebral, with a frequency approximately of 4% per patient-year, of which 15–25% of events are fatal. Thus, bleeding complications are nearly 10 times more common in patients with mechanical valves than those with bioprostheses.

Platelet deposition dominates initial blood-surface interaction when valves and other cardiovascular devices are exposed to blood at high fluid shear stresses.[32,33] Nevertheless, the sites where thrombi occur on prosthetic valves tend to be associated with local hemodynamic disturbances and regions of static blood flow. Because of this interaction between platelet-mediated and bulk events, valve and other device-associated thrombi can be either composed predominantly of fibrin and erythrocytes (red) or largely platelets (white). The lack of vascularized tissue adjacent to such thrombi retards typical histologic organization. Thus, morphologic determination of duration of a thrombus on a prosthesis is thus frequently impossible, and valve-associated thrombi can be friable for extended periods.

ENDOCARDITIS

Infective prosthetic valve endocarditis is an infrequent but serious problem (1–6% of valve replacement patients, over 50% mortality). Secondary effects include embolization of vegetations, congestive heart failure secondary to valvular obstruction or regurgitation caused by bulky and destructive vegetations, or the consequences of local tissue destruction and ring abscess (Fig. 10.5). Rates of infection are not different for mechanical and bioprosthetic valves, but patients in whom endocarditis necessitated the original surgery are at greater risk.

Prosthetic valve endocarditis occurs most frequently in the first several months postoperatively and has a preponderance of organisms comprising normal skin flora, reflecting perioperative valve contamination or bacteremia. Late infections probably are almost always caused by bacteremic seeding. The high frequency of staphylococcal infection (especially *Staphylococcus epidermidis*), particularly in early prosthetic valve endocarditis, contrasts with the relatively low frequency of such organisms in endocarditis on natural valves. *S. aureus,* streptococci, and gram-negative bacilli and fungi also cause prosthetic valve endocarditis.

Similar to other infections involving biomaterials, prosthetic valve endocarditis is resistant to hose defense mechanisms and antibiotics, and thereby difficult to cure medically. Because the synthetic biomaterials (polymers, met-

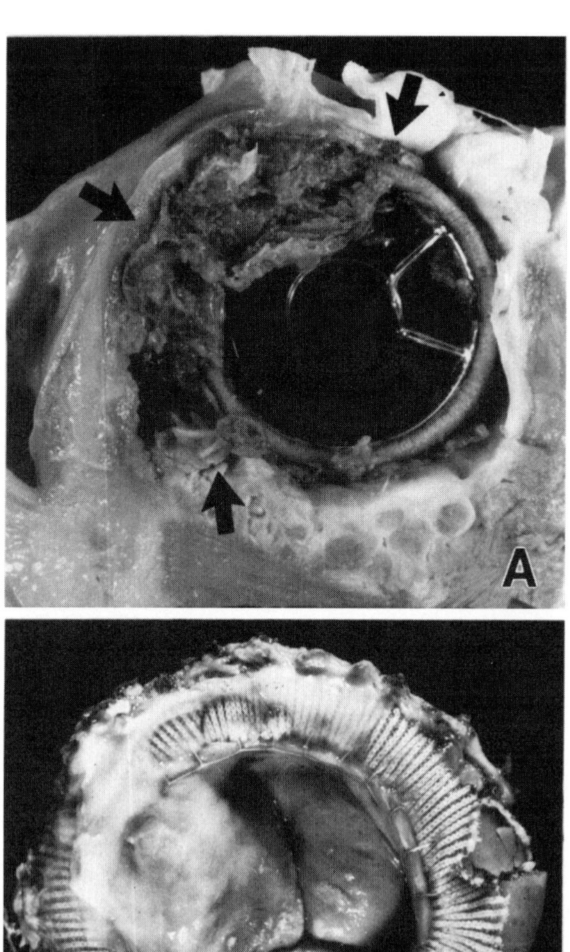

FIG. 10.5. Prosthetic valve infective endocarditis. *A.* Prosthetic valve staphylococcal endocarditis with large ring abscess (*arrows*), demonstrated from ventricular aspect of aortic Bjork-Shiley tilting disk prosthesis in patient who died suddenly. Ring abscess impinged on proximal atrioventricular conduction system. A Reproduced with permission from Schoen FJ. *J Cardiac Surg* 1987;2:65. Bioprosthetic valve endocarditis with cuspal perforation by organism-induced necrosis (*arrow*). B Reproduced with permission from Schoen FJ, et al. *Am J Cardiol* 1983;51:957.

als, carbons) that comprise mechanical prostheses generally cannot support bacterial or fungal growth, infections of these valves are almost always localized to the prosthesis-tissue interface at the sewing ring, causing a *ring abscess* (Fig. 10.5*A*).[34,35] The resultant tissue destruction can induce separation (dehiscence) of the prosthesis from the annulus, with regurgitation of blood around the device (septic paravalvular leak), or cause septic pericarditis, pseudoaneurysm, or complete or partial interference with atrioventricular conduction. In contrast, bioprosthetic valve endocarditis can be either localized to the prosthesis sewing ring and complicated by ring abscess similarly to that of mechanical valves, or confined to the cuspal tissue, often with tearing, perforation, or destruction leading to valve incompetence (Fig. 10.5*B*).[36] Histologic examination of the cusps of infected bioprosthetic valves often demonstrates deep clumps of bacterial or fungal organisms with few inflammatory cells.

The presence of a foreign body potentiates infection in several ways.[37] Through implantation of a device, microorganisms are provided access to the circulation and to deeper tissue by description of natural barriers against infection during implantation or subsequent function of a prosthetic device. Moreover, microorganisms inadvertently may be introduced by contamination of medical devices during manufacture or implantation surgery. A foreign body limits phagocyte migration into infected tissue and interferes with inflammatory cell phagocytic mechanisms, probably by virtue of either release or toxic implant constituents or surface-mediated interactions causing release of lysosomal contents into the adjacent tissues. The cumulative effect is a lessening of the bactericidal ability of these cells, causing local tissue injury and allowing bacteria to survive adjacent to the implant.

STRUCTURAL DYSFUNCTION

Prosthetic valve failure can be precipitated by the limited durability of biomaterials. The modes of degradation vary among valve types.

MECHANICAL VALVES

Contemporary tilting disk designs with pyrolytic carbon occluders, with or without carbon cage components, have generally favorable durability. Fractures of components of the St. Jude Medical and other mechanical valves are rare. However, in a specific cohort of Bjork-Shiley 60 and 70° convexo-concave (C-C) tilting disk heart valves, the welded outlet strut has fractured and separated from the valve, leading to disk escape (Fig. 10.6). Most patients experiencing strut fracture died before a reoperation could be accomplished.

Such fractures are a result of a concurrence of abnormal loads and welding flaws.[38] Detailed analysis of a fractured valve frequently reveals a pronounced flat wear mark on the tip of the strut indicative of an abnormally hard contact of the disk with the tip of the outlet strut during closing. The excessive load induces high bending stresses in the welds joining the outlet strut to the housing. Welds are typically intrinsically brittle because of shrinkage porosity and/or inclusions, and thus are easily fractured.

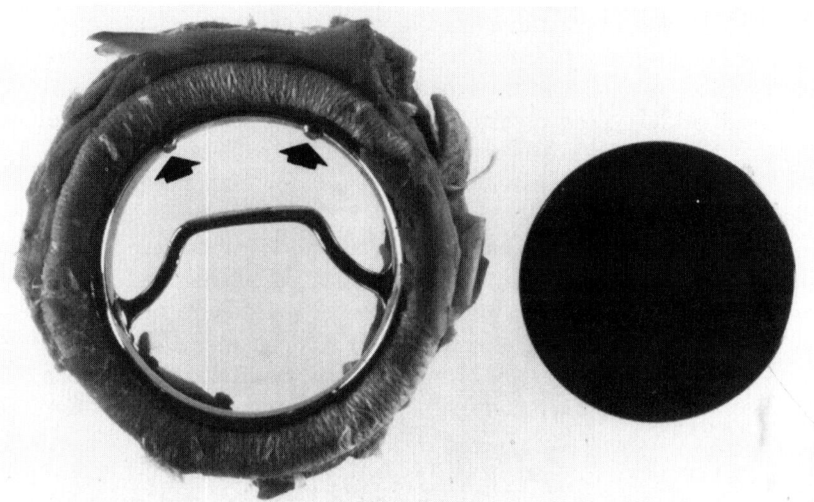

FIG. 10.6. Fracture of the minor outflow strut at its welds to the valve housing (*arrows*) of a Bjork-Shiley tilting disk valve prosthesis. The fractured strut could not be located at autopsy. Reproduced with permission from Ref. 38.

BIOPROSTHETIC VALVES

The major cause of bioprosthetic valve dysfunction is noninfective tissue degeneration, usually related to cuspal mineralization (Fig. 10.7). Primary tissue failure of glutaraldehyde-pretreated porcine bioprostheses is progressive with time. In adults, although less than 1% of valves implanted for 5 years have failed, 20–30% become dysfunctional within 10 years, and more than 50% suffer critical degeneration (less than half are functional) by 15 years postoperatively.[39–41] The failure rate is identical for the Hancock and Carpentier-Edwards types.[42] The risk of structural failure is strongly age-dependent, with younger patients having a much higher rate of failure[40–42] then elderly patients.

Regurgitation through tears forming adjacent to calcific nodules is overwhelmingly the most frequent failure mode of porcine aortic valve bioprostheses. Pericardial bioprostheses also frequently suffer calcific degenerative failure in both adults and children. However, noncalcific cuspal perforations and tears most frequently cause failure of clinical pericardial bioprostheses. Defects usually occur near the cuspal attachments, adjacent to the stent posts.[43,44]

Degenerative cuspal calcific deposits in bioprosthetic valves form within the cusps (intrinsic mineralization), and are composed of calcium phosphates, with a composition and crystal structure closely related to that of physiologic bone mineral (hydroxyapatite).[45] Generally predominating at the cuspal commissures and basal attachments, the calcific deposits are grossly visible as nodular gray/white masses that often ulcerate through the cuspal tissue. Experimental investigations of calcification, particularly those using a rat subcutaneous im-

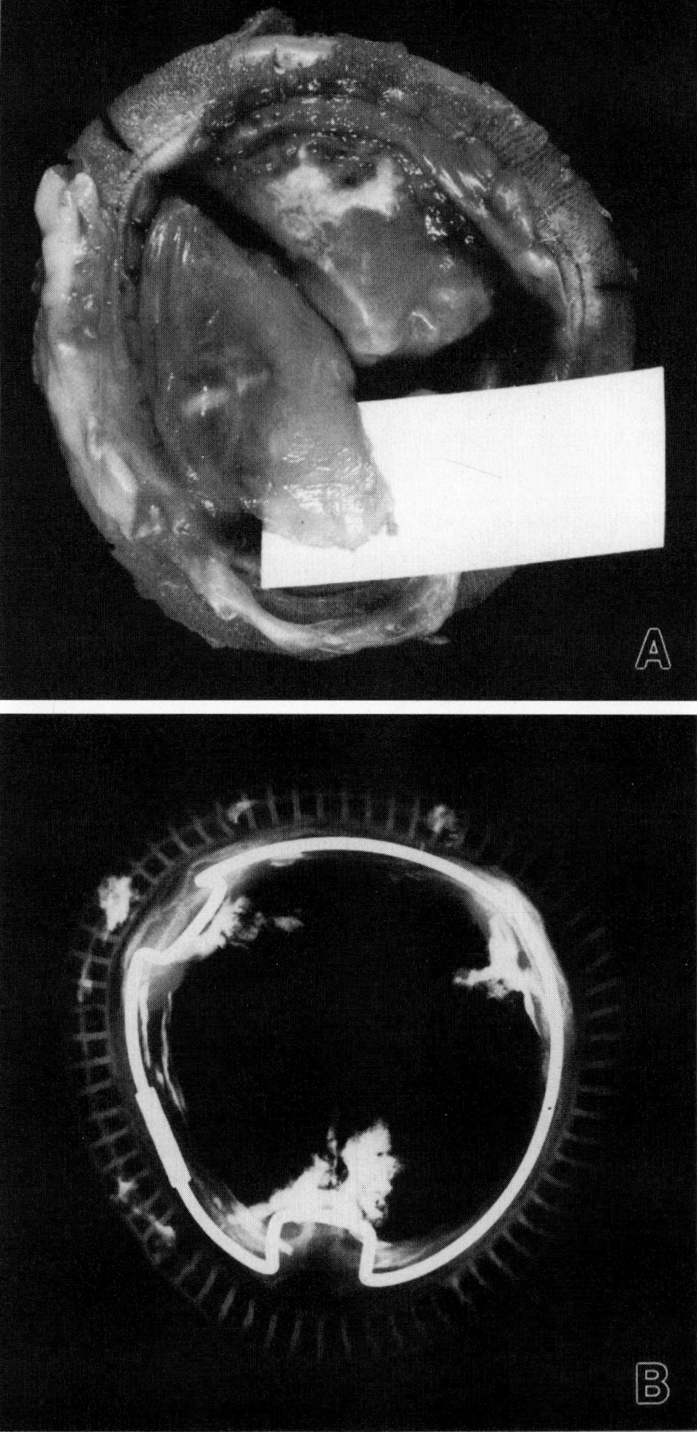

Fig. 10.7. Primary tissue failure due to calcification with secondary cuspal tear leading to severe regurgitation of a porcine bioprosthetic valve. *A*, gross photograph; *B*, specimen radiograph. Dense calcific deposits are apparent at the commissures. Reproduced with permission from Ref. 27.

plant model, have demonstrated that the most important mechanism of calcification in bioprosthetic valve tissue is cell-mediated, with mineral deposits being nucleated largely at the membranes and in organelles of the transplanted cells (Fig. 10.8).[46,47] Although calcification of circulatory implants is accelerated and most pronounced in areas of leaflet flexion, where deformations are maximal (*i.e.,* cuspal commissures and bases), dynamic mechanical stress and strain

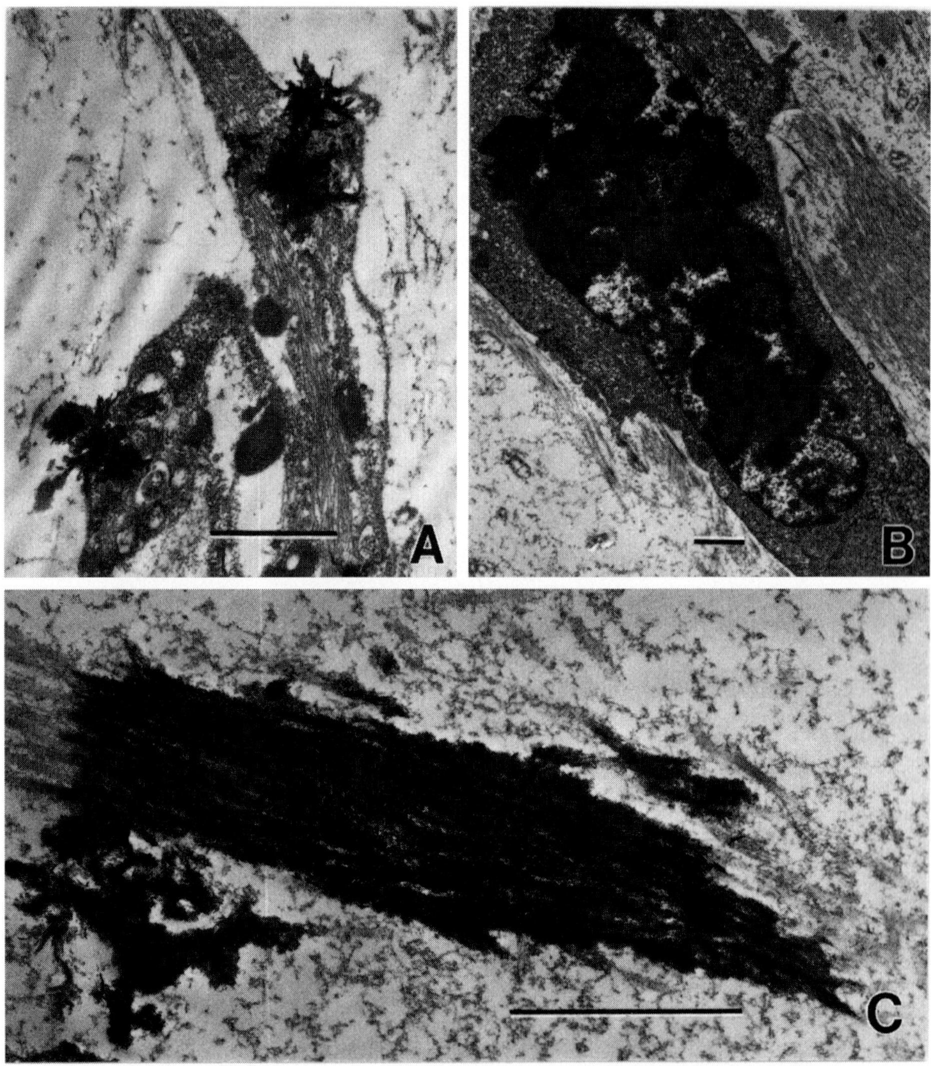

FIG. 10.8. Ultrastructure of porcine connective tissue and collagen-associated calcific deposits in subcutaneous bioprosthetic tissue implants. *A.* Focal deposits at cell surface and cytoplasm (48 hr). *B.* extensive intranuclear calcification (72 hr). *C.* collagen calcification (21 days). Bar = 1 μm. (*A,* reproduced with permission from Schoen FJ et al. In: Waller BF, ed. *Contemporary issues in cardiovascular pathology,* Philadelphia: F.A. Davis, 1988;289. *B* and *C,* reproduced with permission from Ref. 46.

are not prerequisites for calcification. Immunological and inflammatory factors appear unimportant. In rat subcutaneous implants, calcification requires pretreatment of tissue with an aldehyde cross-linking agent; nonpreserved cusps do not mineralize. Glutaraldehyde-treated porcine aortic valve and bovine pericardium calcify comparably with respect to kinetics, extent, and morphology. These data suggest that the fundamental mechanisms of bioprosthetic tissue mineralization depend on specific biochemical modifications of implant microstructural components that are induced by aldehyde pretreatment.[16,38]

The critical event, reaction of calcium derived from plasma with the membrane-associated organic phosphorus, is hypothesized to occur as follows[47]: Normal cells have an approximately 10,000-fold gradient of calcium from outside to inside; low intracellular calcium concentrations are maintained by energy-requiring pumps at the cell membranes. In cells rendered nonviable by glutaraldehyde fixation or autolysis, energy is unavailable, membranes are disrupted, and calcium exclusion is impaired. This allows high concentrations of calcium in the fluid bathing the tissue to react with membrane phosphorus. Collagen calcification occurs later.

NONSTRUCTURAL DYSFUNCTION

Nonstructural dysfunction of a valve prosthesis comprises a heterogeneous group of complications that are based on interactions of an otherwise structurally intact prosthesis with its environment. Paravalvular leak, extrinsic interference, and hemolysis are the most common problems in this group.

PARAVALVULAR LEAK

Early dehiscence is often the result of separation of sutures from a pathologic annulus when valve replacement was done for endocarditis with ring abscess, myxomatous degeneration of the mitral valve, or calcified aortic valve or mitral annulus. In contrast, small paravalvular leaks are usually caused by tissue retraction from the sewing ring between sutures during healing (Fig. 10.9) or, in some cases, late infection (see *Endocarditis,* above). Small periprosthetic defects are often clinically inconsequential; large leaks can aggravate or cause hemolysis or heart failure. In surgical pathology specimens, a valve removed for paravalvular leak usually appears normally functioning. Detection of a periprosthetic healing defect at autopsy may require careful probing.

EXTRINSIC INTERFERENCE

Prosthetic valve stenosis or regurgitation can be promoted by factors extrinsic to a prosthesis. For example, retained valve remnants, unraveled or excessively long ends of sutures or a large mitral annular calcific nodule, exuberant overgrowth of fibrous tissue, or septal hypertrophy can prevent full excursion of a tilting disk valve occluder (Fig. 10.10). Sutures may be looped around bioprosthetic valve stents, particularly with pericardial bioprostheses, thereby restricting cuspal motion, and suture ends cut too long may perforate a bioprosthetic valve cusp.

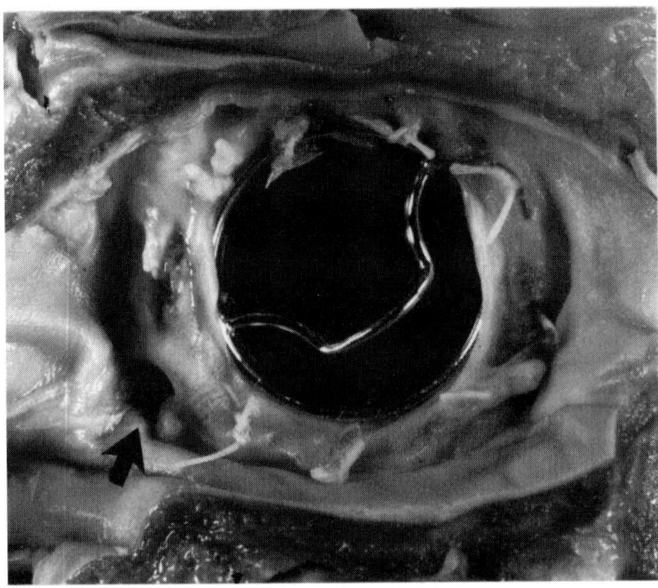

FIG. 10.9. Late paravalvular leak adjacent to a mitral valve prosthesis (*arrow*).

HEMOLYSIS

Some red blood cell destruction by the turbulent flow in prosthetic heart valves is common, but hemolysis is generally slight and well compensated. Severe hemolytic anemia is unusual. However, when a high-velocity jet of blood is forced through a paravalvular leak or when valvular dysfunction occurs, severe hemolytic anemia can ensue. Pathologic markers for hemolysis include elevated serum lactate dehydrogenase (LDH), a blood smear with schistocytes and other evidence of erythrocyte fragmentation and renal tubular hemosiderosis in kidney tissue specimens.

ALLOGRAFT VALVES

Homograft/allograft aortic valves have excellent hemodynamic performance, nearly equivalent to that of the natural aortic valve, and an exceedingly low rate of thromboembolism without anticoagulant therapy.[29,30] They are particularly advantageous for young patients with aortic valve disease or those requiring pulmonic valve or pulmonary artery replacement for congenital heart disease. Current interest is directed toward cadaver-derived allografts that are cryopreserved in liquid nitrogen at −196°C, using dimethyl sulfoxide as a protective agent. The limiting factor that prevents uniform long-term success is late failure resulting from progressive degeneration. The mode of failure is generally incompetence caused by either cuspal rupture, distortion with retraction, or perforations, whereas stenosis is most frequently a result of somatic growth of the recipient, with or without calcification of the cusps or distal aortic wall in children who have right ventricular to pulmonary

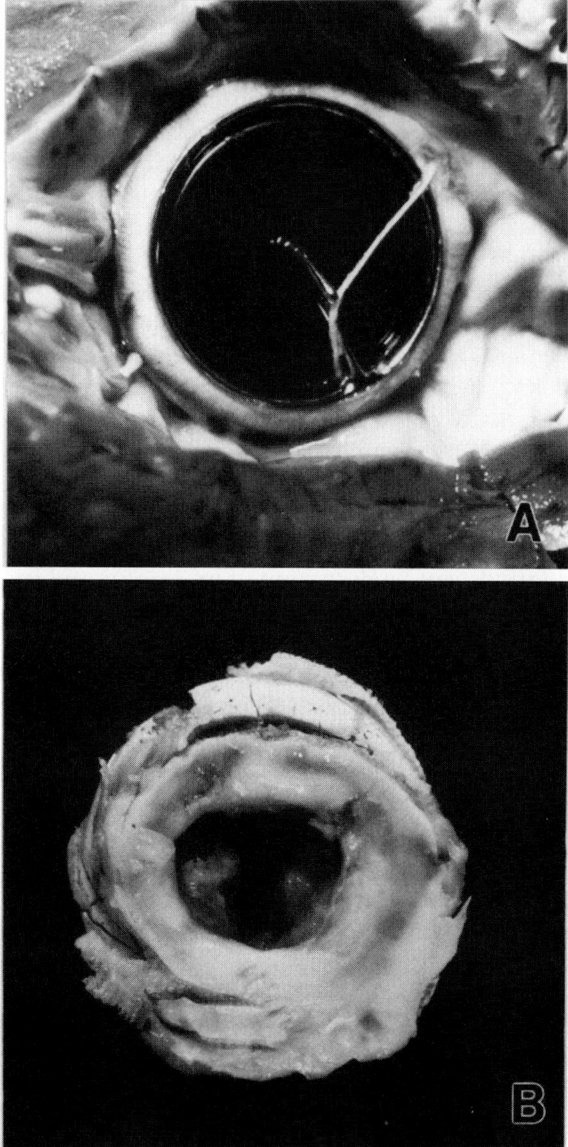

FIG. 10.10. Extrinsic interference with function of prosthetic heart valve. *A.* Suture looped around central strut of a Medtronic-Hall tilting disk valve causing disk immobility. (Photo courtesy of Office of the Chief Medical Examiner, New York City). *B.* Tissue overgrowth compromising inflow orifice of porcine bioprosthesis. Reproduced with permission from Ref. 3.

artery conduits. The rate of failure is equivalent to or slightly superior to that of bioprosthetic valves.[29–31]

Pathologic features noted in removed failed or nonfailed aortic valve allografts are summarized in Table 10.2 (R. N. Mitchell and F. J. Schoen, unpublished observations). Late explants frequently have variable amounts of proximal intimal fibrous sheath, cuspal hematoma, aortic wall calcification, and, occasionally, cuspal calcific deposits. Calcification of the contiguous aortic wall prominently involves elastic elements. Valves removed after various periods of implantation are largely acellular, being devoid of surface endothelium and deep connective tissue cells of both valve cusps and aortic wall. Inflammatory cellularity is variable. The cusps are usually bland and virtually featureless at the light microscopic level, but special stains for elastin and collagen as well as electron microscopy demonstrate substantial preservation of the essential connective tissue elements. Residual fragments of nonviable cuspal cells are noted by electron microscopy. They often comprise sites of early calcification. Despite both frequent crossing of major blood groups between donor and recipient and lack of therapeutic immunosuppression, immunological rejection does not seem to be a limitation.

PATHOLOGIC ANALYSIS OF CONTEMPORARY VALVE SUBSTITUTES

Valve-related failure can be documented by careful and informed examination by surgical and autopsy pathologists of artificial valves, either removed or *in situ*. Although the anticipated pathology and thus the detailed protocol for analysis depends in large part on the type of prosthesis under consideration, generalized approaches to dissection of heart valve prostheses and documentation of their most important findings have been described.[1,2]

In brief, a prosthesis at either autopsy or surgical removal is photographed from all pertinent aspects and examined for thrombi, vegetations, exuberant tissue overgrowth, and structural defects. Autopsy specimens are carefully probed for paravalvular leaks. The specific type and model of the prosthesis are identified using radiographic and morphologic keys as necessary.[1,11,16,48] A serial number placed by the manufacturer that uniquely identifies each valve is usually hidden under the sewing ring at the valve base. Mechanical heart valve prostheses are also checked for adequacy of poppet excursion and seating, defects and fractures of components, asymmetries, sites of abrasive wear, and poppet swelling or distortion. Bioprostheses are gently palpated to assess

---

TABLE 10.2   ALLOGRAFT VALVE MORPHOLOGIC FEATURES

Variable cuspal distortion and tears
Loss of cuspal connective tissue cells
Loss of endothelium
Variable inflammatory cellularity
Variable aortic wall calcification
Variable cuspal calcification
Mural thrombus
Cuspal hematomas

cuspal excursion and visually inspected for the presence of fenestrations, tears, cuspal hematomas, calcific nodules, and central migration of struts. Routine morphologic analysis of bioprostheses includes radiography (we use the Faxitron, Hewlett Packard, McMinnville, OR; 0.8, 1 min × 35 KV), that aids identification of the prosthesis type and assessment of calcific deposits. Calcification is semiquantitatively graded[49] and the location of calcific deposits noted (with respect to cuspal bodies, commissures, basal attachment sites, and at the free cuspal edges). Specimens of cuspal and adherent tissue are specifically labeled, oriented in cross-section, and embedded (preferably in a hard embedding medium such as glycolmethacrylate) for histologic analysis. Embedding in glycolmethacrylate allows sectioning of undecalcified bioprosthetic valve specimens with good morphological preservation. Histologic analysis is directed toward determination of the morphology of tissue-prosthesis interactions, cuspal degeneration, and the degree and specific morphology of calcific deposits. The key morphologic findings sought in examination of a prosthesis are summarized in Table 10.3. Specialized approaches and analyses are appropriate to answer specific questions regarding mechanisms of failure or other patient-prosthesis interactions.[49–52]

VASCULAR GRAFTS

Coronary arterial bypass and other vascular grafts are frequently encountered by pathologists. The specific complications that occur and pathological considerations in analysis vary with graft type and location. Vascular grafts in any site of implantation can become complicated by thrombosis or thromboembolism, infection, periprosthetic fluid collection, pseudoaneurysm (particularly due to disruption of an anastomosis), and/or structural degeneration (most commonly due to fabric degeneration with fragmentation or graft dilatation) (Table 10.4). Despite several potential complications that occur uncommonly, Dacron (polyethylene terephthalate) grafts in current use gener-

TABLE 10.3   PATHOLOGICAL FEATURES OF RETRIEVED SUBSTITUTE HEART VALVES

Gross examination	Radiography
Tissue overgrowth	Valve identification
Thrombi	Calcification
Vegetations	Degree
Cuspal stiffness	Location
Cuspal hematomas	
Calcification	Histologic examination
Fenestrations/tears	Vegetations/organisms
Cuspal abrasion	Thrombi
Cuspal stretching	Inflammation
Strut relationships	Degeneration
Mechanical dysfunction	Calcification
Extrinsic interference/damage	Degree
	Location
	Morphology
	Endothelialization

TABLE 10.4. MAJOR COMPLICATIONS OF VASCULAR GRAFTS

	Large Dacron Graft	Small Synthetic Graft	Autogenous Saphenous Vein
Thrombus/thromboembolism		X	X
Infection	X	X	
Perigraft seroma		X	
Erosion into adjacent structure	X		
Anastomotic pseudoaneurysm	X	X	X
Intimal fibrous hyperplasia		X	X
Atherosclerosis			X
Degradation with fragmentation or dilation	X		

ally perform well in large-diameter, high-flow locations such as the aorta and the iliac and proximal arteries of the lower extremities. The 10-year patency rate is nearly 100% at the aortic bifurcation, approximately 75–80% in the aortofemoral position, and 50% in the above-knee femoropopliteal position. In contrast, small diameter fabric vascular grafts (<6–8 mm in diameter) have lower flow rates and generally perform less well. The most widely used small vessel replacements are reversed autogenous saphenous vein and (expanded polytetrafluoroethylene (ePTFE), essentially a microporous Teflon), of which Gore-Tex is a widely used type. Patency of above-knee femoropopliteal autologous saphenous vein bypass grafts and ePTFE grafts is comparable with that of Dacron, but more distal ePTFE bypass grafts have a 3–4 year patency rate of only 30–50%.

Failure of small-diameter vascular prostheses is most frequently due to occlusion by thrombus formation or generalized or anastomotic intimal hyperplasia (Fig. 10.11). Intimal hyperplasia is an exaggeration of the normal arterial healing response, arising from the intimal migration and proliferation of medial smooth muscle cells, derived from the host vessel with a synthetic vascular graft, and from either host vessel or the graft itself when the graft has potentially viable cells (such as an autogenous saphenous vein).[53] Thus, whereas synthetic vascular prostheses develop intimal hyperplasia and resultant stenoses predominantly at or near anastomoses, intimal hyperplasia is often diffuse in vein grafts, leading to narrowing of the entire graft length.

Vascular graft healing has complex determinants (Fig. 10.12). The blood contacting surface lining a vascular graft could hypothetically arise from (1) host vessel-derived tissue growth across anastomotic sites, (2) transinterstitial tissue migration, or (3) deposition of cells from blood. However, healing of the inner capsule of contemporary vascular grafts primarily involves endothelial cells and smooth muscle cells derived from the artery adjacent to the anastomosis (Fig. 10.12*A*).[54] In contrast, transinterstitial growth occurs only under special circumstances (*e.g.,* high porosity), and deposition of cells from blood capable of differentiating into vascular wall cells probably never occurs. Except under specialized circumstances, the ability of humans to endothelialize synthetic cardiovascular prostheses is limited, with endothelial cells ultimately extending only 10–15 mm or less across an anastomosis. The blood-con-

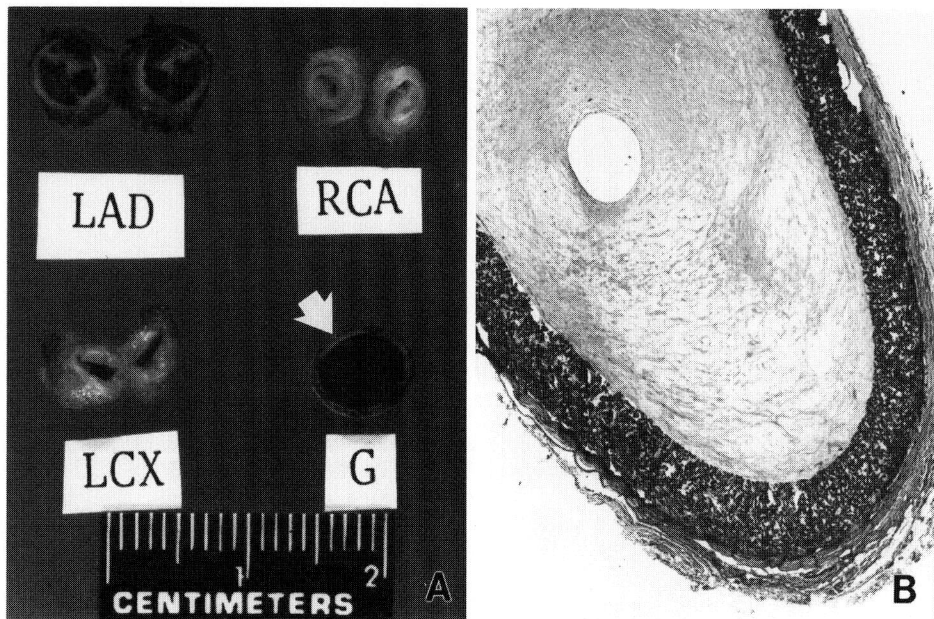

FIG. 10.11. Complications of small diameter vascular grafts. *A.* Gross photo of a thrombosed Gore-Tex small diameter graft used as an aortocoronary bypass graft (*arrow*). Thrombosis occurred within the first several days postoperatively. Reproduced with permission from Ref. 1. *B.* Intimal hyperplasia of a Gore-Tex graft that nearly occluded the lumen several years following femoro-popliteal bypass. (Reproduced by permission from *Robbins Pathologic Basis of Disease,* 5th ed. Philadelphia: WB Saunders, 1994.)

tacting surface of the graft is best termed *neointima* if the surface is truly endothelialized (Fig. 10.12*B*), but *pseudointima* if the surface is composed of fibrin, collagen, platelets, or smooth muscle cells. Why endothelialization is limited and why different materials facilitate healing to different degrees are controversial subjects of active investigation (Fig. 10-12*C*).

Vascular grafts are widely used in aortocoronary bypass graft surgery. The American Heart Association estimates that 265,000 patients had aortocoronary bypass in 1991.[56] The small caliber of these grafts presently necessitates that either autogenous saphenous vein or internal mammary artery is used. A small fraction (perhaps 5–10%) of saphenous vein grafts used as aortocoronary bypass vessels occlude within 1 month, approximately 10–20% occlude within 1 year, and by 10–12 years postoperatively, only approximately 50–60% remain patent. Three pathologic processes are primarily responsible for graft occlusion: thrombosis (early closure), intimal hyperplasia (a few months to a few years), and atherosclerosis (usually after at least 3 years).[57] The risk of early thrombotic occlusion is increased with low vein graft blood flow and small luminal size of the grafted artery, both correlates of poor run-off.

Atherosclerosis, the major cause of late vein graft occlusion, yields lesions that in this context have high potential for disruption and embolization.

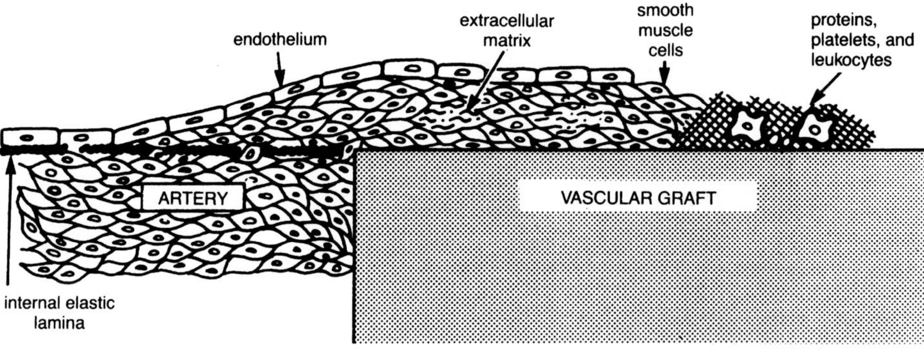

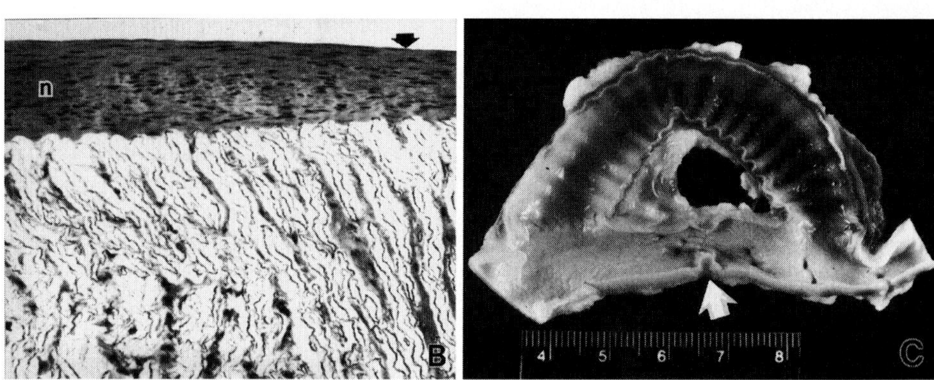

FIG. 10.12. Vascular graft healing. *A.* Schematic diagram of pannus formation, the major mode of graft healing with currently available vascular grafts. Smooth muscle cells migrate from the media to the intima of the adjacent artery and extend over and proliferate on the graft surface; the smooth muscle cell layer is covered by a proliferating layer of endothelial cells. *B.* Neointima (*n*), consisting of smooth muscle cell proliferation, covered by endothelium, in experimental ePTFE graft in the rabbit aorta. Blood-contacting surface is indicated by arrow. Hematoxylin and eosin, magnification X150. *A* and *B* reproduced with permission from Ref. 1. *C.* Experimental composite vascular graft composed of two separate materials anastomosed together, used to bypass a surgically created stenotic segment in the sheep aorta (*arrow*). The extent of healing is vastly different on the two prosthetic materials. On the left is a gelatin-sealed graft, on the right an albumin sealed graft. (Reproduced with permission from Ref. 55.)

Plaques that occur in grafts typically have poorly developed fibrous caps, and the necrotic core and the secondary dystrophic calcific deposits that develop may be adjacent to the lumen rather than deep to the surface, as in typical native arterial atherosclerosis. As in native arteries, secondary thrombosis may be initiated by plaque rupture.

The autologous internal mammary artery, with its proximal origin from the subclavian artery maintained intact, has been used increasingly as an aorto-coronary bypass conduit with highly favorable results. Late patency of internal mammary artery conduits is approximately 90% after 10 years, and pathologic analyses of such vessels have revealed a low frequency of significant postoperative pathologic changes.[1]

CIRCULATORY ASSIST DEVICES AND ARTIFICIAL HEARTS

The use of cardiac-assist devices and artificial hearts has been increasing, particularly to provide support to end-stage heart failure patients who are transplant candidates until a donor organ becomes available ("bridge to transplant").[58] The major complications with blood pumps have been local problems, especially hemolysis, thrombus, infection (intraluminal and periprosthetic), durability limitations (fractures, calcification), thermal compression effects, and other implant-related injury); and distant or systemic effects (especially embolic, septic, and immunologic).[59–64]

Thromboembolism is a major potential complication of clinical circulatory assist. Thromboembolism has occurred in most patients having implantation of the Jarvik-7 artificial heart for temporary or permanent support and in approximately one-third of patients with the Novacor ventricular-assist device. Pathologic examination of several device types reveals thrombi associated with valves, connections of conduits, and other components to each other and to the natural heart and the pumping bladders (Figure 10.13).[59,64] Infectious complications, particularly those associated with percutaneous pneumatic drive lines, have been a major limiting factor in the prolonged use of mechanical hearts, affecting virtually all the long-term recipients for the Jarvik-7 artificial heart and many patients supported with ventricular-assist devices. The complications of the various forms of cardiac assist in potential transplant recipients do not differ widely from those encountered in the use of permanent artificial hearts or in the use of temporary assist devices in other patients.

PACEMAKERS AND DEFIBRILLATORS

More than 100,000 pacemakers are implanted each year in the United States. Cardiac pacing is achieved by a system of interconnected components, including 1) a pulse generator (a power source and associated electrical circuitry that initiates the electrical stimulus and may have sensing functions), 2) one or more electrically insulated conductors leading from the pulse generator to the heart, 3) an electrode at the distal end of each conductor, and 4) a tissue or blood and tissue interface between electrode and adjacent stimulatable cardiac myocytes. The pacing leads connect pulse generator and heart through a long wire conductor and distal electrode(s). The generator is usually placed subcutaneously on the chest; the leads are advanced transvenously through the subclavian vein, with the electrode terminating at the endocardial surface of the right ventricle (Fig. 10.14). Alternatively, the electrodes may be surgically attached to the epicardial surface via the transthoracic route.

The pacing threshold (*i.e.,* the strength of the pacing stimulus needed to initiate a wave of depolarization through the myocardium, thereby initiating contraction) is affected by a variety of factors, including the position of the electrode relative to stimulatable tissue and the thickness of the tissue response to the electrode. Late complications are usually related to the pacemaker pack

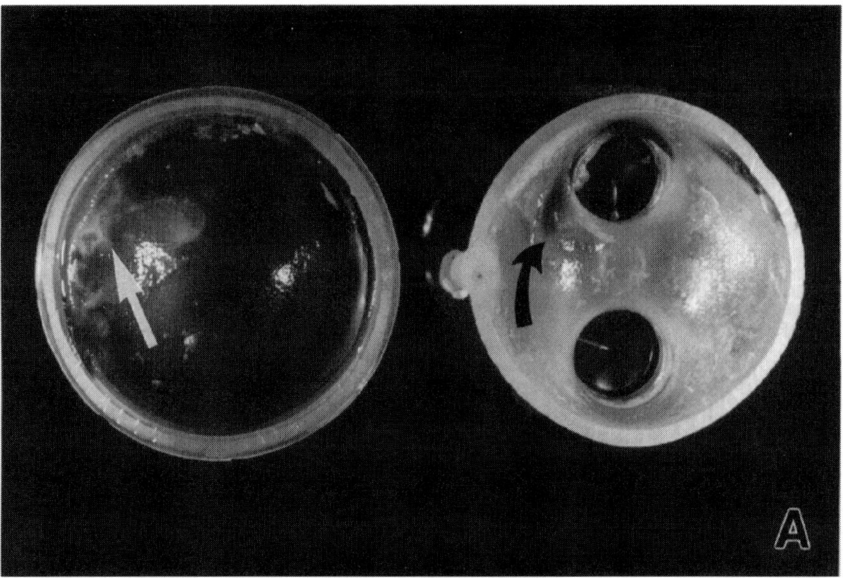

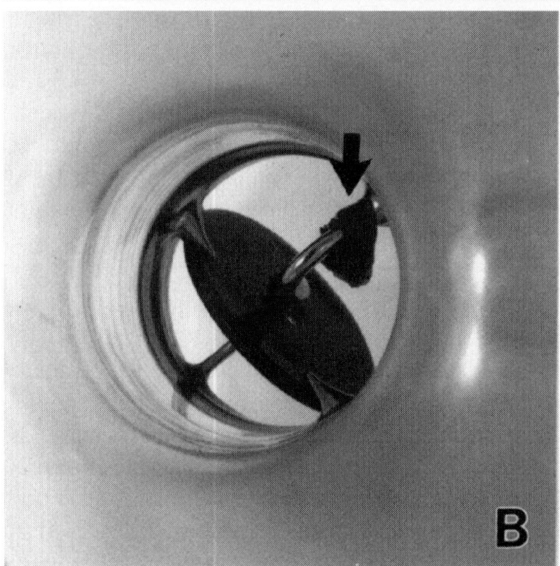

FIG. 10.13. Thrombus associated with ventricular assist devices. *A*. Thrombus associated with pumping bladder (*white arrow*) and housing near valve (*dark arrow*) of Symbion assist device. *B*. Thrombus associated with valve strut (*arrow*). Reproduced with permission from Ref. 59.

and its implantation site, or to the pacing lead or electrodes, including damage to the tricuspid valve or right atrial or ventricular free walls, including perforation, electrode dislodgement, lead fracture, thrombosis and thromboembolism, infection, myocardial penetration or perforation, electrode corrosion and insulation failure, and an unduly high pacing threshold. The pacemaker pulse generator can have electrical failure or complications of the surrounding

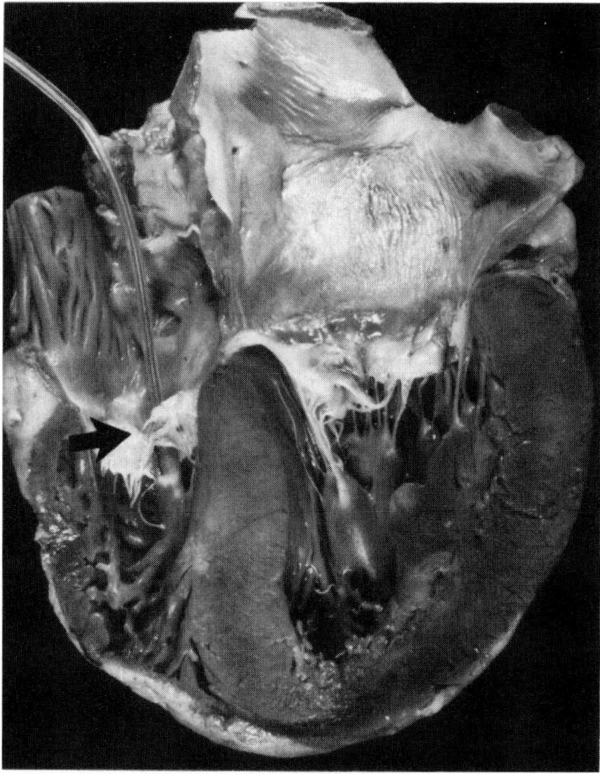

FIG. 10.14. Four-chamber view of heart in patient with longstanding transvenous pacemaker properly positioned in the right ventricular apex, but intertwined with and fibrosed to the tricuspid valve (*arrow*).

tissue. Some degree of thrombus formation is inevitable with either silicone rubber or polyurethane lead coatings. Organization of thrombus can cause adhesions to the endocardium. Serious thrombotic or embolic complications occur in 2% of patients with permanent transvenous pacemakers, but inconsequential thrombosis of small veins in the upper arms and shoulders is more frequent. Endocarditis associated with a pacer lead, an infrequent complication, usually is initiated in the pacemaker pocket with subsequent extension to the pacemaker wire. Alternatively, infection may originate on the pacer lead or adjacent traumatized endocardium. When infection occurs, mortality is high unless the pacing apparatus is removed. Early complications of epicardial insertion include nonseptic pericarditis and ventricular laceration.

Approximately 10,000 automatic implantable cardioverter defibrillators have been implanted worldwide. This device has proved highly effective for terminating lethal arrhythmias and enhancing survival of cardiac arrest survivors and patients with drug-refractory ventricular tachycardia.[65] With cardioverter-defibrillator systems, the more extensive hardware (relative to pacemakers) may increase the frequency of infection and late accumulation of serosanguinous pleural fluid. The leads are applied to the epicardium, which involves opening the pericardium and allowing communication between pericardial and pleural spaces. Complications are related to the surgical procedure used for implantation, the number and size of leads, the size of the generator, and the limitations of the system used for arrhythmia detection and termination.[66,67] Moreover, hardware located in the pericardial and pleural space may cause local irritation. Other complications are relatively uncommon but include mechanical and sensing problems, short battery life, generator erosion through the overlying skin, and infection of the power pack, mediastinum, or patch electrodes (the latter about 5%).

STENTS

The success of percutaneous transluminal coronary angioplasty (PTCA) is limited by acute closure (3–5% of patients) and restenosis (25–40% of patients). Intravascular stents may reverse the untoward effects of PTCA by acting as a scaffold to support the intimal dissections that occur as a mode of PTCA luminal expansion, mechanically prevent vascular spasm, and increase blood flow, all of which could minimize thrombus formation, and reduce the impact of postangioplasty intimal proliferation. Recent studies have suggested that permanent metal prosthetic coronary arterial stents reduce the incidence of clinical restenosis, as compared with standard angioplasty.[68]

The short-term and long-term morphologic effects of several types of intravascular stents have been described.[69–72] Pathological studies suggest that intravascular stents can act as a scaffold to hold open the vessel after the injury produced during PTCA. However, early thrombotic occlusion occurs in some patients, necessitating intensive anticoagulation and antiplatelet therapy that induces a substantial risk of hemorrhage. In vessels that are maintained patent, stent wires are initially covered with a variable platelet-fibrin coating (Fig. 10.15). Within 2–3 weeks, stent wires become covered by neointima. Where stent wires are not firmly embedded into the vessel wall, thrombosis may occur and reendothelialization does not take place, possibly because of movement of the stent wires. Some medial compression and thinning but little inflammatory response to the stent wire have been noted. Nevertheless, the neointima may thicken, and proliferative restenosis is not prevented by stenting.[69] Moreover, important questions remain relative to the potential for late complications of endovascular stents, such as migration, perforation, or infection.

CONCLUSIONS

Cardiovascular medical devices are used widely and the pathologist is likely to encounter substitute heart valves, vascular grafts, cardiac-assist devices, pacemakers/defibrillators, and intravascular stents with increasing frequency. In general, these devices serve their recipients well for extended periods. However, generic late complications are frequent, including thrombotic and thromboembolic problems (and problems of the therapy to prevent them), device-associated infection, structural deterioration, and other nonstructural but device-specific problems. In particular, the modes of failure of substitute heart valves illustrate well the major concepts. The formulation, characterization,

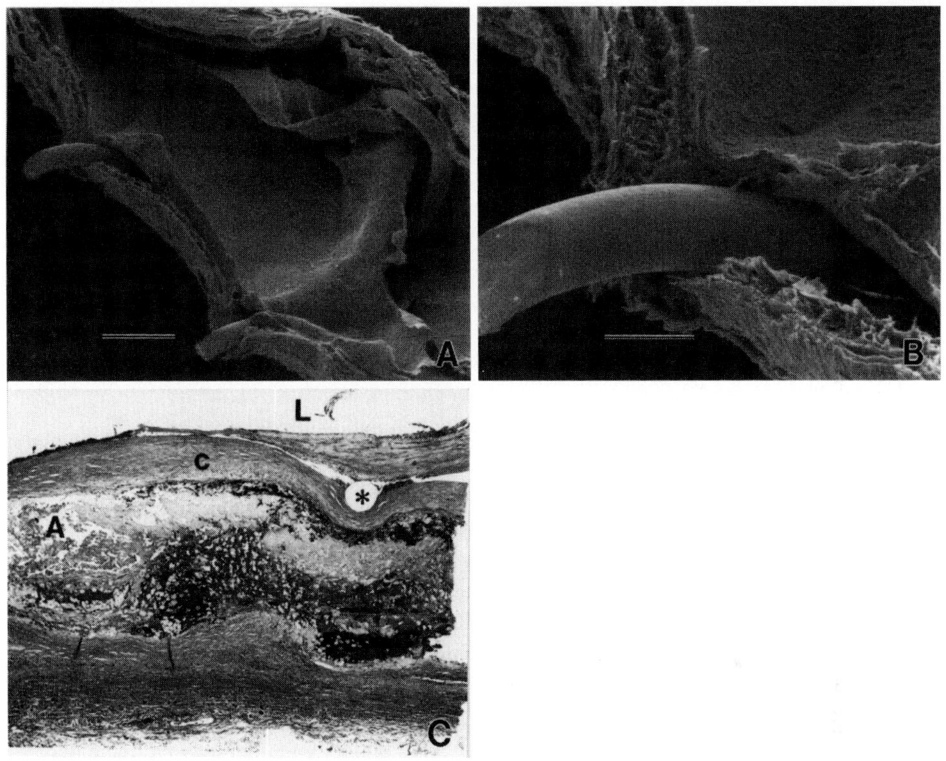

FIG. 10.15. Balloon-expandable metallic flexible coil vascular stent. *A*. Low-power scanning electron microscopic view showing the stent wires (*arrow*) covered by neointima. The neointima covering the stent wires has pulled away from the vessel wall during processing. Bar = 500 μm. *B*. Higher-power scanning electron photomicrograph showing the stent embedded in the media (*M*) of the vessel. The neointima covering the stent wire is lined by endothelial cells (*E*). Bar = 150 μm. *C*. Photomicrograph of longitudinal section of a stent in an aortocoronary saphenous vein bypass graft demonstrating an atherosclerortic lesion within the wall of the vessel (*A*) that is covered by a fibrous connective tissue cap (*c*). The hole left by the stent wire (*) indents the fibrous cap and holds it against the plaque. The neointima consists of smooth muscle cells and fibrous extracellular matrix. Hematoxylin and eosin, magnification ×20. Reproduced with permission from Ref. 70.

and explant-evaluation of new and modified biomaterials and medical devices for cardiovascular application present exciting challenges to pathologists, bioengineers, and other biomaterial scientists and practitioners.[73]

REFERENCES

1. Schoen FJ. *Interventional and surgical cardiovascular pathology: clinical correlations and basic principles.* Philadelphia: WB Saunders, 1989.
2. Schoen FJ. Special considerations for pathologic evaluation of explanted cardiovascular prostheses. In: von Recum AF, ed. *Handbook of biomaterials evaluation.* New York: MacMillan, 1986:412–435.
3. Anderson JM. Cardiovascular device retrieval and evaluation. *Cardiovasc Pathol* 1993;2(Suppl):199S–208S.
4. Savage RA. New law to require medical device injury reports. *CAP Today* 1991;July:40.
5. Kahan JS. The Safe Medical Devices Act of 1990. *Med Dev Diagn Ind* 1991;Jan:67.
6. Morse D, Steiner RM, Fernandez J, eds. *Guide to prosthetic cardiac valves.* New York: Springer Verlag, 1985.
7. Bodnar E, Frater R, eds. *Replacement cardiac valves.* New York: Pergamon Press, 1992.
8. Harker LA, Ratner BD, Didisheim P, eds. *Cardiovascular devices and biocompatibility: A guide to the study of blood-tissue-materials interactions. Cardiovasc Pathol* 1993;2(Suppl): 1S–216S.
9. Schoen FJ, Levy RJ. Pathology of substitute heart valves: New concepts and developments. *J Cardiac Surg* 1994;9(Suppl):222–227.
10. Jamieson WR. Modern cardiac valve devices-bioprostheses and mechanical prostheses: state of art. *J Cardiac Surg* 1993;8:89–98.
11. Morse D, Steiner RM. Cardiac valve identification atlas and guide. In: Morse D, Steiner RM, Fernandez J, eds. *Guide to prosthetic cardiac valves.* New York: Springer Verlag, 1985:257–346.
12. Silver MD, Wilson GJ. Pathology of mechanical heart valve prostheses and vascular grafts made of artificial materials. In: Silver MD, ed. *Cardiovascular pathology,* 2nd ed. New York: Churchill Livingstone, 1991:1487–1545.
13. Yoganathan AP, Reamer HH, Corcoran WH, Harrison EC, Shulman IA, Parnassus W. The Starr-Edwards aortic ball valve: flow characteristics, thrombus formation, and tissue overgrowth. *Artif Organs* 1981;5:6–17.
14. Yoganathan AP, Corcoran WH, Harrison EC, Carl JR. The Bjork-Shiley aortic prosthesis: flow characteristics, thrombus formation and tissue overgrowth. *Circulation* 1978;58:70–76.
15. Kouchoukos NT, Davila-Roman VG, Spray TL, Murphy SF, Perrillo JB. Replacement of the aortic root with a pulmonary autograft in children and young adults with aortic-valve disease. *N Engl J Med* 1994;330:1–6.
16. Schoen FJ. Pathology of bioprostheses and other tissue heart valve replacements. In: Silver MD, ed. *Cardiovascular pathology,* 2nd ed. New York: Churchill Livingstone, 1991: 1547–1605.
17. Ferrans VJ, Hilbert SL, Fujita S, Jones M, Roberts WC. Abnormalities in explanted bioprosthetic cardiac valves. In: Virmani R, Atkinson JB, Fenoglio JJ, eds. *Cardiovascular Pathology,* Philadelphia: WB Saunders, 1993:373–398.
18. Flomenbaum MA, Schoen FJ. Effects of fixation back pressure and antimineralization treatment on the morphology of porcine aortic bioprosthetic valves. *J Thorac Cardiovasc Surg* 1993;105:154–164.
19. Schoen FJ, Titus JL, Lawrie GM. Autopsy-determined causes of death after cardiac valve replacement. *JAMA* 1983;249:899–902.
20. Rose AG. Autopsy-determined causes of death following heart valve replacement. *Am J Cardiovasc Pathol* 1987;1:39–46.
21. Hwang MH, Burchfiel CM, Sethi GK, et al. Comparison of the causes of late death following aortic and mitral valve replacement. *J Heart Valve Dis* 1994;3:17–24.
22. Burke AP, Farb A, Sessums L, Virmani R. Causes of sudden cardiac death in patients with replacement valves: an autopsy study. *J Heart Valve Dis* 1994;3:310–316.

23. Edmunds LH, Clarke RE, Cohn LH, Miller DC, Weisel RD. Guidelines for reporting morbidity and mortality after cardiac valvular operations. *J Thorac Cardiovasc Surg* 1988;96:351–353.

24. Bloomfield P, Wheatley DJ, Prescott RJ, Miller HC. Twelve-year comparison of a Bjork-Shiley mechanical heart valve with porcine bioprostheses. *N Engl J Med* 1991;324:573–579.

25. Hammermeister KE, Sethi GK, Henderson WG, Oprian C, Kim T, Rahimtoola S. A comparison of outcomes in men 11 years after heart-valve replacement with mechanical valve or bioprosthesis. *N Engl J Med* 1993;328:1289–1296.

26. Turina T, Hess OM, Turina M, Krayenbuehl HP. Cardiac bioprostheses in the 1990s. *Circulation* 1993;88:775–781.

27. Schoen FJ, Hobson CE. Anatomic analysis of removed prosthetic heart valves: Causes of failure of 33 mechanical valves and 58 bioprostheses, 1980 to 1983. *Hum Pathol* 1985;16:549–559.

28. Schoen FJ. Surgical pathology of removed natural and prosthetic heart valves. *Hum Pathol* 1987; 18:558-567.

29. Cleveland DC, William WG, Razzouk AJ, et al. Failure of cryopreserved homograft valved conduits in the pulmonary circulation. Circulation 1992;86(Suppl II):II-50–II-53.

30. Kirklin JK, Smith D, Novick W, et al. Long-term function of cryopreserved aortic homografts. *J Thorac Cardiovasc Surg* 1993;106:154–66.

31. Grunkemeier GL, Rahimtoola SH. *Artificial heart valves. Annu Rev Med* 1990;41:251–263.

32. Anderson JM, Schoen FJ. Interactions of blood with artificial surfaces. In : Butchart EG, Bodnar E, eds. *Thrombosis, embolism and bleeding.* London: ICR Publishers, 1992.

33. Hanson SR. Device thrombosis and thromboembolism. *Cardiovasc Pathol* 1993;2(Suppl): 157S–165S.

34. Arnett EN, Roberts WC. Prosthetic valve endocarditis. Clinicopathologic analysis of 22 necropsy patients with comparison of observations in 74 necropsy patients with active infective endocarditis involving natural left-sided cardiac valves. *Am J Cardiol* 1976;38:281–292.

35. Anderson DJ, Bulkley BH, Hutchins GM. A clinicopathologic study of prosthetic valve endocarditis in 22 patients: morphologic basis for diagnosis and therapy. *Am Heart J* 1977;94: 324–332.

36. Ferrans VJ, Boyce SW, Billingham ME, Spray TL, Roberts WC. Infection of glutaraldehyde-preserved porcine valve heterografts. *Am J Cardiol* 1979;43:1123–1136.

37. Gristina AG. Biomaterial-centered infection: microbial adhesion versus tissue integration. *Science* 1987;237:1588–1595.

38. Schoen FJ, Levy RJ, Piehler HR. Pathologic considerations in replacement cardiac valves. *Cardiovasc Pathol* 1992;1:29–52.

39. Bortolotti U, Milano A, Mazzucco A, et al. Extended follow-up of the standard Hancock porcine bioprosthesis. *J Cardiac Surg* 1991;6:544–549.

40. Jamieson WRE, Allen P, Miyagishima RT, et al. The Carpentier-Edwards standard porcine bioprosthesis. A first generation tissue valve with excellent long-term clinical performance. *J Thorac Cardiovasc Surg* 1990;99:543–561.

41. Burdon TA, Miller DC, Oyer PE, et al. Durability of porcine valves at fifteen years in a representative North American patient population. *J Thorac Cardiovasc Surg* 1992;103:238–252.

42. Sarris GE, Robbins RC, Miller C, et al. Randomized, prospective assessment of bioprosthetic valve durability. *Circulation* 1993;88(Suppl II):II-55–II-64.

43. Walley VM, Keon WJ. Patterns of failure in Ionescu-Shiley bovine pericardial bioprosthetic valves. *J Thorac Cardiovasc Surg* 1987;93:925–933.

44. McGonagle-Wolff K, Schoen FJ. Morphologic findings in explanted mitroflow pericardial bioprosthetic valves. *Am J Cardiol* 1992;70:263–264.

45. Tomazic BB, Brown WE, Schoen FJ. Physicochemical properties of calcific deposits isolated from porcine bioprosthetic heart valves removed from patients following 2–13 years function. *J Biomed Mater Res* 1994;28:35–47.

46. Schoen FJ, Levy RJ, Nelson AC, Bernhard WF, Nashef A, Hawley M. Onset and progression of experimental bioprosthetic heart valve calcification. *Lab Invest* 1985;52:523–532.

47. Schoen FJ, Tsao JW, Levy RJ. Calcification of bovine pericardium used in cardiac valve bioprostheses. *Am J Pathol* 1986;123:134–145.

48. Mehlman DJ. A guide to the radiographic identification of prosthetic heart valves: an addendum. *Circulation* 1984;69:102–105.

49. Schoen FJ, Kujovich JL, Webb CL, Levy RJ. Chemically determined mineral content of explanted porcine aortic valve bioprostheses: correlation with radiographic assessment of calcification and clinical data. *Circulation* 1987;76:1061–1066.

50. Schoen FJ, Titus JL, Lawrie GM. Durability of pyrolytic carbon-containing heart valve prostheses, *J Biomed Mater Res* 1982;16:559–570.

51. Schoen FJ, Goodenough SH, Ionescu MI, Braunwald NS. Implications of late morphology of Braunwald-Cutter mitral heart valve prostheses. *J Thorac Cardiovasc Surg* 1984;88:208–216.

52. Schoen FJ, Schulman LJ, Cohn LH. Quantitative anatomic analysis of "stent creep" of explanted Hancock Standard porcine bioprostheses used for cardiac valve replacement. *Am J Cardiol* 1985;56:110–114.

53. Clowes AW. Intimal hyperplasia and graft failure. *Cardiovasc Pathol* 1993;2(Suppl):179S–186S.

54. Clowes AW. Graft endothelialization: The role of angiogenic mechanisms. *J Vasc Surg* 1991;13:734–737.

55. Kadoba K, Schoen FJ, Jonas RA. Experimental comparison of albumin-sealed and gelatin-sealed knitted Dacron conduits. *J Thorac Cardiovasc Surg* 1992;103:1059–1067.

56. *Heart and stroke facts.* 1994 Statistical Supplement. American Heart Association.

57. Virmani R, Atkinson JB, Forman MB. Aortocoronary saphenous vein bypass grafts. In: Waller BF, ed. *Contemporary issues in cardiovascular pathology.* Philadelphia: F A Davis Co, 1988:41–62.

58. Pae WE. Ventricular assist devices and total artificial hearts: A combined registry experience. *Ann Thorac Surg* 1993;55:295–298.

59. Fyfe B, Schoen FJ. Pathologic analysis of 34 explanted Symbion ventricular assist devices and 10 explanted Jarvik-7 total artificial hearts. *Cardiovasc Pathol* 1993;2:187–197.

60. Bolman RM III, Cox JL, Marshall W, et al. Circulatory support with centrifugal pump as a bridge to cardiac transplantation. *Ann Thorac Surg* 1989;47:108–112.

61. Schoen FJ, Anderson JM, Didisheim P, et al. Ventricular assist device (VAD) pathology analyses: Guidelines for clinical studies. *J Appl Biomat* 1990;1:49–56.

62. DeVries WC. The permanent artificial heart. *JAMA* 1988;259:849–859.

63. Eidelman BH, Obrist WD, Wagner WR, Kormos R, Griffith B. Cerebrovascular complications associated with the use of artificial circulatory support services. *Neurol Clin* 1993;11:463–474.

64. Wagner WR, Johnson PC, Kormos RL, Griffith BP. Evaluation of bioprosthetic valve-associated thrombus in ventricular assist device patients. *Circulation* 1993;88:2023–2029.

65. Rosenthal ME, Josephson ME. Current status of antitachycardia devices. *Circulation* 1990;82:1889–1899.

66. Singer I, Hutchins GM, Mirowski M, et al. Pathologic findings related to the lead system and repeated defibrillations in patients with the automatic implantable cardioverter-defibrillator. *J Am Coll Cardiol* 1987;10:382–388.

67. Kelly PA, Cannom DS, Garan H, et al. The automatic implantable cardioverter-defibrillator: efficacy, complications and survival in patients with malignant ventricular arrhythmias. *J Am Coll Cardiol* 1988;11:1278–1286.

68. Topol EJ. Caveats about elective coronary stenting (Editorial). *N Engl J Med* 1994;331:539–541.

69. Serruys PW, Strauss BH, Beatt KJ, et al. Angiographic follow-up after placement of a self-expanding coronary artery stent. *N Engl J Med* 1991;324:13–7.

70. Anderson PG, Bajaj RK, Baxley WA, Roubin GS. Vascular pathology of balloon-expandable flexible coil stents in humans. *J Am Coll Cardiol* 1992;19:372–81.

71. van Beusekom HMM, van der Giessen WJ, van Suylen RJ, Bos E, Bosman FT, Serruys PW. Histology after stenting of human saphenous vein bypass grafts: observations from surgically excised grafts 3 to 320 days after stent implantation. *J Am Coll Cardiol* 1993;21:45–54.

72. Anderson PG. Pathology of intravascular stents in man and experimental animals. In: Waller BF, ed. *Coronary artery stenting.* Cambridge: Blackwell Scientific Publications,Inc. 1994, in press.

73. Peppas NA, Langer R. New challenges in biomaterials. *Science* 1994;263:1715–1720.

Index

Page references followed by *t* or *f* indicate tables or figures, respectively.